DISTRIBUTION OF RESOURCES IN THE NIGERIAN HEALTH CARE SYSTEM

DISTRIBUTION OF RESOURCES IN THE NIGERIAN HEALTH CARE SYSTEM

Ethical Considerations And Proposals Applying Catholic Social Teaching

ANTHONY OKECHUKWU NNADI

Dedication

This work is dedicated to my mother Mrs. Bridget Ngozi Nnadi.

Acknowledgements

I wish to thank Almighty God, creator and giver of life and human wisdom for all that He has endowed me.

My gratitude goes to my mother Mrs Bridget Nnadi, and to my father Tobias Nnadi, who is resting in the Lord. I thank my siblings.

Prof. Dr. Maurizio Pietro Faggioni (o.f.m) has led me, step by step to where I am today in terms of acquiring knowledge and the correct way of analysing bioethics. He also guided me patiently during the course of this dissertation. I thank him immensely for all he has done in the past and thank him for any assistance he may offer in the future.

Prof. Alberto García Gómez carried out his duty as the second moderator in a fraternal manner. His indications and suggestions based on a profound knowledge of the subject, of which I remain in awe, assisted me while writing this thesis.

My study of bioethics was enriched by my lecturers at the Faculty of Bioethics, Ateneo Pontificio Regina Apostolorum, Roma. My special thank you goes to Prof. Gonzalo Miranda of the Faculty of Bioethics and Mr. Gennaro Casa the Secretary of the Faculty.

Rt. Rev. Giovanni Santucci, the Bishop of Massa Carrara-Pontremoli merits my sincere gratitude for his moral and spiritual support throughout the period of my studies. I wish to thank Bishop Eugenio Binini, the bishop emeritus of the above-mentioned diocese, for making himself available to help out right from the beginning of my spiritual, human and intellectual formation in Italy.

My special thanks goes to Archbishop Anthony Obinna (Archbishop of the Catholic Archdiocese of Owerri, Nigeria).

I express my sincere gratitude to all who have assisted me in my spiritual, human and intellectual formations right from the junior seminary (St. Peter Claver Seminary Okpala, Imo State Nigeria), especially Rev. Dr. Anthony Onyeocha, and all my lectures at Seat of Wisdom Seminary, Owerri Imo State, Nigeria.

My sincere gratitude goes to my rectors in the major seminaries of the Diocese of Massa Carrara-Pontremoli and Archdiocese of Pisa, Bishop Alberto Silvani, Bishop Gugliemo Borghetti, Bishop Roberto Fillipini and Don Severino Pizzanelli. I thank my lecturers at the Studio Teologico Interdiocesano Camaiore (LU), affiliate of Faculty of Theology of central Italy, Florence.

I thank Bishop Martin Uzokwu, Bishop Mathew Hassan Kukah, Bishop William Avenya, Bishop Giovanni Mosciati, Rev. Fr. Dr. Raph Madu, Rev. Fr. Dr. Jude Ike and Don Alvaro Marabini for their encouragement.

I thank Dr. Kelechi Ofurum, Dr. Maureen Jones, Mr. Christopher Lock and Mr. James McHugh for proofreading my work. I also thank all friends, my family members, the family of Giovanni Strani and my parishioners who accompanied me on my journey to where I am today. May the God Almighty continue to grant everyone good health of mind and body. Amen.

Abbreviations

AIDS	Acquired Immune Deficiency Syndrome
ANC	Antenatal Care
ART	Anti-Retroviral Therapy
ARV	Anti-Retroviral Drugs
ARI	Acute Respiratory Infections
BCG	Bacillus Calmette-Guérin
BHSS	Basic Health Service Scheme
BHCPF	Basic Health Care Provision Fund
BMJ	British Medical Journal
BP/CR	Birth Preparedness and Complication Readiness
CBCN	Catholic Bishops' Conference of Nigeria
CBHIS	Community-Based Health Insurance
CFR	Confer
CHEWs	Community Health Extension Workers
CHOs	Community Health Officers
CPR	Contraceptive Prevalence Rate
CRF	Consolidated Revenue Fund
DRACC	Daughters of Divine Love Retreat and Conference Centre
ECA	Excess Crude Account

ECP	Emergency Contraceptive Pill
ED	Editor
EDS	Editors
EFCC	Economic and Financial Crimes Commission
FATF	Task Force on Money Laundering
FGM	Female Genital Mutilation
FGC	Female Genital Cutting
FIGO	International Federation of Gynaecology and Obstetrics
FMoH	Federal Ministry of Health
GCE	General Certificate of Education
GDP	Gross Domestic Product
GE	General Electric
HREC	Health Research Ethics Committee
DOTS	Directly Observed Therapy Short Course
DPT	To prevent diphtheria
GAPPD	Global Action Plan for Pneumonia and Diarrhoea
GDP	Gross Domestic Product
HCT	Haematocrit
HIV	Human Immunodeficiency Virus
IBBSS	Integrated Biological Behavioural Surveillance Survey
ICPD	International Conference on Population and Development
ICPC	Independent Corrupt Practices Commission
IPOB	Indigenous People of Biafra
IPTp	Intermittent Preventive Treatment
ITNs	Insecticide-Treated Nets
IUD	Intrauterine Contraceptive Device
JCHEW	Junior Community Health Extension Worker
JAMB	Joint Admission and Matriculation Board
LAP	LAMBERT Academic Publishing
MCH	Maternal and child health
MDGs	Millennium Development Goals
MDCN	Medical and Dental Council of Nigeria
MNCH	Maternal, Neonatal and Child Health Services
MMR	Maternal Mortality Ratio
MOH	Medical Officer of Health

MTSS	Medium Term Sector Strategy
NACA	National Agency for the Control of AIDS
NAFDAC	National Agency For Food and Drug Administration and Control
NARHS	Reproductive Health Survey
NARHS	National HIV/AIDS and Reproductive Health Survey
NBS	National Bureau of Statistics
NCNC	National Council of Nigeria and the Cameroons
NHA	National Health Accounts
NHIS	National Health Insurance Schemes
NHREC	National Code of Health Research Ethics
NMCN	Nursing and Midwifery Council of Nigeria
NMEP	National Malaria Elimination Programme
NMIS	Nigeria Malaria Indicator Survey
NNPC	Nigerian National Petroleum Company
NPC	North People's Congress
NPHCDA	National Primary Healthcare Development Agency
NHIS	National Health Insurance Scheme
NPopC	National Population Commission
NPI	National Programme on Immunization
NRN	Nigerian Registered Nurse
NSF	National Strategic Framework
OPEC	Organisation of Petroleum Exporting Countries
ODA	Official Development Assistance
OTC	Over The Counter
PABA	Para-Aminobenzoic Acid
PCN	Pharmaceutical Council of Nigeria
PHC	Primary Health Care
PLHIV	People Living with HIV/AIDS
PMTCT	Prevention of Mother-To-Child Transmission
PPMVs	Proprietary Patent Medicine Vendors
PRIMASYS	Primary Care Systems Profiles & Performance
QALY	Quality Adjusted Life Year
SHDP	State Health Development Planning level
SOGON	Society of Gynaecology and Obstetrics of Nigeria

SP	Sulphadoxine-pyrimethamine
STD	Sexually Transmitted Diseases
TB	Tuberculosis
TBAs	Traditional Birth Attendants
THE	Total Health Expenditure
UHC	Universal Health Coverage
UN	United Nations
UNICEF	United Nations International Children's Emergency Fund
USAID	United States Agency for International Development
USCCB	United States Conference of Catholic Bishops
UHC	Universal Health Coverage
U5MR	Under-5 child mortality rate
VAPP	Violence Against Persons Prohibition
VHWs	Volunteers Health Workers
VVF	Vesico-Vaginal Fistula
WAEC	West African Examination Council
WASH	Water Sanitation and Hygiene
WDC	Ward Development Committees
WHO	World Health Organisation
WHS	Ward Health System
WPV	Wild Poliovirus
WHS	Ward Health System

Contents

General Introduction

This dissertation examines the healthcare system in Nigeria in the light of the Catholic social teaching. The allocation of health care resources is not only matter of organization, but also an ethical problem[1]. Many Nigerians "cry foul" because they believe their right to basic health needs and other social conditions are not respected. This results in the loss of many lives, in particular, those of the poorest and most vulnerable who die needlessly everyday from curable diseases. The debacles and failure of the Nigerian health system, as our work reveals, depend on many factors ranging from lack of will to implement the right policies on the ground, corruption among the leaders, lack of justice, lack of respect for the dignity of every human person, mismanagement to insufficient consideration and application of the ethical principles in the administration of common good, especially in the distribution of health care and social resources. For the distribution of health care resources, this doctoral dissertation suggests that priority be given to the basic health care needs of the Nigerian citizens especially those who have no means of acquiring these needs themselves. In this context, we affirm that great attention needs to be paid to ensuring that the principle of human dignity is respected in its entirety in each and every policy in this important area.

---

[1]   Cfr. G. BOGNAR – I. HIROSE, *The Ethics of Health Care Rationing – An Introduction*, Routledge, London and New York 2014, 31.

The scope of this doctoral thesis is to study the Nigerian health care system in the light of the Catholic social teaching. It is an ethical vision of the social reality in Nigeria. Proposing the person-centred Catholic principles as a possible way forward in the distribution of health care resources in Nigeria does not imply substituting the economic, political and health experts in offering technical solutions in their areas of competence. The latter is never our aim. We are convinced that healthcare allocation is an ethical issue and it needs to be governed by ethical principles.

The key motivating factors for choosing this dissertation are based on our knowledge of the deplorable condition of the health care system in Nigeria and our desire to save human lives. Distribution of health care and other social resources in Nigeria has been plagued with failures and this provides proof of lack of application of ethical principles focused on the person. Anyone conversant with the present health and economic conditions of Nigeria will agree that something needs to be done urgently. In this respect, we have decided to study the problem, hoping to contribute through this doctoral thesis towards the realization of an ethical health care system for the wellbeing of Nigerians. Furthermore, we believe that if academicians and those who should draw attention to the unjust situations keep quiet, their silence could be termed a "complicit silence". Hence, we are convinced of our moral responsibility to dig deeper to the root of ethical problems in health care allocations in Nigeria and to demand fair treatment for those who cannot speak for themselves.

We are all stewards of human life. This implies the moral obligation to protect the dignity of the human person, which is inseparable from protecting human life. These ethical injunctions cannot be ignored by any country because "the issue of morality is one which deeply touches every person; it involves all people, even those who do not know Christ"[2]. A Professor of Medical Ethics in the University of Oxford affirms: "There is no health care system in the world that has sufficient money to provide the best possible treatment for all patients in all situations, not even those that spend relatively large sums on health care"[3]. This affirmation is true

---

[2] JOHN PAUL II, «*Veritatis splendor* Encyclical Letter Regarding Certain Fundamental Questions of the Church's Moral Teaching (1993)», in J. M. MILLER (ed.), *The Encyclicals of John Paul II*, Our Sunday Visitor Publishing Division – Our Sunday Visitor Inc., Huntington, Indiana 673-771.

[3] T. HOPE, *Medical Ethics. A very short introduction*, Oxford University Press 2004, 29.

but cannot justify the health situation in Nigeria. We hold tenaciously to the affirmation that "the quality and quantity of thousands of people's lives will be affected by the answers that we give"[4] by applying the Catholic principles to the distribution of health care resources in Nigeria. For this reason, the basis of our dissertation shall be the dignity of the human person.

This doctoral thesis will be presented in four chapters. In the first chapter, we will take a general overview of Nigeria from the geographical, socio-cultural, economic, political and historical points of view. Together with this, we will consider Nigeria's key health indicators and major causes of death and main pathologies in Nigeria to enable us to have an appropriate knowledge of the factors that affect the life of the people, especially their health situation. The study of the general background of Nigeria in chapter one reveals that Nigeria is a country blessed with natural and human resources, but because of poor political practices and bad leadership which mark its political history, the country's huge wealth does not reflect on the health of the people, who die of hunger and poverty related diseases every day. These results indicate that the objectives of the Sustainable Development Goals (SDGs) are far from being obtained in Nigeria.

We will study the ethical issues regarding sexual and reproductive health in Nigeria. Some of these practices as we will see are harmful and capable of provoking reproductive ill health. However, the first chapter also bears a positive note regarding the gallantry of the Nigerian Health system in combating the Ebola diseases which erupted in 2013 in Guinea, arriving in Nigeria in July 2013.

Chapter two gives insight into the Nigerian health care system. A brief historical outline of health care in Nigeria discloses its Christian origin and the deviation of the Nigerian health care system from the spirit that was at its origin. We will also treat in this chapter the laws, plans, and strategies guiding the administration of the Nigerian health care system. Study of the structure and administration of the Nigerian health care system reveals that it is fashioned according to the three-tier system of government practiced in Nigeria. This chapter highlights the primary health care as the 'key system' of the Nigerian health care systems. In connection with that, it stresses how the primary health care is underfunded and how this

---

[4]   Ibid., 29.

has affected the performance of the entire health care system in Nigeria. The consequences are borne by the poor and vulnerable.

In chapter three, we are going to consider how the societies of the world react to the problem of health care resource allocation. In the distribution of health care resources, it is difficult to satisfy the health care needs of every member of society. Nevertheless, it is morally imperative to give decent-minimum care to everyone, especially to the poor and most vulnerable. This has to be done in order to realize a just health care system.

In this context the third chapter studies the response of society to the health needs of the people. Thus, it examines the concept of justice and some of the major theories and approaches of justice employed to seek solution to the problems that arise from health care resource allocation. The same Chapter Three discloses that in the application of these theories and approaches, there is a gap that needs to be filled. There is a group that 'cries foul' because, the procedures of the theories and approaches studied do not respect its rights to health and access to care. For instance, the legitimate complaints made in favour of the poor and the vulnerable who are marginalized and denied their rights due to their social, economic and health conditions. Therefore, in an attempt to straighten up the procedures of these theories and approaches, we will present a brief description of the main features of an ethical health-care system that are contained in the Catholic principles proposed in the fourth chapter.

Chapter four bears the major purpose of this dissertation: application of Catholic principles to the distribution of resources in the Nigerian health care system. It is an ethical approach to the problems relative to the Nigerian health care system. The Catholic principles of distributive justice this dissertation is proposing are: principle of the dignity/integrity of the human person; common good and solidarity; preferential option for the most vulnerable; and subsidiarity. This chapter highlights the personalist approach which characterizes our main arguments in this thesis.

The Catholic social doctrine proclaims that the dignity of the human person is founded on the fact that every human being is created in the image and likeness of God[5]. The Church is clear in its teaching that such dignity must be safeguarded from conception to death and it is non-negotiable. The Catholic notion of the common good implies that people

---

[5] Cfr. THE CATECHISM OF THE CATHOLIC CHURCH, n. 1934, Pauline's Publications-Africa, Nairobi, Kenya 1995, 461.

either as groups or individuals should be provided with all the social conditions which will enable them realize their fulfillment more fully and more easily[6]. Solidarity as conceived by the Catholic social teaching confirms "the intrinsic social nature of the human person, the equality of all in dignity and rights and the common path of individuals and peoples towards an ever more committed unity"[7]. Preferential option for the poor and the vulnerable is inspired and guided by charity, which according to the teaching of the Church is the greatest social commandment. The Catholic Magisterium sustains that being poor or vulnerable does not in any way reduce the dignity of the person in this condition. The principle of subsidiarity according to the Magisterium is "the most important principle of "social philosophy"[8]. Subsidiarity in the light of the Catholic teaching implies that societies of a higher order have the duty to help those of the lower order, without substituting them, thus promoting and respecting their dignity[9]. The Pontifical Council for Justice and Peace, affirms that "the principles of the Church's social doctrine must be appreciated in their unity, interrelatedness and articulation"[10]. The Catholic principles do not oppose or contradict one another.

Before the utilization of the Catholic principles in addressing the concrete health and ethical problems pertinent to the distribution of health care resources, we will study them specifically, in the bid to understand them and to underline their theoretical, logical and practical connectedness. Subsequent to the acquaintance of the nature and characteristics of the Catholic principles, our doctoral thesis will use them to critically analyse the health problems of Nigeria examined in chapters one and two of this thesis, thus, demonstrating how their correct applications can obtain the desired results.

This dissertation will adopt a pluri-disciplinary method typical of bioethics. Some parts are descriptive while others are philosophical, analytical and the method typical of applied ethics. The general description of Nigeria from the geographical, socio-cultural, economic, political and

---

[6]   Cfr. Ibid., n. 1906, 457.
[7]   PONTIFICAL COUNCIL FOR JUSTICE AND PEACE, *Compendium of the Social Doctrine of the Church*, n. 192, Libreria Editrice Vaticano, Citta Del Vaticano 2010, 109.
[8]   Ibid., n. 186, 105.
[9]   Cfr. Ibid.
[10]   Ibid., n. 162, 92.

historical perspectives we believe, will facilitate our understanding of its health and other life-threatening problems. The third chapter will use a philosophical method. It considers the various secular theories of distributive justice, confronting them with the main characteristic of a just healthcare system and the principles of distributive justice accustomed to the social teaching of the Catholic Church. The method to be utilized in the fourth chapter is that typical of applied ethics. In this chapter, we will apply the Catholic social teaching to the Nigerian health system. It is a moral vision of social reality of Nigeria especially in the aspect of health care resource allocation. The fourth chapter shows clearly the personalist approach which governs the entire reasoning in this doctoral thesis. In general, we will use the analytical method to identify the problems, their root causes and to find adequate solution(s).

In order to realize this doctoral dissertation, we made use of appriopriate sources to widen our knowledge in our areas of interests. We consulted documents of Ecclesiastical Magisterium relative to our areas of interest (teachings of Popes, documents of the Vatican dicasteries and statements issued by the Episcopal Conferences of Nigeria, USA, England and Wales and Italy). More so, we viewed texts and articles by Nigerian authors on ethics, healthcare, medicine, law and politics in Nigeria. We also read books, articles and internet documents of foreign authors who have treated issues relative to ethics, healthcare, medicine, justice and philosophical and theological questions relevant to study. We painstakingly consulted public documents of the Federal Ministry of Health Nigeria (FMHN), World Health Organization (WHO), United Nations International Children Emergency Fund (UNICEF), World Bank and the Constitution of the Federal Republic of Nigeria.

The novelty of this dissertation lies in the application of Catholic social teaching to the distribution of health resources to the Nigerian health care system. This idea has never been gallantly proposed in Nigeria, may be because of the presence of many religions and cultures, which differ from the Catholic beliefs and practices. For the same reason we envisage difficulties in accepting our proposal in Nigeria. Nonetheless, we are optimistic because the method of approach we are proposing for the Nigerian Health system is a personalist approach, it goes beyond religion, culture and other barriers to defend the dignity of the human person. Hence it could be applied to the Nigerian Health system. The concept of "person" belongs to all human beings of different origins.

The two major religious groups in Nigeria are Christians and Muslims. In order to further consider the adaptability of our proposal in Nigerian and its acceptance by Muslim politicians and population, we will do a comparative analysis of the Catholic and Islamic concepts of distributive justice.

Distribution of health care resources is a bioethical question. It is an issue that is being addressed in Nigeria. This dissertation hopes to contribute to the advancement of bioethics by giving a *Catholic Personalist bioethical vision of social questions like distribution of health care and other social resources in Nigeria* and by *offering to the Catholic Church in Nigeria an analysis and some direction to address these issues.*

Chapter 1

THE GENERAL FRAMEWORK OF THE SOCIO-HEALTH SITUATION OF NIGERIA

Introduction

In this chapter, we shall have an overview of the socio-health situations of Nigeria. This will help us to understand better the social, economic and health situations of the citizens in order to proffer concrete solutions to the various problems at the end of this dissertation. For this purpose, we shall consider Nigeria from the geographical, socio-cultural, economic and political points of view. Understanding the people, her history, her way of everyday life and how she manages her challenges, is necessary to study the various aspects of her life, especially an important aspect like health. This is the first necessary step.

These problems mentioned are highlighted in the 17 Sustainable Development Goals adopted in September 2015 by world leaders during an historic UN Summit[11]. The Goals touch the most important aspects

---

[11]   Cfr. J. WAAGE – C. YAP – S. BELL – C. LEVY – G. MACE – T. PEGRAM – E. UNTERHALTER – N. DASANDI – D. HUDSON – R. KOCK – S. MAYHEW – C. MARX – N. POOLE, «Governing the UN Sustainable Development Goals:

relevant to the socio-health lives of the people. The Goals, which have the aim of transforming our world, target social, geographical, economic and health problems such as: the need to address rising global temperatures, the need to end the various forms of poverty, the need to tackle the problem of lack of education, health, and social protection, the need to create job opportunities and the need to address other issues regarding peace and justice. We are not giving a systematic list of the Goals but will be mentioning some points that we retain to conveniently explain our assertions. Suffice it to mention that among the 17 Sustainable Development Goals, the single health goal that is directly related to health is targeted at "individual and collective wellbeing through improved health and education, ensuring equitable distribution within and between individuals and countries"[12]. Some authors think Nigeria has to solve the problems of poor resource management in the health care system, sequential healthcare worker industrial actions, terrorism and the activities of the Fulani herdsmen in order to be able to significantly advance the Sustainable Development Goals[13].

After this first step, we shall treat some key health indicators of Nigeria such as: life expectancy at birth male/female, maternal mortality ratio and other maternal health indicators, infant and child mortalities (Under 5 mortality rate) and immunisation coverage. Subsequently, we shall study the major causes of death and the main pathologies in Nigeria. Under this section, we intend to consider the following: malaria, childbirth complications, HIV/AIDS, Tuberculosis, Pneumonia and access to potable water, sanitation/dirty or polluted environment. The above issues give a concrete and correct description of socio-health conditions of the Nigerian populace. The results, as we will see in this section, are not encouraging.

Equally, we will study the ways reproductive health care is practiced in Nigeria. The various ideas and methods of practicing reproductive health in Nigeria give rise to moral problems and they evoke the evaluation and

---

Interactions, Infrastructures and Institutions». *THE LANCET Global Health*, 3(2015) PE251-E252. http://doi.org/10.106/S2214-109X(15)70112-9 [9-07-2019].

[12] Ibid.

[13] Cfr. O. O. OLERIBE – S. D. T.-ROBINSON, «Before Sustainable Development Goals (SDG): Why Nigeria failed to achieve the Millennium Development Goals (MDGs) », *The Pan African Medical Journal*, 24(2016), 156.

re-evaluation of some socio-cultural values in Nigeria which according to some authors are not in consonance with the dignity of the human person.

Furthermore, we will see the gallant, efficient and effective reaction of the Nigerian health care system and the Nigerian government to the deadly Ebola Virus Disease (EVD). The success obtained in the "Ebola combat" aroused applause for Nigeria from different parts of the world. This experience stands as a proof that the Nigerian health care system can do well solving other health problems if the right principles are adopted and correctly applied. This is one of the major reasons why our dissertation is proposing the all-inclusive Catholic principles for the distribution of health care resources in Nigeria. We shall see the Catholic principles in the last chapter of this doctoral thesis.

1.1. The Background of Nigeria

1.1.1. Geographical Point of View

A look at the Nigerian geography is very important as it would enable us to understand better some fundamental aspects, such as health, disease and health care in Nigeria, using its geographical information and perspectives. Some scholars such as Philo Christopher, a Professor of geography at the University of Glasgow, affirm that there are some geographical influences, and that the air, water and environment can have an impact on the health of a population[14]. Nigeria is the country with the highest population in Africa. It is geographically located on the west coast of Africa: on the gulf of Guinea, which comprises of the Bights of Benin and Biafra, and of the Atlantic Ocean in the south[15]. The land mass of Nigeria is 98 million hectares. Its territory covers about 725,000 square kilometres[16]. Four Nations surround Nigeria: Republic of Benin in the west, Cameroon in the east, Chad in the north east and Niger in the

---

[14]   Cfr. D. GREGORY – R. JOHNSTON – G. PRATT – M. J. WATTS – S. WHATMORE, (eds.), «Health and Health care», in *The Dictionary of Human Geography*, Wiley-Blackwell, Oxford 2009[5], 325-326.

[15]   Cfr. D. M. N. MCDIKKOH, *The Nigerian health…*, 24.

[16]   Cfr. K. A.-ALLEN, *Nigerian Democracy and Democratic Experience, A Historical, Political, Economic, Social and Religious Analysis*, Kayode Asoga-Allen, Great Britain 2016, 12.

North West[17]. Its territory is 923,768 square kilometres; water cover about 13,000 square[18]. The nation is made up of 36 states spread out in its six major geographical regions which include: south west, south-south, south east, north west, north central, where the administrative capital Abuja is situated and north east.

The climatic conditions in Nigeria differ from the arid north to the equatorial central and the tropical south. The maximum temperatures are 30 to 32 degrees Celsius. The climatic conditions observed in the south are of high humidity, while those in the north are usually of low humidity[19]. The major types of vegetation in Nigeria include: rain forest, savannah, grassland and Sahel. It has especially in the Southern part, two main seasons: the rainy season – from April to August – and the dry season - from September to March[20]. The period between September and March is described as a dry season because there is very low intensity of humidity (less rainfall), while that between April and August is described as a rainy season because there is high intensity of humidity (frequent rainfall).

Clean and polluted water and environment have significant positive or negative effects respectively on the health of the people living within the environment. Some parts of Nigeria are located in a tropical zone and this has a notable influence on the health of the people. In the southern part, the climate is tropical and equatorial. The inland has a lot of vegetation. The issue of mosquitoes and consequently malaria transmitted by them, and some other diseases depend on the tropical-equatorial geographical location of the country and how the people manage their environment. For instance, dirty and stagnant water, unkept and bushy environments can spread diseases and harbour mosquitoes which in turn transmit malaria.

The study of the Nigerian geography will also help us to understand the problems regarding the accessibility of the health care centers, and the distribution of resources in the rural and urban areas of the country. In Nigeria, the health care services often manifest a lopsided pattern with expenditures concentrated in the urban areas, and with the rural areas

---

[17]   Cfr. D. PHILLIPS, *Nigeria*, Chelsea House Publishers, Philadelphia 2004,10.

[18]   Cfr. *Nigerian Fact Sheet 2001,* Published by Nigerian High Commission, New Delhi, 3.

[19]   Cfr. D. PHILLIPS, *Nigeria* ..., 21.

[20]   Cfr. Ibid., 12.

remaining unserved. S. I. Okafor presents thus some of the difficulties and failures of the Nigerian government:

> Health care provision in Nigeria is characterized by two main problems: the problems of limited resources and inadequate spatial organization of facilities. The first problem relates to acute shortages of physical facilities, equipment and personnel, while the second relates to the spatial pattern of available facilities. The problem of spatial organization manifests itself in different forms including interstate variations in the levels of provision and urban-rural disparities. In addition, there is the problem of a poorly developed primary care sector, which is an aspect of medical deprivation in rural areas[21].

The right to health does not mean simply not being sick, but rather having a functional health care system that provides the basic health care services to all, and especially to the vulnerable and those living in underserved areas. Putting this into practice in Nigeria has remained an uphill task owing to various factors such as insufficient health budgets, the large population, and lack of will of those in power to implement the policies and plans on the ground.

1.1.2. Socio-Cultural Point of View

Culture is generally defined as the people's way of life. According to J. Fried, culture is defined as "shared ways of life, common to a group of people and acquired as a member"[22]. The shared way of life of the people that reflects in the life of each individual member of the group, in the thoughts of E. B. Tylor, "includes knowledge, beliefs, art, morals, laws, customs and any other capabilities and habits acquired by man as a member of society.[23]" The definition and description of culture given above portray the general frame of the practices by Nigerians, which are guided by moral codes, customs, and laws, spiritual and cultural values.

---

[21] S. I. OKAFOR, «Spatial Aspects of Health Care Provision in Nigeria», in R. Akhtar (ed.), *Health Care Patterns and Planning in Developing Countries*, Greenwood Press, New York 1991, 263-274.

[22] J. FRIED, *Cultural Anthropology*, Harper's College Press, New York 1976, 41.

[23] Ibid., 46.

These factors influence their worldview, especially their concept of health. Some Nigerian major cultural practices which have some social relevancies include the male circumcision and female genital mutilation, cultural practices in marriage and sexual reproduction, food, the position of women in the society, marriage etc.

Some of the social problems in Nigeria include national identity problems, poverty (More than half of the population live on less than $1 a day and are unable to afford the high cost of health care in the country[24]), corruption, poor health care services, inequality, terrorism, high-level child and maternal mortality (Nigeria Demographic and Health Survey, 2013 reveals: "Infant and under-5 mortality rates in the past five years are 69 and 128 deaths per 1,000 live births, respectively. At these mortality levels, one in every 15 Nigerian children die before reaching age 1, and one in every eight do not survive to their fifth birthday"[25].), unemployment, poor education, tribalism and home violence. We are treating briefly some of these points in this part of the work since most of them will be treated in detail in the subsequent parts.

A Nigerian author, D. M. N. McDikkoh underlines how the social problems can have notable impact on the people's health:

> The socio-cultural aspect of a society influences the health system and the way that services in it are delivered, even more so than the economic impact. Sure, the economy enables and maintains the viability of services, but so are the social-cultural aspects – namely, values, religion, tradition, customs, environment, politics, etcetera – determines the type of policies by the types of laws that would regulate the system[26].

Explaining the position of M.I. Roemer, an already cited Nigerian author asserts that the social, historical, economic, political, and cultural

---

[24]   M. O. WELCOME, «The Nigerian health care system: Need for integrating adequate medical intelligence and surveillance systems», *Journal of Pharmacy and Bioallied Sciences*, 3(2011), 470-478. https://doi.org/10.4103/0975-7406.90100 [6-8-2016].

[25]   NATIONAL POPULATION COMMISSION, Federal Republic of Nigeria Abuja, Nigeria, *Nigeria Demographic and Health Survey 2013*, ICF International, Rockville, Maryland, USA: NPC June 2014.

[26]   D. M. N. McDIKKOH, *The Nigerian health…*, 196.

influences are obviously intermeshed, and together they constantly change and operate in different ways at different times and phases to shape the character of the health service system found in each of the approximately 140 nations of the globe[27].

1.1.3. Economic Point of View

According to R. Akhtar "the political economy of health care is an attempt to specify the ways in which economic interests and political processes structure the provision of services"[28]. It is therefore important to study briefly Nigeria from this point of view because the socio-economic and political forces have great impact on the health service system of any country. Where these forces or aspects are not properly formed and aligned, surely there will be failure in the health care system just as it is the case with Nigeria where these forces are still limping.

An aspect of the economic history of Nigeria reveals that the commercial system of payment that existed in Nigeria before the introduction of money was the trade by barter system; the exchange of goods for goods. Before the arrival of the colonial administration, agriculture was at the centre of its economic activities and the majority of its citizens, about 99.5 percent, were farmers[29]. The Nigerian economic situation started transforming with the arrival of the British colonial masters and the mining of mineral resources such as coal, tin, columbite etc. With the change of the economic situation, the barter system was substituted with the money system. There were more agricultural products as the country started producing also for trade; exporting products for money and foreign exchange.

Under the British Colonial government, agricultural activities grew stronger as there was the emergence of research centres like that of 1893 initiated by Sir Claude McDonald in Lagos, the activities of the British Cotton Growing Association in 1899, which focused more on the experimental work on cotton in Ibadan, Nigeria. To coordinate better the agricultural activities, the Colonial administration in 1912 erected both in

---

[27]   Cfr. M. I. ROEMER, *National Health System of the World*, Oxford University Press, 1991[1], 68.

[28]   R. AKHTAR, Socioeconomic and Political Aspects of Health Care in R. Akhtar (ed.),*Health Care Patterns and Planning in Developing Countries*, Greenwood Press, New York 1991, 73.

[29]   D. M. N. MCDIKKOH, *The Nigerian health…*, 25.

the north and in the south a Department of Agriculture. Between the mid and late 1930s, particular attention was given to the research sector, which was extended and intensified. During this period, the training programmes in agriculture started and students who wanted to study agriculture had access to scholarships for training centres like Yaba Higher College in Nigeria and Imperial College of Tropical Agriculture in Trinidad[30].

Around the late 1940s and early 1950s, the educated and eloquent Nigerians started speaking out for the interest of Nigeria. Their arguments during the constitutional review were geared towards political and economic independence. Nigerians wanted to be in charge of their rich economy. The economic and political elites merged between 1951 and 1959 to achieve this goal. In 1960 when Nigeria acquired her independence from the British Colonies[31], the Federal Department of Agricultural Research was retained. There was a good collaboration between the Federal and the regional ministries in agricultural research activities. The independence of Nigeria officially brought to an end the era of economic exploitation and necessitated for the Nigerian elites, the responsibility to institute economic activities sustained and promoted by Nigerians. More so, there was the need to develop the industrial and other sectors to amplify the ways of economic development and gain more from the potentials of the largely populated nation. More attention was given to the education and skill acquisition sectors. There was a rapid development in the area of infrastructure. Most of the things needed to facilitate the economic development were gradually put in place. The self-sustaining economic enhancement activities of the country at this young stage was often financed with the aid of the big western countries like America and Great Britain.

The Nigerian heads of states within the 1970s and 1980s considered very important, the policies and projects to address the issue of food production. There were projects like that established by General Olusegun Obasanjo tagged "Operation Feed the Nation" and that initiated by President

---

[30] Cfr. O. EFFODUH, «The Economic Development of Nigeria from 1914 to 2014», Academia.edu, citing C. N. NWACHUKWU, «The History of Agriculture in Nigeria from the Colonial Era to the Present Day: Pointing all agricultural programmes», in http://www.onlinenigeria.com/articles/ad.asp?blurb=268, [20-1-2017].

[31] Cfr. J.A. ATANDA - A.Y. ALIYU (eds.) *Proceedings of the National Conference on Nigeria since Independence: Political Development*, Zaria: Gaskiya Corporation, 1985.

Shehu Shagari tagged "Green Revolution". Provision of fertilizers by the government and other initiatives were geared towards encouraging the activities of the local farmers for producing food for the nation. With this, the rate at which food was imported decreased. The period between the early 1960s and late 1970s in Nigeria could be described as a period of economic boom, because there was an increase in the percentage of the national government expenditure from 9 percent in 1962 to 44 percent in 1979. This situation did not last long as there was rapid economic deterioration in the country between the tail end of the1970s and the beginning of the 1980s.

The 1980s also saw a boom in the agricultural sector both at the Federal and State levels where the production of yam, cassava, rice, plantain, sugarcane, palm oil, kernel, groundnut, rubber, cotton, timber and other raw materials for exportation were used to combat hunger and maintain a good standard of living of the citizens. The government invested much to improve this sector and to encourage those involved in the sector. During this period, the Nigerian Agricultural and Co-operative Bank played an important role as it granted loans to farmers. So also did the National Council on Green Revolution, which was instituted in April 1980 and was entrusted with the role of coordinating the activities of the ministries and other stakeholders in the agricultural sectors and of deciphering means of improving this sector, which has fortified and contributed to the growth of the country's economy. A World Bank report regarding this affirms: "this growth has been concentrated particularly in trade and agriculture, which would suggest substantial welfare benefits for many Nigerians"[32]. The paradox of the Nigerian economic situation is obvious in "the puzzle of why a decade of rapid GDP growth by official statistics, concentrated in the pro-poor areas of agriculture and trade, did not bring stronger welfare and employment benefits to the population"[33].

As we have seen, the Nigerian economy was doing well in agriculture but that was not the only economic activity promoted by the country. The iron and steel industries were also growing rapidly alongside that of agriculture. To foster the activities of the steel industry, the government established a steel development authority in 1971 and created the National Steel Council, the Ajaokuta Steel Company Limited and Associated Ores

---

[32]   THE WORLD BANK, *Nigeria Economic Report*, 1 May 2013, 2.

[33]   Ibid., 1.

Mining Company Limited. The year 1979 was the time of the embryonic stage of the Delta Steel industry. The moment was good as the Nigerian manufacturing industry grew from producing goods like beer, soft drinks, cigarettes, shoes and textiles to producing goods like salt, aluminium, sugar, plastics, cements, paper and other goods that were formerly imported. The discovery of oil fields was the apex of the transformation of the economic situation of Nigerian.

The oil sector, which is the most important in the Nigerian economy, has its remote beginning in 1956 when oil was discovered in the Niger Delta by Shell-BP. In 1959, Nigeria was already among the world's oil producers. The progress in this sector of the Nigerian economy continued with the discovery of the EA field in the southeast of Warri in 1965. During the Nigerian-Biafra war 1967-1970, logically the country's economic power declined, but thanks to the rise in the world oil price at the time the war ended in 1970, Nigeria was able to pick up again rapidly and the gain made from this sector was distributed to others to ensure a strong, reliable and diverse economy. Nigeria became a member of the Organisation of Petroleum Exporting Countries (OPEC) in 1971. In 1977, there was the establishment of a company: the Nigerian National Petroleum Company (NNPC), this time not owned by the British or any other foreign country, but by the Nigerian government. In the bid to have a total control of her economy, particularly in the oil sector, the Nigeria government in 1972 issued a decree, which prohibited foreigners from investing in certain businesses and permitted some operations only to the indigenes. Before this decree, the foreigners owned and had an upper hand in the control of trade and activities in the oil sector. Two years before the federal government established the NNPC in 1977, that is in 1975, it acquired about 60 percent of the equity in the marketing affairs of the oil firms operating in its territory and proposed further steps for their complete indigenization, which was not accepted[34].

The profit in the oil business was a major source of the Nigerian economy. In fact, one of the effects of the oil boom was the rapid development of industry and this brought Nigeria in the year 1980, to the important position of being the largest African economy. Suffice it to mention that the Nigerian oil attracted non-indigenous companies from Europe and America, which included Shell-BP, Agip, Chevron, Texaco

---

[34]   Cfr. Oil and Gas 2005, *African Development Bank*, Murrow Prints, 12.

and Mobil, who had business rapport with the Nigerian government. The oil sector was the lifeblood of the Nigerian economic power, and this is evident in the fact that 95 percent of the country's foreign exchange earnings and almost 65 percent of its budgetary revenues were determined by the oil business operations[35]. After touching its apex, the Nigerian economic situation started deteriorating due to the fall in the price of oil on which the country's economy was anchored. However, in 1990, the oil prices and output began to rise again and, consequently, the economy started getting better. The oil sector was in good form again and in 2004, its output touched a daily record level of 2.5 million barrels. The petroleum industry in Nigeria accounts for 80 percent of the Gross Domestic Product (GDP) of Nigeria and more than 90 percent of her total export. Nigeria, just a few years back, was considered 33rd in the world, thanks to its GDP, which was US $2,400 per capita[36].

The problem of Nigeria lies in how its huge wealth is managed. The consequences of the comportment of the Nigerian political leaders is glaringly expressed in the following observation of the World Bank:

> Annual growth rates that average over 7% in official data during the last decade place Nigeria among the fastest growing economies in the world [...] Nevertheless, improvements in social welfare indicators have been much slower than would be expected in the context of this growth. Poverty reduction and job creation have not kept pace with population growth, implying social distress for an increasing number of Nigerians. Progress towards the fulfilment of many of the Millennium Development Goals has been slow, and the country ranked 153 out of 186 countries in the 2013 United Nations Human Development Index[37].

The World Bank Report in a similar analysis underlines the fact that there is a very high geographical concentration as regards economic expansion in Nigeria. It cited Lagos State as an example where the

---

[35] B. PINTO, «Nigeria During and After the Oil Boom: A Comparison with Indonesia», *The World Bank Economic Review*, 1(1987), 419-445, in https://doi.org/10.1093/wber/1.3.419 [6-8-2016].

[36] Cfr. *The Nigerian Petroleum Industry*, in http://www.economywatch.com/worldeconomy/nigeria/ [18- 12- 2016].

[37] THE WORLD BANK, *Nigeria Economic Report…*, 2.

economy is growing rapidly in an exceptional manner and where results have been obtained in the reduction of its poverty headcount from about 44 percent of its population to 23 percent between 2004 and 2010. Whereas in some other states the reverse is the case, because during this moment of economic glory in Lagos, half of the Nigerian States were experiencing increase in the rates of poverty headcount. This is the problem of disparity which the country has to address trying to "unlock rapid growth and job creation in a larger part of the country, as well as to increase standards of education, health, and other social services to enable its citizens to find gainful employment in the emerging great poles"[38]. The report further affirms that:

> Nigeria made a giant step forward during 2004-2009 through the establishment of the Excess Crude Account (ECA) fiscal reserve that successfully insulated the country from the sharp swings in oil prices during this period. But the year 2010 revealed remaining weaknesses in the institutional framework for macroeconomic management. Despite the recovery in oil prices, Nigeria expanded its fiscal stimulus significantly, increasing consolidated spending by an estimated 2.5% of GDP and drawing down the remaining balance of the ECA at the same time that many other oil exporters were building back their reserves. Under this fiscal expansion, the balance of payment remained in deficit, the naira came under pressure, and investor sentiment toward Nigeria became more cautious[39].

The above assertion gives a clear picture of what happens often in the Nigerian economy. The moment of gigantic steps forward in production and trade was an opportunity for other countries involved in oil trade operations to build back their reserves, what those at the helm of economic affairs of Nigeria were not capable of doing. This, as we have seen, landed the country's economy in a problem in 2010. The problem was faced during 2011-2012 through the effort of the government, which strived to reduce its deficit from an estimated 5.7 percent of GDP in 2010 to 2.2 percent in 2011 and a projected 1.9 percent in 2012[40].

---

[38] Ibid.

[39] Ibid.

[40] Ibid.

Part of the reasons for this section of our work is to show how Nigeria has enough wealth that, if distributed very well and according to the right principles we are proposing in this work, it can provide acceptable basic health care for its citizen. The report of the World Bank continues to show concrete evidences of the good economic capacity of the country:

> Nigeria's balance of payments position has strengthened along with oil prices and improved management of fiscal policy. Since September, 2011, the balance of payments has been in surplus most of the time, allowing the Central Bank to build its foreign reserve position from US$ 32 billion naira in mid-2011 to US$ 49 billion by April, 2013 [...] The Government thus has a prime opportunity to make major progress on key reforms and public investments associated with the Transformation Agenda for Job creation, diversification, and more effective governance[41].

The citation above demonstrates how, if sincere efforts are made and selfishness is abhorred, providing basic health care for the citizens would not be a herculean task for the Nigerian Government. The opportunity to do this is not lacking. Maybe what is missing is the good will to do this. The resources are there, but the question is: are they fairly used by those in power? The World Bank report rightly points out that in the distribution of the country's wealth, the realization of minimal standards in health and other social services should be a priority, because the welfare of the greater population largely depends critically on basic educational skills and health. This, according to the report, will go a long way to improve the life of the citizens and the economy of the nation. The World Bank remarks "Despite the high economic growth reported in official statistics, Nigeria is yet to find a formula for translating its resource wealth into significant welfare improvements for the population"[42]. While the economy grows, paradoxically the poverty rate continues to be on the increase and more young people remain unemployed. In fact, the Millennium Development Goals (MDGs) as cited in the 2013 report of the World Bank "has been largely disappointing, with indicators in many areas, resembling those in the poorest countries in Africa"[43]. There are so many signs of contradiction

---

[41]   Ibid., 2-3.

[42]   Ibid., 6-7.

[43]   THE WORLD BANK, *Nigeria Economic Report…*, 7.

in Nigeria. For instance the World Bank observes that: "Poverty rates remain high in Nigeria, particularly in rural areas [...] While the officially reported growth rates of GDP well exceed population growth in the country, the pace of poverty reduction does not"[44].

This implies that the problem of many Nigerians not having access to the basic health care does not really depend on the fact that Nigeria is a poor country as many think, but on the failure on the part of the government to provide it. The right of many Nigerians to basic health care is violated and the access to primary care denied. M. M. Ogbeidi links the above failure to the corruption syndrome. According to him: "Nigeria a country richly endowed with natural resources and high quality human capital is yet to find its rightful place among the community of nations. A major reason that has been responsible for her socio-economic stagnation is the phenomenon of corruption"[45]. This socio-economic quagmire in the interpretation of Robert L. Tignor is linked to the attitude of our political elites: "The political leadership class in Nigeria cannot exonerate itself from the current travails of socio-economic underdevelopment in the country"[46]. Connecting the issue of poverty to the Millennium Development Goals and Sustainable Development, B. Anger affirms that "the evidence suggests that reforms policies have not recorded the spectacular results expected. Thus, poverty alleviation remains a mirage in Nigeria"[47].

1.1.4. Political Point of View: A Brief History of Corruption Among the Nigerian Political Leadership

The state of the various aspects like health, economy, education etc., of Nigeria reflects its condition politically. When politics is done well in a country, logically all the other key sectors function very well, but when politics is poorly done, the key sectors suffer setback. For this reason, we deem it necessary to consider the political aspect of Nigeria in order to understand why the conditions of the aforementioned other aspects, especially the health system in Nigeria, are healthy or poor.

---

[44] Ibid. 9.

[45] M. M. OGBEIDI, «Political Leadership and…».

[46] Ibid.

[47] B. ANGER, «Poverty Eradication, Millennium Development Goals and Sustainable Development in Nigeria», *Journal of Sustainable Development*, 3(2010), 138-144.

In 1861, the territory of Lagos became part of the British Crown colony following an accord with the King of Lagos, Dosumu. Four years later, the British established a Consulate at Lokoja. Between 1887 and 1900, the various parts of the territory that later formed Nigeria were brought under the unique authority of the British colonial rule and was known as Protectorates of Southern Nigeria and Northern Nigeria. The Sokoto Fulani Empire became part of the Northern Protectorate and three years later, i.e., in 1906, the Lagos colony was integrated into to the Southern Protectorate.

In 1914, there was the amalgamation of Nigeria: the unification of the Colony of Lagos and the Northern and Southern Protectorates. The purpose of the unification was economic, rather than political, because it was noticed that, Northern Nigeria Protectorate had a budget deficit, so the colonial administration sought to use the budget surpluses in Southern Nigeria to offset this deficit. So it was done for budgetary and administrative conveniences[48]. The Clifford constitution made it possible for Africans to be eligible to be elected into the Lagos Legislative Council. In 1939, southern Nigeria was divided into Eastern and Western provinces by Governor Bourdillion which later became the Eastern and Western regions. The year 1944 saw the emergence of the National Council of Nigeria and Cameroon. The Constitution of Sir Arthur Richard went into effect in 1946. Between 1949 and 1950 two politically oriented groups were formed; the Northern People's Congress in 1949 and the Action Group in 1950. While the Macpherson Constitution went into effect in 1951, the Lyttleton Constitution went into effect in 1954, bringing Nigeria to a federation of three regions: Eastern, Western and Northern. The election, which was held in 1959, in preparation for the Nigerian independence in 1960, saw the emergence of a coalition government formed by two parties NPC and NCNC. Sir Abubakar Tafawar Belewa emerged as the prime minister.

On October 1, 1960, Nigeria gained her independence from the colonial masters. The first President of Nigeria was Sir Nnamdi Azikiwe from the southern Nigeria, while Sir Abubakar Tafawa Belewa from the northern Nigeria was the first Prime Minister. The political situation in

---

[48]   Cfr. J. D. BARKAN - A. GBOYEGA - M. STEVENS, *State and Local Governance in Nigeria*, Public Sector and Capacity Building Program: Africa Region, August 2, 2001.

Nigeria a little after 1960, when it had its independence was marked by several military coups, war (Nigerian-Biafra war) and other sad experiences of political unrest. In 1963, Nigeria became a republic.

A brief historical overview shows how the corrupt leaders from independence have deprived the citizens of enjoying the wealth of the oil rich country. Corruption started growing wild and wide during the First Republic, which had Sir Abubakar Tafawa Balewa as the Prime Minister, and Nnamdi Azikwe, as the President. This period witnessed an era of Government officials who looted public funds recklessly. The mentality of self-enrichment among the Nigerian politicians started taking root. This selfish attitude of the corrupt leaders during the First Republic warranted the army to take over political power for the first time with the first coup d'état in Nigeria, on 15th January 1966. The coup according to many Nigerians was a wind of change and was welcomed with celebrations, despite the fact that some politicians died during the course. The newly installed military government under the General Aguiyi Ironsi constituted commissions to probe the corrupt politicians of the First Republic. Most of them were guilty of looting and misappropriation of the public funds.

About seven months after the first coup, there was a second coup in July 1966, which ousted General Ironsi and enthroned General Yakubu Gowon. An already cited author explains that:

> The new set of rulers embarked on white elephant projects, which served as a means of looting public funds. The ensuing development clearly showed that the military rulers were not better nor different from the ousted civilian leaders. General Yakubu Gowon ruled the country at a time Nigeria experienced an unprecedented wealth from the oil boom of the 1970s. Apart from the mismanagement of the economy, the Gowon regime was enmeshed in deep-seated corruption[49].

In an attempt to control the widespread corruption in public service General Gowon was overthrown through a coup in July 1975 and, with this, Nigeria had a new military government with General Murtala Mohammed at the helm of affairs. There was a new hope of efficiently fighting corruption because the new military ruler started leading by example, making public every piece of information regarding his assets,

---

[49]   M. M. OGBEIDI, «Political Leadership and…».

and urging other government officials to do the same. He constituted bodies to probe the previous politicians. Through this move, "the Federal Assets Investigation Panel of 1975 found ten of the twelve state military governors in the Gowon regime guilty of corruption. There was the dismissal of the guilty persons from military services with ignominy. They were also forced to give up ill-acquired properties considered to be in excess of their earnings"[50]. But the assassination of General Murtala Mohammed, who was out to unveil and unravel the mystery of corruption among political leaders, quenched the light of hope again. His assassination came just after six months in office. With his death, General Olusegun Obasanjo, who was not interested in continuing the probe move but in a transition of power to a civilian government became the Head of State. In October 1979, he paved the way for the Second Republic led by President Shehu Shagari, a democratically elected president.

The Shagari administration was as corrupt as the past regimes. During his government, embezzlement and fraud were very clear in the claim that "over \$16 billion in oil revenues were lost between 1979 and 1983 during the reign of President Shehu Shagari […] his combative Transport Minister, Alhaji Umaru Dikko, who was alleged to have mismanaged about N4 billion of public fund meant for the importation of rice"[51]. The coup of December 31 1983 truncated the reign of Shagari and brought into power General Muhammadu Buhari. The new government forcibly released Nigerians from the selfish grip of the corrupt leaders. The regime started well with fighting corruption and was efficient in the reinstallation of discipline, with its fight against indiscipline. However, it did not live up to expectations as it failed to respect the human rights and dignity.

After about two years in office, General Ibrahim Babangida toppled General Buhari and became the new Head of State. The coup on August 27 1985 through which Babangida came into office was bloodless. The regimes of Buhari and Babangida lasted for ten years. A prolonged military rule, which saw the increase of corruption in Nigeria, especially during the Babangida's regime. It was because of the corruption among the civilian politicians that the military meddled into politics, to purify Nigeria from corrupt leaders. Unfortunately, with them, instead of decreasing, corruption reached its apex in the Nigerian politics. Describing this situation D.

---

[50]   Ibid.

[51]   Ibid.

M. N. McDikkoh affirms: "Corruption became full-fledged during the Babangida's regime as it had been firmly institutionalized in every aspect of Nigeria's social life and institutions to the point of glamorization, even veneration"[52]. The Babangida administration according to some authors encouraged corruption and rendered futile every effort to fight it. He erased the corruption eradication measures set by his predecessors[53].

The seat of governance became hot with criticisms and demonstrations, after the cancellation of a free and fair election on June 29 1993 won by Chief M.K.O Abiola. This situation led the then Military President to declare that he was stepping aside, handing over power on August 26 1993, to the interim national government composed of military personnel and civilians. The man at the head of the interim national government Ernest Shonekun was a civilian, while the governors of the states were soldiers. The interim national government was mandated to conduct another election and handover to the Third Republic. This dream of Nigerians was cut short on November 17 1993 when the military led by General Sani Abacha took over power from Shonekan, pushing him aside. Things became worse with the Abacha's regime as Nigeria entered another dark tunnel of corruption. M. Ogbeidi, citing the document, "International Centre for Asset Recovery, 2009", writes:

> Abacha's regime only furthered the deep-seated corrupt practices, which already characterised public life since the inception of the Babangida regime. Under General Abacha, corrupt practices became blatant and systematic. General Abacha and his family alongside his associates looted Nigeria's coffers with reckless abandon. The extent of Abacha's venality seemed to have surpassed that of other notorious African rulers, such as Mobutu Sese Seko of Zaire (now called the Democratic Republic of Congo). It was estimated that the embezzlement of public funds and corruption proceeds of General Abacha and his family amounted to USD 4 billion[54].

General Abacha who apart from being a corrupt leader also manifested he was diabolic especially in his sit-tight intention and all that surrounded

---

[52]   D. M. N. McDIKKOH, *The Nigerian health…*, 30.

[53]   M. M. OGBEIDI, «Political Leadership and…».

[54]   Cfr. Ibid.

it. His dictatorship however ended when he died mysteriously in June 1998. Following his death, General Abdulsalami Abubakar became the Head of State. He successfully conducted an election and handed over power in May 1999 signalling the beginning of the Fourth Republic led by General Olusegun Obasanjo (rtd.). The Obasanjo administration mapped out anti-corruption strategies and followed it with diligence. There were two institutions set up by the government in the bid to fight corruption: The Economic and Financial Crimes Commission (EFCC) and the Independent Corrupt Practices Commission (ICPC). The name Nigeria at this moment was notorious for money laundering activities especially by her political leaders. Financial Action Task Force on Money Laundering (FATF) condemned Nigeria for not cooperating with the International community in her anti-money laundering activities. The EFCC, which investigated all cases of Nigerians in every sector living above their means, was a response to this criticism by the International community. In the same vein, the ICPC investigated cases in the public sector relevant to bribery, abuse or misuse of office and other offences under the corrupt practices and other Related Offences Act, 2000[55].

The Obasanjo led government would have been a better opportunity for Nigeria to tackle the problem of corruption, but it failed because the EFCC and ICPC that were established for the eradication of corruption became instruments the president used to hunt his political opponents and other persons who courageously criticized his insatiable quest for power. Another issue that marked the failure in the fight against corruption is that "the political leadership class of the Obasanjo administration from the top to the grassroots were almost entirely entrapped in the snare of corruption, which made the anti-corruption posture of the administration an obvious paradox"[56]. It is really a bizarre idea to think that a corrupt government can lead an anti-corruption campaign. One blind surely cannot lead another.

President Shehu Musa Yar'Adua who took over from Obasanjo as the second president of Nigeria's Fourth Republic had a clean record. While in office, President Yar' Adua fell ill and died from the sickness. Yar'Adua for Nigerians was different from other political leaders. He had a sincere spirit of service and his record was free from corruption and/or ethnic favouritism. The Vice President, Goodluck Jonathan, in accordance

---

[55]   Ibid.

[56]   Ibid.

with the Nigerian constitution, became the new president to complete the four year tenure of Yar'Adua. President Goodluck Jonathan, after completing this tenure, contested in the 2011 election and emerged the winner, thus becoming the president of Nigeria. Goodluck brought the Nigerian economy to be the strongest economy in Africa and, according to many, he improved the economic life of many Nigerians. A gentle man, who unlike some African leaders, congratulated Buhari and accepted defeat when he contested the second time in the presidential election, which saw Muhammadu Buhari emerging the winner.

Muhammadu Buhari, who was the military president of Nigeria from 1983 to 1985, was sworn in on May 29, 2015, and became, for the second time, the president of the Federal Republic of Nigeria, just like the former president, Olusegun Obasanjo. Buhari promised change and promised to free Nigeria from corrupt politicians, but his government is drowning in corruption. This year there will be a general election and Nigerians are hoping and yearning to see a true and positive change.

1.2. Nigeria's Key Health Indicators

1.2.1. Life Expectancy at Birth Male/Female

Life expectancy is described as the length of time expected to be lived by an individual at birth. For the developing countries like Nigeria, Ghana, Tanzania etc., life expectancy is very important in the bid to achieve its goal of socio-economic progress, which is to be realized by making serious investments in important social sectors such as health, education, sanitation and environmental management[57]. Life expectancy at birth male/female in the year 2015 is 53/56. Neonatal mortality rate (per 1000 live births), in 2015 in Nigeria is 34.3 according to WHO. Under-five mortality rate (probability of dying by age 5 per 1000 live births), in 2015 in Nigeria is 108.8[58]. In the bid to have a better life expectancy, the "attainment of 70 years life expectancy by 2020 is one of the millennium development goals

---

[57] Cfr. P. I. SEDE - W. OHEMENG, «Socio-economic determinants of life expectancy in Nigeria (1980-2011) », *Health Economics Review*, 5(2)2015, in https://doi.org/10.1186/s13561-014-0037-z [7-2-2015].

[58] Cfr. WHO: *World Health Organization Statistics 2015.*

in Nigeria"[59]. Life expectancy is an important issue for the "UN 2030 Agenda for Sustainable Development", which underlines its commitments in the extension of life expectancy for all, by achieving universal health coverage and access to quality health care, by reducing new born, child and maternal mortality through the prevention of preventable deaths[60].

A study on life expectancy in Nigeria by P. I. Sede and W. Ohemeng, reveals how government expenditure on health is one of the major determinant factors of life expectancy in Nigeria. The study thus suggests that in order to improve life expectancy in Nigeria, there must be an improvement and a change of attitude on the part of the government by way of increasing qualitatively and quantitatively its health expenditure and tackling convincingly the problem of unemployment. Regarding this, P. I. Sede and W. Ohemeng, affirm: "In Nigeria, as in other developing countries, variation in morbidity and mortality have been associated with a wide variety of measures of socio-economic status including per capita GDP"[61].

In countries where there is even distribution of income, the level of life expectancy is usually high. In Nigeria, the reverse is the case. There is a big gap between the rich and the poor; the tendency of mortality is high. When per capita income is high, it increases the level of health care expenditure and this, if properly done, could have a positive impact on the health status and the life expectancy of the citizens. In Nigeria for instance:

> Although income and health expenditure are increasing [...] life expectancy has been unsteady. An analysis of three deciles average shows that between 1980 and 1989, in Nigeria, life expectancy averaged 45.8 years; 1990 and 1999, it was 45.6 years; and 2000 and 2010, it improved marginally to an average 5.8 6 years[62].

The unsatisfactory state of life expectancy in Nigeria could also be seen in a thirteen year average (1999-2011) data on life expectancy, under five infant mortality rate, per capita income and unemployment rate for

---

59   P. I. SEDE, W. OHEMENG, *Socio-economic determinants…*

60   UNITED NATIONS DEPARTMENT OF ECONOMIC AND SOCIAL AFFAIRS. (2015). «*Transforming our world: The 2030 agenda for sustainable development*», in https:// sustainabledevelopment.un.org/post2015/transformingourworld [6-6-2016].

61   P. I. SEDE, W. OHEMENG, *Socio-economic determinants…*

62   Ibid.

Nigeria, Ghana, Kenya, China and India which demonstrates how Nigeria performed poorly on all these indicators. Most other nations who show more commitments achieved better results[63].

The Nigerian government intends to improve the life expectancy by bringing it to 70 years by 2020. For this, it had right from 1980 established policies and embarked on projects that focused on the reform of the health sector. Some of these policies include the Primary Health Care (PHC), which was put in place to better the rate of life expectancy and the National Health Insurance Schemes (NHIS), which aims at mitigating the cost of access and efficiency in the delivery of health services. Seeing the failure and the unpleasant results of these policies as well as the high level of inefficiencies, some concerned Nigerians have asked questions regarding the extent these health policies have influenced the life expectancy of Nigerians.

> Health policy on its part is government systematic control of important health variable, such as government expenditure on health, so as to make healthy life available and accessible to the individuals. Such policy efforts might have significant influence on life expectancy since they directly help in reducing morbidity and mortality[64].

1.2.2. Maternal Mortality Ratio and other Maternal Health Indicators

In almost all parts of the world, childbirth is an experience that calls for celebration. Expectant mothers are usually curious and at times anxious to see the fruit of their womb. In addition, family members happily wait for the joyful day of deliverance. Nevertheless, this experience is not the same for all. Studies have proved that childbirth is not always a happy event in the developing countries especially for most Nigerian women "who experience childbirth as suffering and tragedy that may end in death"[65].

The average national maternal mortality ratio (MMR) in 2015 according to the United Nation inter-agency estimates was 1,100 deaths per

---

[63]   Ibid.

[64]   P. I. SEDE, W. OHEMENG, «Socio-economic determinants…».

[65]   L. O. OLUSEGUN – T. R. IBE – M. M. IKOROK, «Curbing maternal and child mortality: The Nigerian experience», *International Journal of Nursing and Midwifery*,4(2012), 33-39, in https://doi.org/10.5897/ijnm11.030 [10-9-2016].

100,000 live births, with a lifetime risk of maternal death of 1 in 8. It is sad to note that approximately 1 in every 9 maternal deaths occurs in Nigeria. The World Health Organisation (WHO) makes known that in 2015, 58,000 Nigerian women died due to pregnancy and childbearing complications[66]. This affirms the truth that Maternal and new born mortality are among the major challenges in Nigeria. Some authors following their study retain that "the situation in northern Nigeria is critical where strong cultural beliefs and practices on childbirth and fertility-related behaviours partly contribute significantly to the maternal morbidity and mortality picture compared to southern Nigeria"[67].

Some other Nigerian authors in their study aimed at identifying the factors behind the choice of place of delivery among the pregnant women in Enugu State of Nigeria, discovered that while 52.9% of the women who responded delivered outside health institutions, 47.1% delivered in health institutions. According to this study, prominent among the factors conditioning the above mentioned choice include: promptness of care, the technical capacity of nurses, midwives and doctors, availability and affordability of care, availability and readiness of doctors and the presence of specialist obstetricians[68]. Similarly, a study in 24 local governmental areas in Jigawa State, Northern Nigeria on maternal and child health showed that there was a high demand for health care services but the response does not meet with the level of demand. For instance, the study documented challenges such as low quality of care, uncertain availability of health workers and drug stock-out. These problems, according to the study, are persistent[69].

---

[66]   Cfr. WHO, UNICEF, UNFPA, World Bank Group and the United Nations Population Division. Trends in maternal mortality: 1990-2015. Geneva: World Health Organization; 2015, in http://www.who.int/gho/maternal_health/countries/nga.pdf [07-4-2017].

[67]   H. V. DOCTOR - R. BAIRAGI - S. E. FINDLE – S. HELLERINGER – T. DAHIRU, «Northern Nigeria Maternal, Newborn and Child Health Programme: Selected Analyses from Population-Based Baseline Survey», *The Open Demography Journal*, 4, (2011), 11-21.

[68]   Cfr. H. E. ONAH– L. C. IKEAKO – G. C. ILOABACHIE, «Factors associated with the use of maternity services in Enugu, south-eastern Nigeria», *Social Science & Medicine*, 63(2006), 1870-1878.

[69]   Cfr. V. SHARMA –J. LEIGHT – F. ABDULAZIZ – N. GIROUX – N. M. BJORKMAN, «Illness recognition, decision-making, and care-seeking for maternal and

H. V. Doctor, R. Bairagi, S. E. Findley, S. Helleringer and T. Dahiru did not mince words in their declaration on the condition of maternal and child health in Nigeria. According to them: "Maternal and child health (MCH) outcomes in Nigeria are among the worst in the World"[70]. A study in three states, Kastina, Yobe and Zamfara, located in the Northern part of Nigeria, identified the factors responsible for the high rates of maternal, new born and child mortality and morbidity as: "inadequate health facilities, lack of transportation to institutional care, inability to pay for services and resistance among some populations to modern health care"[71]. Another study with similar results affirms that socio-economic barriers are among the major factors that limit optimal utilization of maternal health services by majority of Nigerians[72]. Some mothers are forced to use traditional medicine because they cannot afford the care offered in the health facilities. In this regard, a study to document the herbal medicine used for common ailments in neonates and infants less than six months in Lagos, Nigeria reveals that medicinal plant species were used for treatment of common ailments such as diarrhoea, abdominal cramps, skin rashes, fever (malaria), jaundice and weight loss in neonates and infants less than 6 months[73]. "Financial concerns are often another major barrier to accessing services. In the Kano study, 25% of study participants cited lack of money as a reason for not using health facilities"[74]. Being able to understand what could be the effect of the actual socioeconomic characteristics of women on maternal health service utilization is very important if Nigeria wants

---

newborn complications: a qualitative study in Jigawa State, Northern Nigeria», *Journal of Health, Population and Nutrition*, 36(2017), 59-63, in https://doi.org/10.1186/s41043-017-0124-y [15-8-2018].

[70] H. V. DOCTOR - R. BAIRAGI - S. E. FINDLE – S. HELLERINGER – T. DAHIRU, «Northern Nigeria Maternal...».

[71] Ibid.

[72] Cfr. B. NUHU – T. BABAYO – I. HADIZA – D. T. KELLY, «Knowledge and Perceptions of Maternal Health in Kaduna State, Northern Nigeria», *African Journal of Reproductive Health*, 14(2010), 71-76.

[73] Cfr. O. NWAIWU – O. B. OYELADE, «Traditional herbal medicines used in neonates and infants less than six months old in Lagos Nigeria», *Nigerian Journal of Paediatrics*, 43(2016), 40, in https://doi.org/10.4314/njp.v43i1.8 [15-8-2018].

[74] B. NUHU – T. BABAYO – I. HADIZA – D. T. KELLY, «Knowledge and Perceptions...».

to improve or maximize health benefits and outcomes for infants and children[75].

According to a report of the World Health Organisation (WHO), an estimated 800 women die every day due to pregnancy and childbirth-related complications in developing countries[76]. For this K. O. Osungbade and O. O. Ayinde affirm the important role of antenatal care utilisation in the bid to achieve the Millennium Development Goals[77]. The World Health Organisation (WHO) is of the same view and, for this reason, it introduced the concept of antenatal care and recommended a minimum of four antenatal visits during pregnancy[78]. Unfortunately, in Nigeria, the rate of antenatal care utilisation is estimated at 50 percent - 60 percent; a rate which does not satisfy the standard of the World Health Organisation[79].

Antenatal care is very important because "every pregnant woman faces the risk of sudden, unpredictable complications that could end in death or injury to herself or her infant"[80]. It is sad to note that several studies reveal that a significant number of pregnant women do not have access to these essential "life-saving" health care services. In this regard, the UNICEF gives an insight on the Nigerian situation:

---

[75]   Cfr. T. O. OYEWALE – T. R. MAVUNDLA, «Socioeconomic factors contributing to exclusion of women from maternal health benefit in Abuja, Nigeria», *Curationis*, 38(2015), 1-11, in https://doi.org/10.4102/curationis.v38il.1272 [16-8-2018].

[76]   WORLD HEALTH ORGANISATION (WHO), Maternal Mortality. Factsheet 348, 2014, in http://www.who.int/mediacecentre/factsheets/fs348/en [10-5-2016].

[77]   Cfr. K. O. OSUNGBADE – O. O. AYINDE, «Maternal Complication prevention: evidence from a case-control study in southwest Nigeria», *African Journal of Primary Health Care & Family Medicine*, 6(2014), 656, in http://dx.doi.org/10.4102/phcfm.v6il.656 [20-5-2017].

[78]   Cfr. WORLD HEALTH ORGANISATION (WHO), *Antenatal care randomised trial: Manual for the implementation of the new model*. Geneva: WHO, 2001.

[79]   Cfr. K. O. OSUNGBADE – O. O. AYINDE, «Maternal Complication prevention...».

[80]   E. A. TOBIN - A. N. OFILI - N. ENEBELI - O. ENUEZE, «Assessment of birth preparedness and complication readiness among pregnant women attending Primary Health Care Centres in Edo State, Nigeria», *Annals of Nigerian Medicine*, 8(2014), 76-81, in https://doi.org/10.4103/0331-3131.153358 [27-5-2017].

> A woman's chance of dying from pregnancy and childbirth
> in Nigeria is 1 in 13. Although many of these deaths are
> preventable, the coverage and quality of health care services
> in Nigeria continue to fail women and children. Presently, less
> than 20 per cent of health facilities offer emergency obstetric
> care and only 35 per cent of deliveries are attended by skilled
> birth attendants[81].

A view at the state of maternal health in Nigerian prompts the declaration that having babies in Nigeria, especially in the rural areas, could be a life-threatening affair, because many women have babies whilst malnourished, in hygienically bad conditions and without access to medical treatment.

1.2.3. Infant and Child Mortalities (Under 5-mortality rate)

The **UNICEF** Report 2006 reveals that nearly 10 million children under five die globally[82]. Going by the **UN** estimates, 1 in every 6 children dies before the age of 5 from childhood related illness[83]. Some aforementioned authors continuing in this trend report that: "Under-five mortality in Nigeria is estimated at 191 per 1000 live births. Almost one million children die in Nigeria more than any other country in Africa, largely from preventable diseases"[84]. The **UNICEF** in a report similar to the aforementioned observes: "The deaths of new born babies in Nigeria represent a quarter of the total number of deaths of children under-five. The majority of these occur within the first week of life, mainly due to complications during pregnancy and delivery as well as maternal care"[85]. When we mention infant mortality rate, we refer to the probability that a child may die on or before one year from the time of birth. The under-5 mortality rate implies the probability of a child dying before the age of five.

---

[81]   UNICEF NIGERIA, «The children, Maternal and child health», in https://www.unicef.org/nigeria/children_1926.html [20-5-2016].

[82]   Cfr. L. O. OLUSEGUN – T. R. IBE – M. M. IKOROK, «Curbing maternal and…».

[83]   Cfr. Ibid.

[84]   Ibid.

[85]   UNICEF NIGERIA, «The children, Maternal and child health», in https://www.unicef.org/nigeria/children_1926.html [20-5-2016].

The performance of the Nigerian health sector in the area of child/infant health, shows the country is still far from the set objectives. The consequences of this failure and debacles could be clearly identified in the high infant, child mortality "and periodical outbreak of the same disease, as well as the long period of time spent for control of the various outbreaks"[86]. Despite its numerous efforts, Nigeria has not improved in the area of child survival and it accounts for a large portion of the global disease portion[87].

O. K. Ezeh, A. K. Emwinyore, M. J. Dibley, J. J. Hall and N. A. Page, commenting on a report of the UNICEF/WHO write: "In 2012, approximately half of the world's estimated 6.6 million deaths in children aged less than 5 years occurred in sub-Saharan Africa and Nigeria accounted for approximately 13% of these deaths"[88]. The study by these authors reveals that the major causes of death among infants and children in Africa are communicable diseases such: as malaria, diarrhoea, measles, cholera and respiratory infections. According to them, these deaths are both preventable and treatable, but the lack of effective health policies has resulted in a high under-5 child mortality rate (U5MR) in Africa, with the majority of cases occurring in Nigeria[89]. The above remark underlines some ethical problems regarding the lives of the vulnerable that are lost carelessly. Children who should be protected, defended, nourished, educated and given care are allowed to die needlessly of diseases that could be treated without spending much.

Some authors identified multiparity as one of the factors that make childbirth dangerous. While "parity indicates how many births a woman

---

[86] M. Osain, «Nigerian health care system: Need for integrating adequate medical intelligence and surveillance systems», *Journal of Pharmacy and Bioallied Sciences*, 3(4), (2011), 470-478.

[87] Cfr. A. Wollum – R. Burstein – N. Fullman – L. D.-Lindgren – E. Gakidou, «Benchmarking health system performance across states in Nigeria: a systematic analysis of levels and trends in key maternal and child health interventions and outcomes», 2000-2013, *BMC Medicine*, 13(2015), 208, in https://doi/10.1186/s12916-015-0438-9 [6-8-2018].

[88] O. K. Ezeh, A. K. Emwinyore, M. J. Dibley, J. J. Hall and N. A. Page, «Risk factors for post neonatal, infant, child and under-5 mortality in Nigeria: a pooled cross-sectional analysis», *BMJ Open*, 5(3), (2015). https://doi.org/10.1136/bmjopen-2014-006779. [8-6-2016].

[89] Ibid.

has already had [...] grand multiparity has been defined by the International Federation of Gynaecology and Obstetrics (1993) as delivery of the fifth to ninth viable pregnancies"[90]. Multiparity is described by some notable authors as "dangerous and an independent factor in maternal and infantile morbidity and mortality"[91]. As reported by a study carried out in Bauchi State, Nigeria, childbirth complications found include "haemorrhage [postpartum/antepartum], uterine rupture, abruptio placentae [1:3%] and malpresentation [0.26%]"[92].

Giving an insight on the issue of infant and child mortality in Nigeria, M. I. Olatubi, O. O. Oyediran, I. O. Adubi and O. C. Ogidan write:

> Even though only 2% of the global population is in Nigeria, the country, with an estimated infant mortality rate of 75 per 1000 live births, child mortality rate of 88 per 1,000 live births, under 5 mortality rate of 157 per 1,000 live births and a maternal mortality ratio of 800 per 100,000 live births, contributes a disproportionate 10% to the global burden of maternal and also infant mortality. Wide regional variation exists in infant and maternal across the zones. Infant and child mortality in the North West and North East zones of the country of the country are in general twice the rate in the southern zones while the maternal mortality in the North West and North West and North East is 6 times and 9 times respectively the rate of 165/100,000 recorded in the South West Zone[93].

The surprising aspect of this is that, while globally child death is reducing, in Nigeria, it has remained a great challenge in the public health, where despite the decrease in the number of deaths, the percentage is still high and the risk of more losing their lives persists. "Nearly one million children under 5 years die in Nigeria annually and more than 60% of these deaths occur between 1 and 59 months of life [...] With this marginal

---

[90]   M. C. Ukwuma, Multiparity and Childbirth Complications in Rural Women of Northeastern Nigerian Origin, «*IOSR Journal of Pharmacy and Biological Sciences*», 2(2012), 1-4.

[91]   Ibid.

[92]   Ibid.

[93]   M. I. Olatubi – O. O. Oyediran – I. O. Adubi – O. C. Ogidan, «Health Care Expenditure in Nigeria and National Productivity: A Review», *South Asian Journal of Social Studies and Economics*, 1(2018), 1-7.

reduction in childhood death, it is more likely that Nigeria will not achieve the Millennium Development Goal target of 76 deaths per 1000 live births by 2015"[94]. This prophesy has come true because now in 2019, the mentioned Millennium Development Goal target for 2015 is yet to be achieved. Child death has not been reduced, as the problem continues to be a notable challenge to the Nigerian Health system. In Nigeria, 16 percent of children die before reaching their fifth birthday. This represents about 10 percent of global child deaths, even though it is just 2 percent of the world's population[95].

1.2.4. Immunisation Coverage

The Child immunization coverage in Nigeria "is provided through routine immunization and catch-up supplemental immunization campaigns (also known as National Immunization Days) organized across the country or sub nationally in selected areas"[96]. Some authors retain immunization to be among the safest and most cost-effective means of preventing child morbidity and mortality[97]. Treating the issue of vaccination of children in Nigeria, some above-cited authors propose the definition of vaccination by the Nigerian Federal Ministry of Health. According to such definition, a child is fully vaccinated "if he or she has received a Bacillus Calmette-Guérin (BCG) vaccination against tuberculosis; three doses of DPT to prevent diphtheria, pertussis (whooping cough), and tetanus; at least three doses of polio vaccine; and one dose of measles vaccine"[98]. Other vaccines include Yellow Fewer, within 9 months of age, hepatitis B, pneumococcus

---

[94]   O.K. Ezeh - A. K. Emwinyore - M. J. Dibley - J. J. Hall - N. A. Page, «Risk factors for …».

[95]   G. Timothy - O. Irinoye - U. Yunusa - A. Dalhatu - S. Ahmed - A. Suberu, «Balancing Demand and Efficiency in Nigerian Health Care Delivery System», *European Journal of Business and Management*, 6 (23), 2014, 50-56.

[96]   C. Z. Olorunsaiye - H. Degge, «Variations in the uptake of Routine Immunization in Nigeria: Examining Determinants of Inequitable Access», *Journal Global Health Communication*, 2(1), (2016), 19-29, in http://dx.doi.org/1 0.1080/23762004.2016.1206780 [3-5-2017].

[97]   Cfr. E. Bbaale, «Immunization status and child survival in Uganda», *African Journal of Economic Review*, 3(2015), 1-20, in https://doi.org/10.3329/jhpn. v3li1.14756 [20-3-2017].

[98]   H. V. Doctor - R. Bairagi - S. E. Findle – S. Helleringer– T. Dahiru, «Northern Nigeria Maternal …».

and rotavirus; administered within the first one year from birth. Vitamin A is administered within 9 and 15 months[99] [100].

The Federal Ministry of Health requests that the above-mentioned vaccinations be completed within one year from birth. This implies that, within one year, every child who has the possibility must have completed his or her immunisations, thus being completely immunised. In Nigeria, "Children in the urban areas have consistently higher immunisation rates than those in the rural areas"[101]. Here we see the problem that marks almost all the sectors of health care services in Nigeria such as inequality between the urban and the rural areas, especially in the distribution of resources. The aforementioned authors affirm that: "Findings on low immunisation coverage underscore the importance of further strengthening the programme's initiatives to raise immunisations through increased community mobilization and outreach to build knowledge and social support for immunisations"[102]. The authors further recommend that more attention be given to the rural areas, especially to offset the educational and urban advantages in term of immunisation knowledge, influences and practices[103].

A report of the World Health Organization in 2015 reveals that at the global level, about 3 million children die every year of diseases, which through vaccine could be prevented[104]. C. Z. Olorunsaiye and H. Degge in their study on immunisation in Nigeria, observe that at the global level, "immunization prevents an estimated 2-3 million deaths among under-5 children, yet in Nigeria, only 25% of children ages 12-13 months are fully immunized"[105]. This is due to many factors in Nigeria. For example, Nigeria, since 1988 has been involved in

---

[99] Cfr. NATIONAL PRIMARY HEALTH CARE DEVELOPMENT AGENCY (2009), *National immunization policy* (rev.), Abuja, Nigeria: Federal Ministry of Health.

[100] E. A., OPHORI - M. Y. TULA - A. V. AZIH- R. OKOJIE - P. E.IKPO, «Current trends of immunization in Nigeria: Prospects and challenges», *Tropical Medicine and Health,* 42 (2), 67-75.

[101] H. V. DOCTOR - R. BAIRAGI - S. E. FINDLE – S. HELLERINGER – T. DAHIRU, «Northern Nigeria Maternal...».

[102] Ibid.

[103] Ibid.

[104] WORLD HEALTH ORGANIZATION (WHO), (2015a) *1 in5 children in Africa do not have access to life saving vaccines,* in http://www.afro.who.int/en/media-centre/afro-feature/item/7620-1-in-5-children-in-africa-do-not-have-access-to-life-saving-vaccines.html [20-12-2016]

[105] C. Z. OLORUNSAIYE, H. DEGGE, «Variations in the...».

the global strategies to eradicate polio. However, in 2003, the "anti-polio" move in the country met an obstacle when three states in the northern part decided to boycott the polio vaccination. According to these states, they believed that the vaccine had some anti-fertility agent and a plan to introduce or diffuse HIV among the inhabitants. This boycott brought about the reintroduction of the wild poliovirus (WPV) into 31 countries that were polio free. Some other factors sabotage the fight against polio in Nigeria. Among these is the attack of the Boko Haram, which in some communities, disrupt the vaccination programme. In some states in the northeast of Nigeria, where the terrorists operate often, there are extremely high proportions of unimmunized children: Borno 73.2%, Yobe 64. 8%, Gombe is 52.3% and Bauchi 43.7%[106] [107]. The result is clear in the fact that "children fully immunized in the north ranges from 6-8 percent, compared with 23 percent nationally"[108].

Other factors that hitch immunization in Nigeria are stated in a study on the variations in the uptake of routine immunization in Nigeria, which describes the child, mother and state variables. According to the study, such variations depend on some factors like the educational background of the women (mothers), their religion, economic capacity, location; urban or rural dwellers etc. The results of the above-mentioned study show that generally the proportion of fully immunized children ages 12-23 months is very low[109]. This is similar to the report of the 2013 of the Nigerian Demographic and Health Survey, which reveals the low proportion of 25%[110] [111] [112]. According

---

[106] Ibid.

[107] WORLD HEALTH ORGANIZATION (WHO). (2013b), Progress towards poliomyelitis eradication Nigeria, January 2012 – September 2013, *Weekly Epidemiological Record*, 51-52(88), 545-556.

[108] G. TIMOTHY - O. IRINOYE - U. YUNUSA - A. DALHATU - S. AHMED - A. SUBERU, «Balancing Demand and…»; Nigeria however, in April 2016 participated in the polio vaccination programme of the World Health Organization.

[109] Cfr. C. Z. OLORUNSAIYE, H. DEGGE, «Variations in the…».

[110] Cfr. NIGERIAN DEMOGRAPHIC HEALTH SURVEY, Abuja, Nigeria 2013, (The proportion of fully immunized children ages 12-23 in Nigeria is comparatively lower than that of the neighbouring countries like Benin, which has 43%, Cameroun, which has 53%, Ghana, which has 77%, and Niger, which has 52%).

[111] Cfr. GHANA STATISTISTICAL SERVICE & ICF MACRO (2015), *Ghana demographic and health survey 2014*, Accra, Ghana.

[112] Cfr. C. Z. OLORUNSAIYE, H. DEGGE, «Variations in the…».

to C. Z., Olorunsaiye and H. Degge: "This comparison suggests that the Nigerian routine immunization program does not reach all vulnerable children with critical life-saving vaccines. Moreover, it is surprising that after several years of supplemental immunization; nearly 21% of Nigeria children were unimmunized"[113]. This comment suggests that much needs to be done in the area of immunization especially of children and generally, to make basic health care accessible to the Nigerian populace especially the most vulnerable whose right to health is being violated every day in Nigeria.

G. E. Erhabor, F. O. Akambi and S. B. Gordon rightly affirmed, "Immunisation coverage in Nigeria is largely dependent on political commitment"[114]. If really immunisation coverage in Nigeria depends on the commitments of the Nigerian political leaders, one does not need to go far in order to discover why the immunisation coverage in the nation is not satisfactory. Some authors regarding this emphasize on how "vaccine-preventable diseases coupled with infectious and parasitic diseases continue to exact a heavy toll on the health and survival of Nigerians"[115].

1.3. Major Causes of Death and Main Pathologies in Nigeria

1.3.1. Malaria

Malaria constitutes a major health problem in Nigeria. It is considered very dangerous especially for women and children because "malaria affects maternal health and pregnancy outcome. It causes anaemia in pregnancy which increases the risk of maternal deaths [...] Malaria in pregnancy also causes low birth weight, preterm delivery, congenital infection, and reproductive loss"[116]. Malaria is endemic in Nigeria. It is one of the major

---

[113]   Ibid.

[114]   M. O. Akanbi, C. O. Ukoli, G. E. Erhabor, F. O. Akambi, S. B. Gordon, «The burden of respiratory disease in Nigeria», *African Journal of Respiratory Medicine*, 8(2013), 10-17.

[115]   G. Timothy, O. Irinoye, U. Yunusa, A. Dalhatu, S. Ahmed, A. Suberu, «Balancing Demand and…».

[116]   A. Auta, «Demographic Factors Associated with Insecticide Treated Net among Nigerian Women and Children», *Nort American Journal of Medical Sciences*, 4(2012), 40-49, in https://doi.org/10.4103/1947-2714.92903

causes of morbidity and mortality in Nigeria and it accounts for 30% and 11% of child and maternal deaths respectively[117].

In 2015 the National Malaria Elimination Programme (NMEP), the National Population Commission (NPopC), and the National Bureau of Statistics (NBS), put into effect the Nigeria Malaria Indicator Survey (2015 NMIS), from October 2015 through November 2015, on a nationally representative sample of more than 8,000 households[118]. During this survey, women between 15 and 49 years from the above-mentioned 8,000 households were interviewed on issues regarding the prevention of malaria during pregnancy and treatment of childhood fevers. Some tests were carried out on the children between 6 and 59 months, and microscopy was done to determine the presence of malaria parasites in the various states and the Federal Capital Territory, and to know specifically their types. The nurses following the appropriate treatment protocols gave all the children who tested positive adequate treatment[119].

The 2015 Nigeria Malaria Indicator Survey sadly remarks that Malaria remains a notable public health problem in Nigeria where its favourite victims are children under age 5 and pregnant women. Africa according to the Survey "still bears over 80 percent of the global malaria burden and Nigeria accounts for about 29 percent of this burden"[120]. The information above consolidates the call for the application of the ethical principles in the handling of the affairs of the Nigerian Health Care System. Malaria is a preventable and treatable illness transmitted by mosquitoes. So if it is preventable, treatable, and the source is well known; mosquitoes, which we

---

[10-9-2016].

[117] Cfr. Ibid; Cfr. S. T. ADEDOKUN – V. T. ADEKANMBI – O. A. UTHAM – R. J. LILFORD, «Contextual factors associated with health care service utilization for children with acute childhood illness in Nigeria», *PLoS ONE*, 12(2017), e0173578, in https://doi.org/10.1371/journal.pone.0173578 [3-8-2018].

[118] Cfr. NATIONAL MALARIA ELIMINATION PROGRAMME (NMEP), NATIONAL POPULATION COMMISSION (NPopC), NATIONAL BUREAU OF STATISTICS (NBS), AND ICF INTERNATIONAL 2016, *Nigeria Malaria Indicator Survey 2015, Key Indicators*. Abuja, Nigeria, and Rockville, Maryland, USA: NMEP, NPopC, and ICF International, 1.

[119] Cfr. NATIONAL MALARIA ELIMINATION PROGRAMME (NMEP), NATIONAL POPULATION COMMISSION (NPopC), NATIONAL BUREAU OF STATISTICS (NBS), AND ICF INTERNATIONAL 2016, *Nigeria Malaria Indicator...*, 1.1-4.

[120] Ibid. 3.

know where they harbour; (stagnant waters and dirty environment), how can Nigeria, the acclaimed "giant of Africa" account for 25 percent of the cases and deaths at a global level?

There are ways through which malaria could be prevented like: using mosquito nets, taking preventive doses of antimalarial drugs, especially during the rainy season, when there is a prevalent presence of mosquitoes, indoor and outdoor spraying with lasting insecticides, doing constant tests and keeping the environment clean and free from stagnant waters. Affirming this A. Auta writes, "Insecticide-treated nets (ITNs) have been shown to be the most cost effective measures in the prevention of malaria. ITNs have been shown to reduce malaria mortality by 17% in children below the age of five"[121]. Commenting on the sources of mosquito nets in Nigeria, the document of "the 2015 Nigeria Malaria Survey Indicator" says that apart from the possibility of purchasing them directly at shops, markets or from hawkers, "the Federal Ministry of Health (FMoH) and other stakeholders have conducted net distribution campaigns between 2009 and 2013 and net replacement campaigns from 2013 to 2015"[122]. Without any intention of doubting this information or denying the Federal Ministry of Health their merits for this plausible gesture, we ask, if this is true, why is it that "Nigeria accounted for up to 25 percent of the cases and deaths" resulting from malaria according to the 2015 edition of the above-cited document?

We are still on the same problem of distribution. Where were the net distribution campaigns made? What were the modalities or principles applied? To what extent did the distributed nets get to the vulnerable, the majority in need? We ask these questions being aware of how complicated distribution could be in Nigeria, owing to several factors like the immensity of its population, tribalism, and the difficulty in reaching those in the remote areas. However, these factors cannot serve as alibi because, where there is the goodwill to act in the way of justice, the mentioned problems could be solved without much qualms because the factors mentioned above are not insurmountable.

---

[121] A. Auta, «Demographic Factors Associated…».

[122] National Malaria Elimination Programme (NMEP), National Population Commission (NPopC), National Bureau of Statistics (NBS), and ICF International 2016, *Nigeria Malaria Indicator…*, 15.

Malaria is the most common cause of the outpatient visits to health facilities in Nigeria. Available results and records from studies and surveys show that at least 50% of the population of Nigeria suffers from at least one episode of malaria each year. As a matter of fact, malaria is affirmed to be responsible for about 45% of all out-patient visits[123] [124] [125]. The major victims of malaria in Nigeria are women and children. According to "the 2015 Nigeria Malaria Survey Indicator": "Pregnant women and young children are particularly vulnerable to malaria. Among pregnant women, the disease adversely affects birth outcomes and can lead to spontaneous abortion, pre-term labour, low birth weight, and stillbirth"[126]. Malaria is preventable and curable but deadly. This has been revealed by the studies done in Nigeria. Its attack is deadlier especially for those who our work has chosen to identify as the most vulnerable: women and children. For this, the above-cited Survey reiterates:

> Pregnant women and children are population of particular interest to programs endeavouring to reduce the burden of malaria, and preventing malaria among pregnant women and children is a key step in reducing malaria-related morbidity and mortality. Among young children, malaria has high rates of mortality; and even when not fatal, it can affect nutrition and growth[127].

The report on the Malaria Survey Indicator in Nigeria, underlines that the World Health Organization recommends for malaria prevention during pregnancy the "intermittent preventive treatment (IPTp) with

---

[123] Cfr. A. J. Istifanus, «A Comparative Analysis of Health Indicators of Nigeria and Rwanda: A Nigerian Volunteers' Perspective», *American Journal of Public Health Research*, 1.7(2013), 177-182, in https://doi.org/10.12691/ajphr-1-7-6 [13-12-2016]; WHO, Practical chemotherapy of malaria, Report of scientific group, *Technical Report Series*.1998, n. 981.

[124] UNICEF, *Childhood under threat. The State of the world's children*. United Nation Children Fund (2006), 118.

[125] Federal Ministry of Health (FMOH), *National Strategic Plan for Roll Back Malaria in Nigeria 2001*, Abuja, Federal Ministry of Health, Nigeria (2001).

[126] National Malaria Elimination Programme (NMEP), National Population Commission (NPopC), National Bureau of Statistics (NBS), and ICF International 2016, *Nigeria Malaria Indicator...*, 18.

[127] Ibid. 15.

sulphadoxine-pyrimethamine (SP) at each antenatal care (ANC) clinic visit (at least 1 month apart) after the first trimester"[128]. This important recommendation for pregnant women may sound as utopia to most Nigerian women who do not visit the clinic before giving birth because they are constrained by factors which we will see later in this work. Women in the rural areas owing to many factors attached to their location have lesser possibility of doing so than those in the urban areas. In fact, the Nigeria Malaria Survey Indicator of 2015 reveals, "women in the urban areas were more likely to have received at least a dose of IPTp (63 percent) than women rural areas (38 percent)"[129].

The document discloses that the change in the economic and educational life of women (their empowerment) can change their vision and attitude towards their health and that of their children. According to the result of the study:

> Receipt of IPTp increases with education; nearly two-third (61 percent) of women with secondary or more education received at least one dose of IPTp, compared with one-third (33 percent) of women with no education. As wealth increases, so does IPTp uptake. Twenty-seven percent of women in the lowest wealth quintile received at least one dose of IPTp, increasing to 65 percent of women in the highest wealth quintile[130].

Some studies show also that the economic impact of malaria in Nigeria is enormous. According to one of these studies, Nigeria loses about N132 billion annually[131]. The government in accordance to the Abuja declaration and its national strategic plan has established policy guidelines for the implementation and scaling-up use of ITNs. Its malaria prevention programme was expected to provide about 60 million ITNs by the end of 2010 because it is believed that the consistent use of the nets is an effective preventive measure against malaria[132]. Malaria until today has continued

---

[128]   Ibid.

[129]   Ibid., 20.

[130]   NATIONAL MALARIA ELIMINATION PROGRAMME (NMEP), NATIONAL POPULATION COMMISSION (NPopC), NATIONAL BUREAU OF STATISTICS (NBS), AND ICF INTERNATIONAL 2016, *Nigeria Malaria Indicator...*, 20.

[131]   Cfr. A. AUTA, «Demographic Factors Associated...».

[132]   Cfr. Ibid.

to present enormous problem in Nigeria and the other parts of sub-Saharan Africa[133]. In Nigeria, its prevalence is higher in the rural areas where some microscopy results manifested that 36 percent of children tested positive compared to 12% in the urban areas[134].

1.3.2. HIV/AIDS

The Federal Ministry of Health Nigeria, in a report issued in 2001 states that "the HIV epidemic is spreading rapidly in Nigeria"[135]. It continues specifying that there is increase in the rate of HIV sero-positive among antenatal clinic clients from 1.4% in 1991/92 to 4.5% in 1995/96 and 5.4% in 1999. The report asserts that in this period, about 2.7 million Nigerians were living with the deadly infection, the rate of the young people infected was high; about 8.1 percent of youths within the ages of 20, and 24 years were infected with HIV. The Federal Ministry of Health reveals that there is a very high probability of contacting the virus through sexual intercourse. In fact, it affirms that about 80 percent of the cases were contacted through this mean. Other means by which one can be infected are through unsterile injections and the "inadvertent transfusion of unsafe blood and body piercing, scarification or cutting"[136]. It has been noted that between 25 and 45 percent of women infected with HIV, pass it to their babies during pregnancy, delivery or through breastfeeding. This shows how HIV poses a threat to the health of the child. On a similar note, many children remain without parents because they die of the dangerous infection. These children are identified with the term "AIDS-orphans"[137].

According to the Federal Ministry of Health, the factors that worsen the HIV situation in Nigeria include:

---

[133] Cfr. A. J. Istifanus, «A Comparative Analysis…», see also WHO. Practical chemotherapy of malaria. Report of scientific group. *Technical Report Series,* 1998, n. 981.

[134] Cfr. National Malaria Elimination…, 25.

[135] Federal Ministry of Health Abuja, Nigeria May 2001, *National Reproductive Health Policy and Strategy to achieve quality Reproductive and Sexual Health for all Nigerians.*

[136] Ibid.

[137] Ibid.

> Ignorance and denial; stigmatisation of the infected people; inappropriate health care practices (including traditional ones); inadequate number of, and lack of access to voluntary testing and counselling facilities; lack of appropriate care for infected people; and false claims about cure. The low level of education among females as indicated by, among others, an adult literacy rate of 40.7 percent compared to 58 percent for males, and generally low social status of women in the Nigerian society also play a part in the rising HIV rate as well as other reproductive problems. Urbanisation, unemployment and poverty have fuelled high-risk sexual behaviours including prostitution and thus contribute to the increasing rate of HIV infection[138].

The Federal Ministry of Health pointing out another class that is affected by this epidemic remark that "the young people are the ones most affected by the HIV/AIDS epidemics"[139]. Citing examples, the Ministry affirms that 60 percent of the 20,334 reported cases of AIDS in Nigeria were found among the youths of 15 to 24 years[140]. Regarding the adolescent reproductive health in Nigeria, it discloses that, there is a very poor status of reproductive health among this category. One of the major factors responsible for this poor situation, according the Ministry is that, there is a high rate of the practice of unprotected sexual intercourse among young people with multiple partners. Citing a study carried out by the Nigeria Demographic and Health Survey (NDHS) in 1990, the Ministry of Health reports that the median age at first sexual intercourse is 16.6 years and one third of the women had their first sexual intercourse already at the age of 15. The document also says that in a study of 5,500 urban youths aged 12 -24 years, it was discovered that 41 percent experienced sexual intercourse; 82 percent of girls and 72 percent of boys had the experience by the age of 19[141].

Among the identified 22 high burden countries, Nigeria the most populous country in Africa had the highest death rates in HIV-negative people in 2014 (97 per 100,000) and a high HIV-positive TB death rate

---

[138] FEDERAL MINISTRY OF HEALTH ABUJA, Nigeria May 2001, National Reproductive Health...

[139] Ibid.

[140] Ibid.

[141] Ibid.

(44 per 100,000)[142] [143]. Nigeria ranks second in the rating of countries with the highest HIV/AIDS burden in the world with an estimated 3,391,546 persons living with HIV[144]. Though the threat remains, the new infections in the country have reduced from an estimated 316,733 in 2003 to 239,155 in 2013. The number of deaths caused by HIV/AIDS related cases in Nigeria declined from 210,031 in 2013 to 174,253 in 2014[145]. The aforementioned figures demonstrate that Nigeria has made progress in terms of achieving universal access to HIV/AIDS services. The country's steady stride towards achieving universal access to HIV/AID prevention, treatment and control is also evident in the fact that, the number of facilities providing HIV/AIDS Counselling and Testing (HCT) in the country has increased eightfold and there are multiple strategies on ground geared towards the increment of access to HCT, like the adoption of community outreaches. With this, in 2014, 6,716,482 people of 15 years and above were counselled, tested and they received their result. This is considered as progress when compared to the 4,077,668 person that received the same services in 2013. The same is applicable to the health facilities that provide Anti-Retroviral Therapy (ART) where the number of adults and children who receive services increased in 2014 to 748,846, and to PMTCT, where there is an expansion in the number of sites providing services. It is recorded that the number of pregnant women who were counselled, tested and received result increases from 1,706,524 in 2013 to 3,067,514 in 2014. A figure representing about 46% of all pregnant women in the country as at 2014[146].

---

[142] Cfr. A. L. ADAMU - M. A. GADANYA - I. S. ABUBAKAR - A. M. JIBO - M. M. BELLO - A. U. GAJIDA - M. M. BABASHANI - I. ABUBAKAR, «High mortality among tuberculosis patients on treatment in Nigeria: a retrospective cohort study», *BMC Infectious Diseases*, 1, (2017), in https://doi.org/10.1186/s12879-017-2249-4 [12-9-2017].

[143] WHO, *Global tuberculosis report 2016*, Geneva: World health Organization, 2016.

[144] Cfr. FEDERAL REPUBLIC OF NIGERIA, National Agency for the Control of AIDS (NACA 2015), *Global Aid Response Country Progress Report*, Nigeria (GARPR 2015), Abuja, Nigeria.

[145] Ibid.

[146] Cfr. FEDERAL REPUBLIC OF NIGERIA, National Agency for the Control of AIDS (NACA 2015), *Global Aid Response...*

The monitoring of the HIV epidemic in Nigeria has been done with the use of program data, surveys and special studies. The following are the surveys used in monitoring HIV epidemic in Nigeria: the Antenatal Care (ANC) Sentinel Survey, the National HIV/AIDS and Reproductive Health Survey (NARHS), the Integrated Biological Behavioural Surveillance Survey (IBBSS) and in line with guidelines from the World Health Organization (WHO), the ANC sentinel surveillance has been adopted as the system for assessing the epidemic[147].

On a similar note, it is on record that Nigeria has policies aimed at reducing the impact of HIV. The National Policy on HIV/AIDS was developed in 2009 to provide regulations and guiding principles on issues related to HIV/AIDS. The National Strategic Plan (NSP), which is derived from the architecture of the National Strategic Framework 2010-15 (NSF II) was articulated to halt and control the spread of HIV infection and to mitigate the impact of HIV/AIDS by 2015. Nigeria has other policies like the National Action Plan on Orphans and Vulnerable Children and the National HIV/AIDS Prevention Plan[148]. These policies nevertheless do not have sufficient positive impacts on the lives of the people living with HIV/AIDS in Nigeria because often they are not translated into concrete actions that protect the right of the citizens. The report of National Agency for the Control of AIDS (NACA), explains this failure:

> In spite of the numerous policies, substantial progress is needed in addressing the human rights and legal issues surrounding HIV/AIDS. This is mainly due to the fact that, in Nigeria, official policy documents do not constitute law and cannot be enforced in the courts of law.[149].

NACA (2015) remarks that despite the noted progress made in curbing and treating HIV/AIDS in Nigeria, there is still much to be done since the challenges persist. HIV/AIDS remains a threat to population health in Nigeria; it continues to strain the struggling health system and reverse many developmental gains of the achievements including maternal and under-five mortality rates. According to the Director General of the NACA, "The proportion of health facilities in the country offering HCT,

---

[147]   Cfr. Ibid.

[148]   Cfr. Ibid.

[149]   Ibid.

ART and PMTCT services is still low with more access in the urban than rural areas. Also, the proportion of the general population that has ever been tested for HIV is slow at 26%"[150]. The shortcomings undermine the tremendous efforts and progress by the Nigerian government in this regard. But the truth remains that the percentage of the population receiving the services shows that only a very few are being served. The following remark explains the big challenge facing the Nigerian health system in the fight against HIV/AIDS:

> Based on the National HIV Sero-prevalence Sentinel Survey (2010), the prevalence of HIV stands at about 4.1 percent in the general adult population. It is estimated that there are 3.14 million PLWHAs. This figure ranks Nigeria third among countries with highest burden of HIV infections in the world after India and South Africa. It is estimated that there are 2.2 million HIV orphans in the country. HIV is also straining the health system[151].

1.3.3. Tuberculosis

Many people suffer tuberculosis in Nigeria, which ranks fourth among the 22 high-burden TB countries in the world. A. J. Istifanus reports that "more than 2 billion cases of tuberculosis are recorded worldwide (1/3 of the world's population); 250-300,000 cases are reported in Nigeria and 50 % are smear positive. Nigeria is the 4th in the world in terms of total cases of TB in 2007"[152] [153]. To confirm the above-mentioned information, a survey by some scholars noted among its findings that "it is estimated that 395,000 cases of TB in Nigeria in 2007 (283 cases per 100,000 population)" [...] the reported incidence of TB has been on the increase during the last 10 years"[154].

---

[150] Ibid.

[151] G. TIMOTHY - O. IRINOYE - U. YUNUSA - A. DALHATU - S. AHMED - A. SUBERU, «Balancing Demand and ...».

[152] A. J.ISTIFANUS, A Comparative Analysis of ...,

[153] WORLD HEALTH ORGANISATION: «Global tuberculosis control – epidemiology of Tuberculosis: Prospects for control», *Seminars in Respiratory and Critical Care medicine*,29, (2008), 481.

[154] M. O. AKANBI - C. O. UKOLI- G. E. ERHABOR - F. O. AKAMBI - S. B. GORDON, «The burden of...».

In 2008, the World Health Organization reported over 14 million cases of tuberculosis worldwide and Nigeria was considered the world's fifth largest TB burden with nearly 450,000, estimated new cases annually[155]. The WHO estimates that 460,000 new cases of all forms of TB occurred in the country in 2009[156]. In year 2010, Nigeria was at the 10th position among the 22 high-burden TB countries in the world and the highest number of cases are found in Lagos, Kano, and Oyo states[157]. According to a study done on the high mortality among tuberculosis patients in Nigeria almost thirty people die of TB every hour. The same study points out that TB prevalence and mortality have been under-estimated in many high burden countries with revised estimates from Nigeria changing global figures in 2013[158]. The 2014 World Health Organization (WHO) Report presented Nigeria as the country with the highest TB cases in Africa and ranked the country 3rd in the whole world[159]. The World Health Organization mentioned Nigeria among the six countries that stand out as having the largest number of incident cases in 2015[160]. P. Erah and W. Ojieabu note that the unsatisfactory political commitment of the Nigerian government in combating tuberculosis among the factors that discouraged a number of external donors who see no reason why they should continue to give funds while the government funding is very limited[161].

Some conditions like the low socio-economic status of the people, poor ventilation in some poor environments and often-careless contact with already infected people, increase the risk and possibility of the development of pulmonary TB. To worsen the issue, the location of hospitals in places very

---

[155]   Cfr. P. ERAH - W. OJIEABU, «Success of the control of tuberculosis in Nigeria: a review», *International Journal of Health Research,* 1(2009), 2, in http://dx.doi.org/10.4314/ijhr.v2i1.55382 [17-2-2016].

[156]   Cfr. G. TIMOTHY, O. IRINOYE, U. YUNUSA, A. DALHATU, S. AHMED, A. SUBERU, «Balancing Demand and...».

[157]   Cfr. O. AKINGBADE, «Perspectives on Community Tuberculosis Care in Nigeria», *International Journal of Tropical Disease & Health,* 16(2016), 1-13, in https://doi.org/10.9734/ijtdh/2016/23447 [10-3-2017].

[158]   Cfr. A. L. ADAMU - M. A. GADANYA - I. S. ABUBAKAR - A. M. JIBO - M. M. BELLO - A. U. GAJIDA - M. M. BABASHANI - I. ABUBAKAR, «High mortality among...».

[159]   Cfr. O. AKINGBADE, «Perspectives on Community...».

[160]   Cfr. WHO, GLOBAL TUBERCULOSIS REPORT 2016, Geneva 2016.

[161]   Cfr. P. ERAH - W. OJIEABU, «Success of the...».

far from most citizens limits their chances of being treated[162]. In existence in Nigeria also is the problem of the emergence of multi-drug resistant TB, which constitutes a herculean task that maims the past efforts to combat tuberculosis in Nigeria. "Burden of drug resistant TB" according to some authors "is high in Nigeria, with an estimated 29,000 (16 per 100,000) new cases in 2015"[163]. Some authors identify other obstacles as lack of qualifies pharmacists and the corrupt attitude of health professional involved in the distribution of drugs, who "frequently divert the drugs to patent and propriety medicine store license holders for sale"[164]. Similarly, enumerating the factors that contribute to the spreading of tuberculosis in Nigeria, A. J. Istifanus writes: "In the case of TB, the issues are ignorance about the diseases, poor access to treatment due to poverty (despite the fact that the drugs are free), poor contact tracing, people defaulting from treatment, ingestion of unpasteurized cow milk…"[165]. O. Akingbade indicates that, the case detection rate for all forms of TB in Nigeria is about 16%, one of the lowest case detection rates in the world[166].

1.3.4. Pneumonia

Pneumonia is an acute respiratory infection that can affect either one of the lungs or both of them. The infection is more serious among the elderly and the children. The UNICEF tags pneumonia and diarrhoea the leading killers of children under age 5. The reports of the cited organ of the United Nations claim that pneumonia is responsible for the death of 29 per cent of children aged between 1 and 5 worldwide. The number of lives lost is highly concentrated in the poorest and developing countries and among the most vulnerable members of the society[167]. Similarly, F. Shann observes:

---

[162] Cfr. P. Erah - W. Ojieabu, «Success of the…».

[163] A. L. ADAMU - M. A. GADANYA - I. S. ABUBAKAR - A. M. JIBO - M. M. BELLO - A. U. GAJIDA - M. M. BABASHANI - I. ABUBAKAR, «High mortality among…».

[164] Ibid.

[165] A. J. ISTIFANUS, «A Comparative Analysis of…».

[166] Cfr. O. AKINGBADE, «Perspectives on Community…».

[167] Cfr. UNICEF: «*Pneumonia and diarrhoea, Tackling the deadliest diseases for the world's poorest children*», in http://www.childinfo.org/publication [10-6-2017].

> The World Health Organization has estimated that 25 to 33% of deaths in children, or 4 to 5 million child deaths per year, are caused by acute respiratory infections. Similarly the United Nations Children's Fund (UNICEF) has estimated that "over 3 million" children die from pneumonia each year[168].

A survey carried out in some parts of Nigeria reveals that: "Between the year 2000 and 2003 it was estimated that pneumonia accounted for 20% of deaths in children under the age of 5 years in Nigeria"[169]. Describing the effect of Pneumonia in the health and life of the Nigerian children, O. Daodu, M. Crockett, A. G. Falade, present the report of the 2008 pneumonia estimate, which confirms that about 177,000 children under the age of five years died of pneumonia in Nigeria. Pneumonia according to this report represents the third most common cause of the 1 million deaths among children in the nation[170].

A UNICEF report laments that most children as it is the case in Nigeria, die due to some diseases which are highly preventable[171]. Indicating how to tackle pneumonia, UNICEF suggests that: "timely recognition of key pneumonia symptoms by caregivers followed by seeking appropriate care and antibiotic treatment for bacterial treatment is lifesaving"[172]. Most poor families in Nigeria start with "self-medication", because of their inability to meet with the economic demands or inaccessibility of the health centres. Regarding this, the UNICEF affirms, "Child survival impact is thus reduced when key interventions miss these vulnerable children at greatest risk of dying from pneumonia"[173].

Disease such as pneumonia and diarrhoea should not be a herculean task for a country like Nigeria because according to the UNICEF "the solutions

---

[168] F. SHANN, «Etiology of severe pneumonia in children in developing countries», *The Paediatric Infectious Disease Journal*, 5(1986), 247-252, in https://doi.org/10.1097/00006454-198603000-00017 [10-7-2016].

[169] M. O. AKANBI- C. O. UKOLI - G. E.ERHABOR - F. O. AKAMBI - S. B. GORDON, «The burden of...».

[170] Cfr. O. DAODU - M. CROCKETT - A. G. FALADE, «Supportive Care in the Management of Severe Pneumonia in Nigerian Children using Oxygen Concentrators», *JSM Allergy Asthma*, 2(2017), 1008.

[171] Cfr. UNICEF: «*Pneumonia and diarrhoea...*».

[172] Ibid.

[173] Ibid.

to tackling pneumonia and diarrhoea do not require major advances in technology"[174]. The UNICEF emphasized that many children die because services are provided slowly and those most at risk are deprived of care because they are not reached. Often the use of effective interventions remains too low. This is evident in the report, which reveals, "Only 39% of infants less than 6 months are exclusively breastfed while only 60% of children with suspected pneumonia access appropriate care. Moreover, children are not receiving life-saving treatment; only 31% of children with suspected pneumonia receive antibiotics..."[175]. This affirmation was not referred directly to the Nigerian situation, but thorough investigations done on various diseases that claim the lives of many vulnerable in Nigeria show that these words are true about the health situation in the country. "Children who are poor, hungry and living in remote areas are most likely to be visited by these "forgotten killers" and the burden placed by pneumonia and diarrhoea on families and health systems aggravates existing inequalities"[176]. These words give a true image of the condition of many Nigerian children. Unfortunately, their "silent scream" is not heard and they die because of poverty.

Pneumonia is considered a deadly disease because it affects seriously the lungs, the organ through which oxygen gets to the body and the brain in particular. When the brain remains without oxygen for 3 minutes, this could lead to death. Many Nigerians believe that pneumonia is caused by cold weather and drinking very cold liquids since the symptoms such as cough, fever and shortness of breath could easily occur when the weather is cold. But the truth is that pneumonia is caused by germs contracted under poor sanitation and hygiene. People should also be helped to live in clean environments, as this will help to check the harm caused by this severe disease. Studies make known that the primary health care could help in halting the threats to the lives of the vulnerable. According to one of these studies, if "the disease is recognised early and adequate treatment given at the primary care level [...] this can dramatically reduce the mortality and morbidity associated with pneumonia"[177].

---

[174] UNICEF: «Ending Preventable Child Deaths from Pneumonia and Diarrhoea by 2025 – The integrated Global Action Plan for Pneumonia and Diarrhoea (GAPPD) », *UNICEF*, (2013), 5.

[175] UNICEF: «Ending Preventable Child...», 5.

[176] Ibid., 5.

[177] W. B. R. JOHNSON - A. A. ABDULKARIM, «Childhood pneumonia in developing countries», *African Journal of Respiratory Medicine*, 8(2013), 4-9.

1.3.5. Access to Potable Water, Sanitation/
Dirty or Polluted Environment

Water is very essential for every type of life: human life, animal life, plants life and in almost all human activities. The 2030 Agenda for Sustainable Development adopted at the United Nations Summit on 25 September 2015 states: "We are determined to end poverty and hunger, in all their forms and dimensions, and to ensure that all human beings can fulfil their potential in dignity and equity and in a healthy environment"[178]. In the above-mentioned summit, the United Nations declared its promise to strive in order to assure a world with equitable access to health care and its commitments regarding the human right to safe drinking water and sanitation and improved hygiene. The conditions of most Nigerians testify to the validity of the declaration by the UN Summit 2015: "People who are vulnerable must be empowered"[179].

In the bid to solve the issue of lack of access to potable water, there was an impact evaluation from January to June 2014 by the Royal Tropical Institute on the Water Sanitation and Hygiene WASH programme organized by the Nigerian government with the support of the UNICEF. The programme took place in six states in Nigeria. The WASH programme was aimed at ensuring increased access to safe water sources, improved sanitation and the promotion of good hygiene practices. The programme had among its major targets, the rural areas and the vulnerable populations. The evaluation shows that the access to improved water sources by the poor/vulnerable is low because they live very far from the sources and children walk a long distance in order to fetch water. The water is taken untreated, because they have no instruments and are not capable of treating it. When they treat the water, they use the traditional methods that are most often not reliable. We know how dangerous this could be to the health of these people. In the few places where there are public good water sources, children wait for their turn, for about two hours before fetching water[180].

---

[178] UNITED NATIONS DEPARTMENT OF ECONOMIC AND SOCIAL AFFAIRS, (2015), *Transforming our world: The 2030 agenda for sustainable development*, in https://sustainabledevelopment.un.org/post2015/transformingourworld [10-03-2017].

[179] Ibid.

[180] Cfr. UNICEF, *Final Report, Impact Evaluation of Water, Sanitation, and Hygiene (WASH) within the UNICEF Country Programme of Cooperation, Government of*

A report of the UNICEF affirms that a sustainable access to clean water and proper sanitation is unquestionably linked to a healthy and productive life of any population as well as environmental sustainability. The World Health Organization (WHO) estimates that about 2.2 million people, most of whom are children, in developing countries die annually from diarrhoea. Also that approximately 88% of diarrhoeal diseases are caused by unsafe water supply as well as poor sanitation[181].

Akin to the view of the World Health Organisation is that of UNICEF precisely in reference to Nigeria: "The Nigerian situation mirrors the sub-Saharan African situation where out of an estimated population of 160 million, approximately 63 million still lack access to safe water supply and 113 million people lack access to basic sanitation facilities"[182]. The issue of water and sanitation is a sensitive one, because it has been proven by studies that, children are more vulnerable to health hazards linked to unimproved water supply and sanitation. This is evident in the fact that approximately 1.4 million children die every year globally due to unimproved water and sanitation. These children are exposed to more dangers also because they play in contaminated spaces and their immune, respiratory, and digestive systems are still developing. "Children aged between 1 and 4 years old living in households with access to both an unimproved source of water and sanitation facilities had a greater risk of child mortality"[183]. The Nigerian government in order to combat this problem and improve the lives of the vulnerable embarked on projects and policies like the National Water Policy, Presidential Water Initiative, and National Economic Empowerment and Development Strategy[184].

A Global Report on sanitation and drinking water affirms that while approximately 109 million Nigerian citizens lack access to basic sanitation facilities, 66 million do not have improved drinking water[185]. The WHO and the UNICEF consider unimproved water and sanitation

---

Nigeria and UNICEF, 2009-2013, 29 August 2014, Abuja, Nigeria.

[181] Cfr. Ibid.

[182] Ibid.

[183] O. K. EZEH - K. E. AGHO - M. J. DIBLEY - J. HALL - A. N. PAGE, «The Impact of...».

[184] Cfr. Ibid.

[185] Cfr. UNICEF/WHO, *Report of the Joint Monitoring Programme: Progress on Sanitation and Drinking Water*, New York, USA 2013.

among the major causes of diarrhoea[186]. Some experts in this area affirm that: "In Nigeria, as in many low and medium income countries, the majority of well-equipped hospitals and health centres are located in urban areas"[187]. The just cited authors affirm that children under 5 years of age in households with access to unimproved water source and unimproved sanitation facilities had more risk of neonatal, post-neonatal, and child death than children in areas with access to improved water sources and sanitation[188]. With the following assertion, they suggest some ways forward: "Water and Sanitation community-based interventions are needed to prevent child deaths, and that such interventions should target low socio-economic households in Nigeria"[189]. In the same vein, some other scholars believe that at least about 85% of the burden of disease preventable by water supply is caused by faecal-oral contaminants, especially diarrhoeal diseases. These diseases are responsible for many child mortalities in Africa[190].

The importance of sanitation for the improvement of the health was proved during a poll of readers of the *British Medical Journal*, where sanitation was voted the greatest advance in public health in the last century[191]. An evaluation of the health impact of water supply, sanitation and hygiene interventions in Nigeria is poor. This shows how the nation needs to apply the right principles in order to get closer to the Sustainable Development Goals "that relate to the production, distribution, and delivery of goods and services including food, energy, clean water, and waste and sanitation services in cities and human settlements"[192]. Hand hygiene for instance

---

[186]   Cfr. UNICEF/WHO, Diarrhoea: Why Children are still Dying and What Can Be Done, UNICEF/WHO; Geneva, Switzerland 2009.

[187]   O. K. Ezeh - K. E. Agho - M. J. Dibley - J. Hall - A. N. Page, «The Impact of…».

[188]   Cfr. Ibid.

[189]   Ibid.

[190]   Cfr. S. Cairncross - C. Hunt - S. Boisson - K. Bostoen - V. Curtis - I. CH Fung - W. P. Schmidt, «Water, Sanitation and hygiene for the prevention of diarrhoea», *International Journal of Epidemiology*, 39(1), (2010), 193-205, in https://doi.org/10.1093/ije/dyq035 [17-10-2016].

[191]   Cfr. Ibid.

[192]   J. Waage – C. Yap – S. Bell – C. Levy – G. Mace – T. Pegram – E. Unterhalter – N. Dasandi – D. Hudson – R. Kock – S. Mayhew – C. Marx – N. Poole, «Governing the UN …».

is a very good method, but it becomes difficult to do this where there is no water or where the water people have to use is already a means of transmitting diseases, since it is already contaminated. In fact, "a Water and Sanitation Program (WAP) reported that 70 million Nigerians use unsanitary or shared latrine; 32 million have no latrine at all and they defecate in the open and the poorest quintile is ten times more likely to practice open defecation than the richest"[193].

The just mentioned latrine system is among the many bad habits in Nigeria, which contribute to the pollution of water and of the environment. In many crowded settlements in Nigeria for instance, (Douglas road, Owerri, Imo State during the tenure of Rochas Okorocha as the governor), it is usual to find refuse dumped at odd places, unhygienic disposal of human waste, stagnant waters in dirty gutters and open sewages and the littering of toxic waste all over, where they should not be. In some villages, rivers and streams serve as sources of drinking water and as well as places for taking bath, swimming, washing clothes, and processing some agricultural products. Some dwellers wash motorcycles in the same rivers, thereby introducing soap and petroleum materials to the water sources. It becomes very difficult, if not impossible, to expect the water from these sources to be potable.

Related to the above treated issue is the problem of health care waste. Some of the health hazards in some parts of Nigeria are caused by poor management of healthcare waste (HCW) such as: sharps, non-sharps, blood, body parts, chemicals, pharmaceuticals, medical devices and radioactive materials. Many infections, diseases and epidemic outbreaks suffered by Nigerians are associated to environmental pollutions[194]. Such insufficient handling of the by-products of healthcare exposes health workers, patients and inhabitants of areas where these waste products are disposed to infections, toxic effects and injuries. Hence, A. S. Oyekale and T. O. Oyekale reveal that "solid waste management is one of the major

---

[193]   S. O. OYENIYI - J. O. OLOYEDE, «A Comparative Analysis of Safe Water and Sanitation in Selected Urban and Rural Areas of Osun State, Nigeria», *Donnish Journal of Research in Environmental Studies*, 3(2016) 8-16.

[194]   Cfr. O. AWODELE – A. A. ADEWOYE – A. C. OPARAH, «Assessment of medical waste management in seven hospitals in Lagos, Nigeria», *BMC Public Health*, 16(2016), 269, in https://doi.org/10.1186/s12889-016-2916-1 [30-7-2018].

challenges facing many developing countries"[195] especially Nigeria[196]. Some of the above-cited scholars agree that in Nigeria, there several constraints that hamper the adequate management of health care waste. In view of that, they note:

> It is sad to however realize that many healthcare facilities in Nigeria do not comply with professional ethics of HCW management, thereby compromising some internationally acceptable standards [...] absence of functioning platforms for monitoring compliance with ethical standards in HCW disposal, ignorance of assigned staff on some safety practices and deliberate violation of prescribed ethical procedures subject to higher risk of pollution from HCW[197].

The just cited authors maintain that "adequate management of healthcare waste (HCW) is a prerequisite for efficient delivery of healthcare services"[198]. Efforts should be made by the government, the environmental sanitation agencies and members of the society to improve the management of healthcare waste in Nigeria. This should be done through awareness on the dangers the poor handling may cause and the advantages of better management may bring. Surely, when there are workable and sustainable means of managing the large spectrum of wastes that are daily generated from the urban health care and public/private health care facilities, utmost environmental and human safety can be guaranteed. Some aforementioned authors think that "ensuring adequate supply of power and water is critical for HCW management in Nigeria [...] several processes that are associated with waste disposal would require regular supply of water"[199]. It is important to note that there is a strong link between the health and wellbeing goals and other goals[200]. According to some cited authors "the institutional

---

[195] A. S. OYEKALE – T. O. OYEKALE, «Healthcare waste management practices and safety indicators in Nigeria», *BMC Public Health*, 17(2017), 740 in https://doi.org/10.1186/s12889-017-4794-6 [30-7-2018].

[196] Cfr. E. N. ANYIKA, «Challenges of implementing sustainable health care delivery in Nigeria under environmental uncertainty», *Journal of Hospital Administration*, 3(2014), 113-126.

[197] A. S. OYEKALE – T. O. OYEKALE, «Healthcare waste management...».

[198] Ibid.

[199] A. S. OYEKALE – T. O. OYEKALE, «Healthcare waste management».

[200] Cfr. J. WAAGE – C. YAP – S. BELL – C. LEVY – G. MACE – T. PEGRAM – E.

structures for delivering wellbeing goals stem from the historical role of states in providing health, education, and welfare"[201].

1.4. Reproductive Health Care in Nigeria

During the International Conference on Population and Development (ICPD) held in Cairo in 1994, reproductive health was recognised as an essential part of an individual's wellbeing, which is critical and central to human development. This recognition according to the Federal Ministry of Health Nigeria make individual health and rights the centre of policies, programmes and implementation of plans[202]. The Federal Ministry of Health Nigeria agrees that reproductive health includes sexual and reproductive rights. Thus it conceives the reproductive rights concept as "the basic rights of all couples and individuals to decide freely and responsibly the number, spacing and timing of their children and to have the information and means to do so without discrimination, coercion and violence, as expressed in human rights documents"[203].

The Cairo Conference defined reproductive health as "a state of complete physical, mental and social well-being, and not merely the absence of disease or infirmity, in all matters related to the reproductive system and to its functions and processes"[204]. With this Conference which saw Nigerian as one of the participant countries, focus was shifted from population and development programmes to reproductive health. Nigeria thus set a goal "to improve the quality of all Nigerians, men, women and children through enhanced reproductive health"[205]. To achieve the set goal, the Nigerian government decided to offer reproductive healthcare services, which will focus attention on the following priorities: safe motherhood,

---

UNTERHALTER – N. DASANDI – D. HUDSON – R. KOCK – S. MAYHEW – C. MARX – N. POOLE, «Governing the UN ...».

[201] Ibid.

[202] Cfr. FEDERAL MINISTRY OF HEALTH ABUJA, Nigeria, National Reproductive Health Strategic Framework and Plan, 2002-2006, Federal Ministry of Health Abuja 2002, 9, in http://www.policyproject.com/pubs/countryreports/nig_rhstrat.pdf [10-04-2018].

[203] Ibid., 19.

[204] Ibid.

[205] Ibid., 6.

family planning, adolescent reproductive healthcare, STIs, HIV/AIDS, harmful practices, reproductive rights and gender issues, tumours of reproductive organs, infertility and sexual dysfunction and menopause and andropause[206].

An already cited document of the Federal Ministry of Health Nigeria sadly remarks that according the 1999 NDHS record, only 31 percent of deliveries took place within health facilities. It also reveals that maternal mortality in Nigeria is very high. Citing some figures of the reproductive health indicators in Nigeria, the Federal Ministry of health indicates that the maternal mortality in Nigeria is estimated to be 1,000 maternal deaths per 100,000 live births. It further reveals that an estimated 40 percent of pregnant women experience pregnancy-related health problems during or after pregnancy and childbirth[207].

Concerning family planning, the Federal Ministry of Health Nigeria observes that due to factors such as socio-cultural beliefs and norms, negative impact of myths and rumours about family planning methods, poor access to services especially in rural areas and for specific target groups such as adolescents and males, low quality of services due to inadequate skills of providers and inadequate and irregular supply of commodities and low status of women, the fertility level in Nigeria is constantly high at a national average of about 6 children per woman. For the aforementioned Ministry of Health, "these factors have resulted in low contraceptive prevalence rate of 8.6% and a large pool of people whose needs are unmet [...] Among adolescents and young persons, contraceptive use is very low, resulting in high prevalence of undesired pregnancies, unsafe abortions and hence high abortion-related morbidity and mortality"[208].

Thus, for family planning projects in Nigeria, the Federal Ministry of Health reveals that "the contraceptive logistics and management section was developed and relevant staff were trained"[209]. The Federal Ministry of health Nigeria promotes new initiatives on the supply and distribution of condom and availability of some commodities and services relating to implants and long term or permanent contraception. To this effect, it deems it wise to give the opportunity especially to adolescents and young adults to

---

206 Cfr. Ibid., 6-7.
207 Cfr. Ibid., 8.
208 Ibid., 14.
209 Ibid., 15.

have access to permanent contraception and Emergency Contraceptive Pill (ECP)[210]. There is an obstinate insistence on the utilisation of contraceptive devices by the government rather than on the moral principles and values. For this we find it necessary to introduce the Catholic principles in the Nigerian health care system to inculcate the system with reliable moral values.

Some of the solutions proffered by the Federal Ministry of Health in Nigeria are such that give rise to ethical debates. They are false solutions, considering the concrete reproductive health and other health problems in Nigeria. The solutions to the main reproductive health problems of the Nigerian women are not contraception and abortion. They need empowerment through education, which does not mean educating them on the utilisation of contraceptives and practicing abortion. This type of knowledge does not help in the empowerment of women it rather impoverishes and enslaves women. It is not a culture that respects and considers the Nigerian woman globally as a person, but rather, one that see her as a body simply for sex and pleasure. Otherwise, there is no reason why those responsible should sweep the major family planning problems of women in Nigeria under the carpet, while they pursue projects of contraception and abortion sponsored by the multinationals for their interests, which are very far from the interests of the Nigerian women. The Nigerian woman has to be considered as a person with dignity that must be respected; as a mother, as such giving her the possibility of responsibly having children and seeing to their upbringing.

There are some practices in Nigeria, which contribute to reproductive ill health because they are harmful and violate the reproductive rights of the human person. The Federal Ministry of Health, regarding this writes:

> A number of traditional practices in Nigeria infringe on the reproductive rights of the Nigeria woman and girl-child. The commonest of these include female genital cutting (FGC), forced early marriage, traumatic puberty initiation rites, gender-based violence, wife inheritance with widowhood rites. A national survey in 1988 showed that 32% of household in Nigeria practice FGM[211].

---

[210] Cfr. Ibid.

[211] Ibid., 17.

Other non-traditional practices in Nigeria violate the reproductive health rights of the Nigerian Child and woman are abortion and the use of contraceptives.

1.4.1. Safe Motherhood, Access to and Utilisation of Reproductive Health in Nigeria

The rate of access to and utilisation of quality reproductive health information and services in Nigeria is very low. There is also a highly limited access to reproductive health and service especially to the vulnerable groups and the adolescents. This reflects the poor quantity and quality of health facilities in Nigeria. Safe motherhood means that there are the necessary conditions for the woman to go through the period of pregnancy and childbirth without suffering any injury or losing her life or that of the child[212]. Concerning the situation of safe motherhood in Nigeria, the Federal Ministry of Health reports that about 60,000 women die annually from complications of pregnancy or childbirth. Some women according this report suffer long term and often debilitating illness. The paradox of these situations is that most of the maternal and child death are caused by "preventable/treatable conditions of haemorrhage, obstructed labour, unsafe abortions, pregnancy induced hypertension, sepsis and malaria"[213]. The Federal Ministry of Health sadly remarks that in most cases factors such as poor maternal and child health services, uneven and often weak access to emergency obstetric care, low status of women, weak coordination of activities, poor access to and quality of service and collapse of referral system, supervision, monitoring and evaluation of activities, contribute to high maternal and child mortality in Nigeria. The Federal Ministry of Health also laments, "The contraceptive prevalence rate remains very low at 8.6%"[214].

The lack of access to proper sex and reproductive health information and education causes the young people to learn about human sexuality from the wrong sources. This has negative impacts mostly on the teenager. The government is part of the problem. The issue of moral decadence has to be addressed and the lives of the youths must be protected. These cannot be achieved by the distribution of condoms and the promotion of abortion.

---

[212] Cfr. Ibid., 12.

[213] Ibid.

[214] Ibid., 12-13.

The policies in the Nigerian health system that are connected to the reproductive health include: The National Policy on Population for Development, Unity, Progress and Self Reliance (1988); Maternal and Child Health Policy (1994); National Adolescent Health Policy (1995); National Policy on HIV/AIDS/STIs Control (1997); National Policy on the Elimination of Female Genital Mutilation (1998); and Breastfeeding Policy (1994). The National Adolescent Reproductive Health Policy of 1995 was revised in 2002. L. Omo-Aghoja indicates that these policies are not translated into practice and the various consequences: "Despite these pronouncements and seeming efforts, the status of SRH of Nigerians remains abysmally poor and available data tend to suggest worsening indices"[215].

1.4.2. The Practice of Female Genital Mutilation in Nigeria

The female genital mutilation/cutting is widely practiced in the Nigeria. It has many complications and is associated with some negative reproductive consequences such as Psychological consequences, recurrent urinary tract infections, sexual dysfunction, chronic pelvic infection, infertility, prolonged obstructed labour, vesico-vaginal and recto-vaginal fistulae. Reproductive health in Nigeria is intertwined with cultural practices such as female genital mutilation, childhood marriages, widowhood rites and wife inheritance. These cultural practices violate the rights and dignity of the human person. Most of them take root from the mentality of inequality between men and women typical of African culture. Female Genital Mutilation (FGM) is a strong cultural practice, which notably interferes with the health of the woman. FGM includes procedures that intentionally alter partially or totally or cause injury to the female genital organs for non-therapeutic reasons[216]. In Nigeria it is done more for cultural rather than any other reason. According to WHO, the FGM has no health benefits for the girls and women but rather inflicts injuries

---

[215]   L. O.-AGHOJA, «Sexual and reproductive health: Concepts and current status among Nigerians», *African Journal of Medical and Health Science*, 12(2013), 103-113, in https://doi.org/10.4103/2384-5589.134906 [25-8-2017].

[216]   Cfr. WORLD HEALTH ORGANIZATION, Female Genital Mutilation: An overview, Geneva: World Health Organization 1998.

both physical and psychological. It leads to complications in childbirth and often leads to child mortalities[217].

This procedure is widely practiced in Nigeria[218], which accounts for the highest number of FGM globally. Before 2015, there was no explicit and strong federal law banning FGM in Nigeria. Nevertheless, some agree on the need to eradicate FGM in Nigeria. Others who believe in the cultural impact think the procedure should continue[219]. In 2015, the Nigerian President Goodluck Jonathan enacted a law called the Violence Against Persons Prohibition (VAPP) Act, meant to stop FGM and other related practices. FGM is practiced according to those that sustain it as an initiation ceremony of young girls into womanhood. Some claim that the practice ensures virginity and curbs promiscuity, protecting female modesty and chastity. There is a claim that the practice is done for aesthetic reasons like making the female genital organ look neat and good.

However, these reasons do not obscure the fact that girls and women are physically injured, tortured physically and psychologically and that their rights are infringed by the practice of FGM which is a non-therapeutic surgical alteration of children's genitals. For this, some authors believe that giving opportunities of education and enlightenment in Nigeria can be an effective intervention strategy to change the concept and behaviour of those who are naive and misinformed on the issue of FGM[220]. A study in some states in Nigeria reveal that about 99% of people with tertiary education would not recommend FGM for their daughters. Their level of education some authors think has probably empowered them "to resist the cultural norms/pressure to circumcise their children"[221]. There is also a view that "the government should involve the religious leaders and influential personalities in the community for the prevention of negative

---

[217] Cfr. Ibid.

[218] Cfr. E. EBOMOYI, «Prevalence of female circumcision in two Nigerian communities», *Sex Role*, 17(1987), 139-151.

[219] Cfr. T. K. OKEKE – U. S. B. ANYAEHIE – C. C. K. EZENYEAKU, «An Overview of Female Genital Mutilation in Nigeria», *Annals of Medical and & Health Sciences Research*, 2(2012), 70-73. https://doi.org/10.4103/2141-9248.96942 [20-12-2017].

[220] Cfr. I. JEREMIAH – D. G. B. KALIO – C. AKANI, «The Pattern of Female Genital Mutilation in Port Harcourt, Southern Nigeria», *International Journal of Tropical Disease & Health*, 4(2014), 469-476.

[221] Ibid.

and harmful traditional practices including female circumcision"[222]. Another view thinks it is necessary to involve not only religious both other groups because according to this view "in Nigeria, just as in other African countries FGM "crosses all religious, racial and social boundaries [...] FGM is widespread and a highly valued ritual"[223]. In the same vein, I. O. Iyiola argues:

> Considering the diversity of ethnic and religious values in Nigeria, it is therefore not surprising a recurrent element in the narrative on healthcare rights in the nations is the role of social, cultural and religious norms in either enhancing or impeding access to and delivery of health services[224].

1.4.3. The Practice of Abortion in Nigeria

Another problem relevant to the reproductive health in Nigeria is the practice of abortion. There are two different laws for abortion in Nigeria: 1) The Criminal Code of 1916 is in effect in the Southern states. 2) The Penal Code Law No. 18 of 1959 is in effect in the Northern states. The laws are part of Colonial heritage. The Codes have nothing to do with religion. Both Codes ban abortion in Nigeria and they apply similar criminal penalties for noncompliance in both regions. The major difference between the two Codes is that while the Criminal Code applies to anyone acting with the intent of procuring abortion, whether or not the woman is with child, the Penal Code applies to those cases where a woman is in fact with child. Abortion may be legally performed in Nigeria if it is necessary for saving the life of the pregnant woman. In February 1988, Nigeria adopted a population policy; new abortion policy, which takes into consideration the idea that apart from saving the life of the pregnant woman, abortion, may also be illicitly practiced in Nigeria to preserve physical health, and

---

[222] L. O. A.-RAHMAN – O. I. MUSA – G. K. OSHAGBEMI, «Community-based study of circumcision practices in Nigeria», *Annals of Tropical Medicine and Public Health*, 5(2012), 231-235.

[223] I. JEREMIAH – D. G. B. KALIO – C. AKANI, «The Pattern of Female...».

[224] I. O. IYIOHA, Pathologies, Transplants and Indigenous Norms: An Introduction to Nigerian Health Law and Policy, in I. O. IYIOHA I. O. IYIOHA – R. NWABUEZE (eds.), *Comparative Health Law and Policy – Critical Perspectives on Nigerian Global Health law*, ASHGATE, England 2015, 5.

to preserve mental health. In Nigeria, abortion may be legally performed for eugenic reasons[225]. Thus, induced abortion is illegal in Nigeria unless it is practiced to save the life of the woman, to preserve her physical and mental health, or is performed for eugenic reasons.

Some people have the opinion that the ban placed on abortion in Nigeria has worsened instead of ameliorating the situation. Some authors that share this critique of the law state:

> A woman who has an illegal abortion is liable to a jail term of up to seven years. Neither the Criminal nor the Penal Code prevents the large number of abortions that are performed clandestinely in Nigeria, but they do greatly increase women's vulnerability to unsafe abortion and are a major impediment to the improvement of the sexual and reproductive health and rights of Nigerian women[226].

Similarly, some authors maintain illegal abortion should continue to take place in Nigeria because of what they describe as unwanted pregnancy[227]. For them the unwanted pregnancy occurs because of the low knowledge and usage of contraceptives and pills among the adolescents and adult men and women in Nigeria. According to some of these authors "an estimated 1.25 million induced abortions occurred in Nigeria in 2012, equivalent to a rate of 33 abortions per 1,000 women aged 15–49"[228].

---

[225] Cfr. I. OKAGBUE, «Pregnancy termination and the law in Nigeria», *Studies in Family Planning*, 21(1990), 197-208, in https://doi.org/10.2307/1966614 [12-1-2017].

[226] Cfr. B. A. O-Adeniran – C. M. Long – I. F. Adewole, «Advocacy for Reform of the Abortion Law in Nigeria», *Journal of Reproductive Health Matters*, 12(2004), 209-217.

[227] Cfr. O. A. ABIODUN – J. SOTUNSA – O. JAGUN – B. FATUROTI – F. ANI – I. JOHN – A. TAIWO – O. TAIWO, «Prevention of unintended pregnancies in Nigeria ; the effect of socio-demographic characteristics on the knowledge and use of emergency contraceptives among female university students», *International Journal of Reproduction, Contraception, Obstetrics and Gynaecology*, 4(2015), 755-764, in https://doi.org/10.18203/2320-1770.ijrcog20150087 [17-8-2018].

[228] A. BANKOLE – I. F. ADEWOLE – R. HUSSAIN – O. AWOLUDE – S. SINGH – J. O. AKINYEMI, «The Incidence of ...».

The above statements reveal that the law or the legal ban alone is not enough. There is need to apply ethical principles we are proposing in this dissertation to rightly guide the people. The ethical principles can get to the conscience of the people to bring them to a change of mentality. When people know that by performing abortion, they are killing another human person, that can make them to rethink and desist from such practice. This, our view, is similar to a minority opinion in Nigeria which recommends the involvement of right and balanced religious doctrines in treating health matters. This position observes that there is a strong belief in Nigeria that religion contributes to health care and with its contributions, religion remains relevant to Nigeria's health system. This assertion is true "oftentimes health policies are based mainly on medical sciences whereas there are other complementary dimensions such as the religious approach"[229].

1.4.4. Adolescent Sexual and Reproductive Health in Nigeria

A. Adepoju, O. Ogunjuyigbe and A. Adepoju, identify the following as the major adolescent reproductive health problems in Nigeria: "Teenage pregnancy, sexually transmitted infections (STIs) and illegal abortion, high and early entry into sexual activities among adolescents, and a lack of adequate information"[230]. A study in Nigeria by above-mentioned authors reveals that:

> A small proportion of the adolescents aged under 15 claimed knowledge of most contraceptive methods. A significant proportion of these who knew about these methods also indicated that they had at one time or the other used them. For this group, the most well-known method was using a condom; though a few others, especially girls, claimed knowledge of the pill[231].

---

[229] A. J. OLUWABAMIDE – J. O. UMOH, «An assessment of the relevance of religion to health care delivery in Nigeria: case of Akwa Ibom State», *Journal of Sociology and Anthropology*, 2(2011), 47-52.

[230] A. ADEPOJU – O. OGUNJUYIGBE – A. ADEPOJU, *Adolescent Sexual and Reproductive Health in Nigeria, Behavioural Patterns and Needs*, iUniverse, United States of America 2006, 8.

[231] Ibid., 48.

In a report on unwanted pregnancy in Nigeria, G. Sedgh, A. Bankole, B. O.-Adeniran, I. F. Adewole and R. Hussain write: "Studies have consistently indicated that large numbers of Nigerian women experience unwanted pregnancies and births"[232]. The major reason why many pregnancies are named "unwanted" and the primary reason for seeking abortion in Nigeria according to a study is premarital sex. According to the aforementioned study "more than half of women who sought to end their last unwanted pregnancy cited being unmarried when they became pregnant as a primary"[233] reason for their choice. Some authors affirm this, stating that: "Data from Nigeria show that adolescents 15 to 19 year engage in high sexual risk behaviour: 64.7% of sexually active boys and 71.4% of sexually active girls had had unprotected sex with a sexual partner who was neither spouse nor co-habiting partner"[234]. Many adolescents are afraid of pregnancy. The girls entertain fear more than the boys because getting pregnant at a very young age can damage their social reputation and their future, create tension between them and their parents, make them drop out of school and other inconveniences that accompany getting pregnant out of marriage and at adolescent ages. This is why abortion is higher among the adolescents than the adults.

L. Omo-Aghoja supports the motion that sexual right means giving everyone the right and opportunity to engage in sex that is enjoyable and safe, to decide with whom, how and when to do[235]. Hence, he believes that reproductive and sexual right implies that young people, women and men should have access to clear and accurate information about sexuality and contraception and safe abortion should be affordable and accessible to all who desire them[236]. According to the author, "a huge number of women and girls wanting to practice birth control cannot gain access to contraceptives"[237]. The above view is similar to those of the multinational,

---

[232] G. SEDGH – A. BANKOLE – B. O.-ADENIRAN – I. F. ADEWOLE – R. HUSSAIN, «Unwanted Pregnancy and Associated Factors Among Nigerian Women», *International Perspectives on Sexual and Reproductive Health*, 32(2007), 175-184.

[233] Ibid.

[234] M. O. FOLAYAN – B. HAIRE – A. HARRISON – M. ODETOYINGBO – O. FATUSI – B. BROWN, «Ethical Issues in Adolescents Sexual and Reproductive Health Research in Nigeria», *Developing world bioethics*, 15(2015), 191-198.

[235] Cfr. L. O.-AGHOJA, «Sexual and reproductive...».

[236] Cfr. Ibid.

[237] Ibid.

some governmental and non-governmental agents and organisations who are accused of imposing reproductive health models that contradict the African culture and ethics in order to supply and sell their goods. While some authors identify the following as factors that significantly influence contraceptive use among women of reproductive age in Nigeria: "Age of women, marital status, religion, educational status of women, level of knowledge of women about family planning, socioeconomic status of women"[238].

We think that educating rightly the adolescents on reproductive health issues is very important because many are dying due to ignorance and information from the wrong sources. Some people make grave mistakes on sexual and reproductive health issues either because they educated wrongly or because they are without any form of enlightenment. The family must play a major role in educating the adolescents and youths on the right ways to handle sexual and reproductive issues. Parents should not shy away from their duty of talking with their children about sexual and reproductive health. When this link is missing, the adolescents and youths fill it up by talking with and learning from their peers, who are inexperienced and incapable of giving the right sexual and reproductive health advice. Schools can be of great help for creating awareness successfully. The schools are good channels because the age for first sexual experience for adolescents in Nigeria is 15 years. Most of them start having such experience between 13 and 17[239]. The government is invited to embark on enlightenment programmes for the adolescents, youths and the entire public and health reproductive facilities in locations easily accessible[240]. Some aptly think, "The government should do more to improve the life of adolescents rather than encourage them to commit abortion"[241].

---

[238] Cfr. C. B. Duru – O. F. Emelumadu – A. C. Iwu – I. Ohale – C. C. Agunwa – E. Nwaigbo – E. N. Ndukwu, Prevalence, Pattern and Determinants of Contraceptive Use among Women of Reproductive Age (15-49) In Rural Communities in Imo State, Nigeria, *International Journal of Science and Healthcare Research*, 3(2018), ISSN: 2455-7587.

[239] Cfr. A. Adepoju – O. Ogunjuyigbe – A. Adepoju, *Adolescent Sexual and…*, 67.

[240] Cfr. Ibid., 65.

[241] Ibid., 53.

1.5. Nigeria's rapid and efficient response to the 2014 Ebola outbreak

On the "origins of the 2014 Ebola epidemic", the World Health Organisation affirms: "A "mysterious" disease began silently spreading in a small village in Guinea on 26 December 2013 but was not identified as Ebola until 21 March 2014"[242]. A report of the World Health Organisation states that when Ebola virus which entered Lagos, Nigeria on 20 July 2014, was confirmed and announced on 23 July 2014, "the news rocked public health communities all around the world"[243]. Some Nigerian authors describes it origin and dissemination thus: "The 2014 Ebola virus disease (EVD) outbreak remains unprecedented both in the number of cases, deaths and geographic scope"[244].

On July 20 2014, a symptomatic air traveller from Liberia, who contracted Ebola virus from a sister who died from the same virus, arrived in Lagos, Nigeria with Ebola. He arrived at a private hospital in Lagos where he told the staff that he was suffering from malaria. There was no alarm because malaria is not transmitted from person to person. Fear started gripping the health workers when the protocol officer who escorted the Liberian died of Ebola and 9 doctors were subsequently infected, 4 of whom died[245]. The world was afraid because the nature of Lagos as a chaotic and densely populated city, was seen as a possible obstacle to an effective contact tracing and control of the virus. Another issue created global panic:

---

[242] WORLD HEALTH ORGANIZATION, «One year into the Ebola epidemic: a deadly, tenacious and unforgiving virus - One year into the Ebola epidemic. January 2015 -», in https://www.who.int/csr/disease/ebola/one-year-report/nigeria/en/ [13-01-2019].

[243] Ibid.; Cfr. D. OGOINA – A. S. OYEYEMI – O. AYAH – A. A. ONABOR – A. MIDIA – W. T. OLOMO – E. ONYAYE KUNLE-OLOWU, «Preparation and Response to the 2014 Ebola Virus Disease Epidemic in Nigeria—The Experience of a Tertiary Hospital in Nigeria», *PLoS ONE* 11(2016): e0165271, in https://doi.org/10.1371/journal.pone.0165271 [13-02-2019].

[244] A. OUT – S. AMEH – E. OSIFO-DAWODU – E. ALADE – S. EKURI – J. IDRIS, «An account of the Ebola virus disease outbreak in Nigeria: implications and lessons learnt», *BMC Public Health*, 18 (2018), 18: 3. https://doi:10.1186/s12889-017-4535-x [13-01-2017].

[245] Cfr. WORLD HEALTH ORGANIZATION, «One year into...»

When a close contact of the index case entered the country's oil hub, Port Harcourt, on 1 August. A doctor who treated him developed symptoms on 10 August and died of Ebola on 23 August. An investigation undertaken by Nigerian and WHO epidemiologists revealed an alarming number of high-risk and very high-risk exposures for hundreds of people[246].

The world remained astonished when the speculated disaster was prevented by the Nigerian government and its health agencies. On how Nigeria was able to do this, an already cited WHO's report affirms:

> That explosion never happened, thanks to the country's strong leadership and effective coordination of an immediate and aggressive response [...] Nigeria had a first-rate virology laboratory, affiliated with the Lagos University Teaching Hospital, that was staffed and equipped to promptly diagnose a case of Ebola virus disease [...] The government generously allocated funds and dispersed them quickly. Isolation facilities were built in both cities, as were designated Ebola treatment facilities. Contact tracing reached 100% in Lagos and 99.8% in Port Harcourt[247].

The effective and efficient intervention of Nigeria to halt the spread of the virus that shocked the world was described as a "spectacular success story", because "the country held the number of cases to 19, with 7 deaths" and was declared free of Ebola virus transmission by the World Health Organisation on 20 October, 2014[248].

---

[246] Ibid.

[247] WORLD HEALTH ORGANIZATION, «One year into...».

[248] Cfr. Ibid., WORLD HEALTH ORGANIZATION, «WHO declares end of Ebola outbreak in Nigeria», in http://www.who.int/mediacentre/news/statements/2014/nigeria-ends-ebola/en/ [13-01-2019]; FEDERAL MINISTRY OF HEALTH, «Status of Ebola Virus Disease in Nigeria», in http://www.health.gov.ng/index.php/component/content/article/9-uncategorised/201-the-declarationof-nigeria-as-ebola-virus-free-hon-minister-s-address [13-01-2019].

Conclusion

We have seen the general socio-economic, political and health profile of Nigeria. This has helped us to have an insight of the health situations of the citizens of the most populated country in Africa. This chapter has been able to clearly demonstrate that Nigeria is naturally blessed with natural and human resources. The question to ask is this: What is the effect of these resources and the Nigerian economy on the life and activities of her citizens, especially on the access to their basic health needs? According to a World Bank Report, the "Nigerian economic statistics reveal a puzzling contrast between rapid economic growth and quite minimal welfare improvements for much of the population"[249]. The above-cited Report makes it clear that the procedure of distribution of resources in Nigeria is not fair. For there to be fair distribution, there must be the right application of some principles and approaches of justice that we will consider in chapter three of this work. These principles as we will see in both chapters three and four, need to stand on the catholic principles in order ensure distribution of health care resources that is just and fair.

Our study has revealed that Nigeria is richly endowed with wealth, natural and human resources, but the health conditions of its members do not reflect this richness, owing to some phenomena, which could be described as "Nigerian factors". The issues presented in this chapter on Nigeria's key health indicators and the major causes of death and main pathologies in Nigeria, show how the country is far from recognizing the right to health of her citizens. There is very little impact of the Nigerian wealth on the people's lives. The majority of the citizens, especially the vulnerable and those living in underserved areas, lack a functional health care system and basic health care services. This as we have seen, is not because Nigeria is a poor country, but rather, because of insufficient health budgets, lack of will on the political leaders to implement existing policies and act in the best interest of the people. The loss of human lives is among the worst impacts of this nonchalant attitude. The respect for the dignity of the human person and the sacredness of human life seems to be lacking in the entire political system of government. This is among the major reasons why we consider the Catholic principles, proposed in the fourth chapter of this work, as a necessary rescue measure for the Nigerian populace.

---

[249] THE WORLD BANK, *Nigeria Economic Report...*, 2.

Many Nigerians belong to the poor class and they are denied access to primary care needs. This does not show seriousness on the part of a country that wants to achieve an appreciable life expectancy which is one of the major aims of the UN 2030 Agenda for Sustainable Development. What is done to prevent deaths that are preventable is insufficient. With this, it will be difficulty to realize the dream of the Nigerian government to bring life expectancy to 70 years by 2020. We are in 2019; only one year remains and the latest news on life expectancy in Nigeria is not encouraging. We still hear of a country threatened by high infant/child mortality, maternal mortality, malaria, poor access to potable water and sanitation/polluted environment.

Other problems of Nigeria, as we have seen, are relevant to the moral questions about wrong orientation and education about human sexuality and some life-threatening practices, like abortion, use of contraception and female genital mutilation. How these issues are addressed in Nigeria give the impression of a nation where human life and dignity especially of the woman are not respected. The dignity of the human person with the sacredness of life as we will see in chapter four are principles necessary in sex education and practices concerning human sexuality and reproductive health in Nigeria.

The issue is not solely with distribution within the health sector, it has to do also with the general distribution and management of the country's resources. The Nigerian populace live in poverty, not just because the economy is stagnant but, because of some other factors like corruption among the leaders, mismanagement of public funds, etc. According to M. M. Ogbeidi, "The political leadership of the country since independence is responsible for entrenching corruption in Nigeria and, by extension, had impeded meaningful socio-economic development"[250]. The standard of human and moral values in Nigeria is very low. This reflects on the life-styles and the *modus operandi* of the political leaders and most of the governmental and non-governmental agents. The principles we are proposing in this dissertation will address corruption and some other related moral issues, especially among the political leadership of Nigeria. Corruption is an enemy of civil society, it is a destroyer of human prosperity, it is an enemy of the poor. Thus, corruption is considered the enemy of common good. The

---

[250] M. M. OGBEIDI, «Political Leadership and Corruption in Nigeria Since 1960: A Socio-economic Analysis», *Journal of Nigeria Studies*, 1(2012), 1-25.

principle of common good, as our work will demonstrate in the last chapter is a good arm for fighting corruption. We believe that if the principle of common good with the other correlated Catholic principles is properly applied, corruption will be eradicated from the minds of many Nigerians.

It is indeed sad to note that the campaigns for the 2019 elections in Nigeria are still centred on fighting corruption and alleviating poverty. Just as we have partly considered in this chapter and as we will see in the subsequent chapter, the Millenium Development Goals were not achieved and the target has passed since 2015. The UN 2030 Agenda for Sustainable Development has been inaugurated since 2015, but the Nigerian situation, especially on health care resource allocation, is still too bad; having little to show for these life-improving plans. This implies that something important is lacking. The present doctoral dissertation will demonstrate in chapters three and four, how the Catholic principles can help Nigeria achieve her aim of ameliorating the life of her citizens especially in the aspect of provision of health needs and health care needs.

On a positive note, the way Nigeria reacted to the Ebola Virus Disease (EVD) attracted credibility to the Nigerian government and her health care system. This demonstration of capability by the Nigerian government which was described as "spectacular success story" by the World Health Organisation made many Nigerians believe that our health care system can rise again. We also believe like other Nigerians and we see this dissertation as one of the instruments for the revival of the Nigerian health care system.

For this, the object of the next chapter is the administration of the Nigerian health care system; to have an idea of how the country's resources, especially those related to health care are distributed. Chapter two will enable us understand how Nigeria reacts to the citizens' quest for health care services through the activities of the three sectors of her health system.

Chapter 2

THE NIGERIAN HEALTHCARE SYSTEM

Introduction

The World health report (2000) defines 'health system' to include all activities whose principal purpose is to promote, restore or improve health[251]. "The health sector is crucial to the growth and development of a nation"[252]. As we have seen in the previous chapter, understanding the background of Nigeria from the geographical, socio-cultural, economic and political viewpoints, is very important to understanding the socio-health situations in Nigeria. The key health indicators of Nigeria and the major causes of death and main pathologies in Nigeria, give a profound and concrete knowledge of the Nigerian health conditions and the various tasks facing the Nigerian health care system. After this useful acquaintance from chapter one, the second chapter logically explores the identity of the Nigerian health system, identifing and studying the instruments and modes

---

[251] Cfr. WORLD HEALTH ORGANIZATION, *The World health report, Health Systems: improving performance*, Geneva: WHO 2000.

[252] G. TIMOTHY – O. IRINOYE – U. YUNUSA – A. DALHATU – S. AHMED – A. SUBERU, «Balancing Demand and...».

in which it handles the health challenges.In this part of our dissertation, we are going to study the Nigerian Health care system considering some salient points relevant to firstly its history and evolution; secondly, the National Health Policy, National Health Insurance Scheme, National Health Bill, National Health Act 2014 and National Strategic Health Development Plan; thirdly, the concept of a health care system in Nigeria; fourthly, its nature, structure and administration (giving more attention to the primary health care system, which is considered the foundation of the general health system and vital to the efficient realization of the purpose of every health system); fifthly, the various health workers in Nigeria; and lastly, health care financing in Nigeria. These points we believe will be necessary for a good knowledge of how government and society respond to the health needs of the Nigerian people.

2.1. History and Evolution of Healthcare in Nigeria

The scientific and modern medical health care services in Nigeria exist thanks to the contacts with the west and western civilization of about five hundred years ago. D. M. N. McDikkoh affirms it would be wrong to talk about the Nigerian health care system without mentioning the important contributions of the catholic missionaries. According to him:

> The efforts of the Christian missionaries played a key role for the efforts of education in Nigeria [...] Equally true is the fact that the missionaries contributed to building hospitals and health centres [...] They were first in erecting hospitals along the coastal areas with the very first hospital in Sao mine in 1504, at Abeokuta in 1860s, in Lagos and Calabar in 1888 [...] The colonial government arrived at the health scene very late and, rather, as a matter of adjustment than an initiative to improve the health lot of its subjects[253].

At the origin of hospitals in the world's history is Christianity so also in Nigeria. As it appears in the affirmation of D. M. N. McDikkoh, while the colonial masters ventured into health in Nigeria for their selfish interests, Christianity rendered health services with the sole intention of assisting the

---

[253]   D. M. N. McDikkoh, *The Nigerian health...*, 32.

dignity of the human person. This is one of the reasons why we feel it is very important to propose the principles of justice which are basic in the social teaching of the Catholic Church, for the distribution of health care resources in Nigeria. At the origin of health care in Nigeria is the Christian doctrine. M. O. Welcome narrates the development of health care delivery in Nigeria thus:

> Before independence in 1960, a 10-year developmental plan (1946–1956) was introduced to enhance health care delivery. Several health schools and institutions (Ministry of Health, several clinics and health centres) were developed according to this plan. By the 1980s, there had been great development in health care—general hospitals and several other health centres (over 10,000) had been introduced[254].

In Nigeria, it is often the case that things that were started with good intentions end up changing their objectives thus giving a contrary result to that for which they were instituted. This is exactly what happened with the Nigerian Health care system. According to an already cited author, the modern medical care cost:

> Started graduating from the initial free care, especially in the mission facilities, to small charges; then the cost started getting excessively expensive [...] This fact, coupled with the steady decline of both the accessibility and the quality of care delivered in these modern medical facilities, made it necessary for the return to the detested traditional medicine[255].

When modern medicine in some sense failed the people, they resorted to traditional medicine. The high expectation from the health system by the population was never realized because of poor management, selfishness, corruption and lack of the application of the principles of justice. This unimpressive foundation of health care service in Nigeria has continued to produce similar fruits to date. The Nigerian Health care system is ranked among those with very poor performance globally.

In this work, we retain that priority should be given to the primary health care system without ignoring the secondary and tertiary health

---

[254] M. O. Welcome, «The Nigerian health... ».

[255] D. M. N. McDikkoh, *The Nigerian health...*, 39-40.

care systems. The primary health care is the foundation of every health care system. If the foundation is not strong, the entire health care structure will not give concrete and convincing assurance to anyone of its efficient services. For this reason, we want to concentrate more on the history and evolution of primary health care, which we retain, are very important for the attainment of efficient services in the Nigerian health care system.

2.1.1. Evolution of Primary Health Care in Nigeria

As we have mentioned above, the missionary activities in the eighteenth and nineteenth centuries, dominated by the Roman Catholic missionaries started and nurtured the idea of hospitals and other health care facilities in Nigeria. An account by D. M. N. McDikkoh, affirms that the "Roman Catholic missions dominated the missionary efforts in Nigeria with approximately 40 percent of the total number of 118 of mission hospitals by independence in 1960"[256]. The government hospitals then were 101. The Catholic mission hospitals were more in the South and the South-East and the Sudan Interior Mission and Sudan United Mission hospitals were present in the in the Middle Belt and in some areas in the north. With the presence of these hospitals and facilities, it was possible to train some health workers, ways were paved for the acceptance of western or modern medical care and foundation was laid for the evolution of the Nigerian health system[257]. When Nigeria gained its independence in 1960, there was no strong focus on health system development. It was between 1975 and 1980, that Nigeria started a health system development that was initiated with primary health care (PHC) as the fulcrum[258]. Within the same period, following the declaration of the universal target of Health for All in 1978, primary health care (PHC) was adopted and globally considered as the best means towards the achievement of the lofty goal[259].

The Nigerian government adopted the Basic Health Service Scheme (BHSS) based on Primary Health Care (PHC) approach in 1979. With this, the government also set some objectives to serve as a means of arriving at

---

[256] Ibid.,73.

[257] Cfr. Ibid., 74.

[258] Cfr. B. S. AREGBESHOLA – S. M. KHAN, «Primary Health Care …».

[259] Cfr. A. O AIGBIREMOLEM – I. ALENOGHENA – E. EBOREIME – C. ABEJEGAH, «Primary Health Care in Nigeria: From Conceptualization to Implementation», *Journal of Medical and Applied Biosciences*, 6(2014), 35-43.

heath for all[260]. The universal coverage or health for all was a national goal set for the year 2000. With the health indicators of Nigeria in 2017, it is clear that the country did not get close to the achievement of the noble goal. With the National Health Policy of 1988, the Federal Government launched the Primary Health Care, which was intended as the fundamental aspect of the Nigerian Health care system. Primary health care in Nigeria since its adoption has continued to evolve through various significant stages of development.

The National Development Plan (1975 - 1979) was inaugurated to make Primary Health Care accessible and available at the grassroot levels. As a result, primary health care accounted for over 85 percent of the Nigerian health care facilities in 2005[261]. The National Development Plan was structured along basic health units that covered about 20 health clinics across each local government area. Alongside the basic units were four primary health care centers and mobile clinics, each serving approximately 150.000 population[262]. Despite the good intentions, the objectives were not realized, because none of the local communities for which the services were made were involved[263].

The Federal government tried again when Professor Olikoye Ransome-Kuti was the Minister of Health, between 1986 and 1992. The project this time was "characterized by the development of model primary health care in fifty-two (52) pilot local government areas all of which were implementing all eight components of primary health care"[264]. Among the attempts by the federal government to create, an impressive image of the Nigeria health care system during this period was the primary health care plan launched in 1987[265]. This health plan did not give the expected positive result due to the lack of infrastructure, lack of personnel and insufficient public health management[266].

The National Primary Healthcare Development Agency (NPHCDA) was launched in 1992 to make basic healthcare available and accessible at the rudimentary level. The National Primary Health Care Development

---

[260] Cfr. D. M. N. McDikkoh, *The Nigerian Health…*, 91.

[261] Cfr. A. O Aigbiremolem – I. Alenoghena – E. Eboreime – C. Abejegah, «Primary Health Care…».

[262] Cfr. Ibid.

[263] Cfr. Ibid.

[264] Ibid.

[265] Cfr. M. O. Welcome, «The Nigerian health…».

[266] Cfr. Ibid.

Agency (NPHCDA) was a centrally funded agency. It had the duty to encourage the promotion and implementation of high quality and sustainable primary health care at state and local government levels. The NPHCDA in collaboration with the state and LGAs, focused on maternal and child health at the community level[267].

The Ward Health System was established in 2001 to serve as grassroot operational points for primary health care delivery. This Ward Minimum Health Care Package, which was constituted within the project of Ward Health System, was intentionally in line with the millennium development goal (MDG) targets of Nigeria[268]. The good initiatives commenced by Professor Ransome-Kuti were truncated by the military takeover of government in 1993[269]. Since then, the primary health care system in Nigeria has been limping. The rural areas, which are supposed to be covered by the primary health system currently, remain unserved. Assessing the status quo of the primary health care in Nigeria, B. S. Aregbeshola and S. M. Khan, wrote: "The current state of PHC system in Nigeria is appalling with only about 20% of 30,000 PHC facilities across Nigeria working"[270]. The condition of the primary health system is not good and many patriotic Nigerians have blamed this on the government's lack of will to attend to the basic health needs of the citizens, lack of implementation of the policies in place, making policies without considering the situation of the citizens and corruption/selfishness among the political leaders.

2.2. The Nigerian Health System: National Health Policy, National
     Health Insurance Scheme, National Health Bill, National Health
     Act 2014 and National Strategic Health Development Plan

In the course of development of its health care system, Nigeria has taken several reformative steps geared towards the improvement of the quality of life and health of the citizens. One such is Nigeria has the National Health Policy, a framework for realizing the MDGs relative to

---

[267] Cfr. G. Timothy - O. Irinoye - U. Yunusa - A. Dalhatu - S. Ahmed - A. Suberu, «Balancing Demand and…».

[268] Cfr. A. O Aigbiremolem – I. Alenoghena – E. Eboreime – C. Abejegah, «Primary Health Care…».

[269] Cfr. B. S. Aregbeshola – S. M. Khan, «Primary Health Care…».

[270] Ibid.

the health of Nigerians, the National Health Insurance Scheme, National Health Bill, National Health Act, National Strategic Health Development Plan and other sub-sectoral policies, strategies and plans on the private-public health rapport, distribution of human and other health resources, health care financing, maternal and child health, malaria control, HIV/AIDS and drug policies. We are going to examine some of these initiatives by the Nigerian government.

2.2.1. National Health Policy

National Health Policy "means all policies relating to issues of national health as approved by the Federal Executive Council on the advice of the National Council on Health through the Minister"[271]. The National Health Policy lays more emphasis on equity in health care and the goal of achieving health for all Nigerians. For the Policy, health and access to quality and affordable health care is a human right. The policy was propagated in 1988 and revised in 2004. This revision was motivated by the need to respond to the unfolding problems and the necessity to focus on new developments. The purpose of the revised edition of the National Health Policy is to strengthen the national health system to ensure an improved health status for Nigerians[272]. Since the dissemination and revision of the national health policy, there is no doubt that the government has made some efforts towards the realization of the set goals. The health status of Nigerians however, cannot be said to have seen any notable improvement. It is rather retrogressing. This also reflects the condition of the Health policy in Nigeria. According to D. Eboh:

> Health care policy development in Nigeria has suffered from terrible unstable political climate, paralysis of the integrity of healthcare professionals, disempowerment of the public, mono-focus of sources of funding and mass emigration of highly skilled professionally qualified health personnel to other developed nations[273].

---

[271] NATIONAL HEALTH RESEARCH ETHICS COMMITTEE OF NIGERIA (NHREC), *National Code of Health Research Ethics 2006*, Federal Ministry of Health.

[272] Cfr. H. V. DOCTOR – R. BAIRAGI – S. E. FINDLEY – S. HELLERINGER – T. DAHIRU, «Northern Nigeria Maternal…».

[273] D. EBOH, *Strategic Concept for Managing Healthcare in Nigeria. Africa's Health and*

For the national health policy, the Primary Health Care (PHC) is an important instrument for the realisation of its objective to offer the possibility of better health conditions to all Nigerians. The coalition of NPHCDA with the National Programme on Immunization (NPI) in 2007, aided the former to become the most important decision marker in issue of primary healthcare in Nigeria[274]. Practically, how has the government demonstrated its seriousness in the consideration of **PHC** as being crucial? The services of the Primary Health Care services include the provision for health education, supply of potable water, ensuring adequate nutrition, environmental sanitation, access to adequate reproductive health, good immunisation coverage, availability, accessibility and affordability of essential drugs. Health is not just an absence of disease, so the formulation of health policies must not be limited to diseases and strictly health issues[275].

Ensuring a primary health care that is promotive, protective, restorative, preventive and rehabilitative is one of the major objectives of the National Health Policy. It also has as its aim to ensure that individuals and communities, within the available resources, are put in the position of enjoying mental, physical and social wellbeing. "Substantively, whether the state recognizes the human right to health in constitutional and international law affects how the state constructs health policy"[276]. Every State or National health policy is expected to have among its major objectives the protection of the health of every human person from risks. This is to be achieved through the provision of health and other health-related services. It is therefore expected that the Local Governments areas, receive from the Federal and State governments, assistance to make effective the primary healthcare system, increasing the quality and quantity of its services in order to minimize high rate of death from preventable causes[277].

Social Care Management, TamaRe House Publishers Ltd, UK 2008, 32-33.

[274] Cfr. PHARM ACCESS FOUNDATION, Nigerian Health Sector, *Market Study Report...*, 20-21.

[275] Cfr. L. O. AREMU, *GATs and Nigeria's National Health Policy: The Issue for Negotiation*, LAP LAMBERT Academic Publishing, Saarbrucken, Germany 2017, 45.

[276] Ibid., 44.

[277] Cfr. PHARM ACCESS FOUNDATION, Nigerian Health Sector, *Market Study Report...*, 21.

2.2.2. National Health Insurance Scheme (NHIS)

The National health insurance scheme (NHIS) was designed by the federal government to revitalize the dismal state of health in Nigeria. It was instituted in Nigeria in May 1999 for covering government employees, those in the private sector and the informal sector. This scheme was created also for covering children under five. The former Nigerian President Olusegun Obasanjo tried to render this scheme more effective by fortifying its legislative statue in 2004[278]. This scheme was confirmed in 2005 by Decree No. 35 of 1999 provided for the establishment of a governing council with the responsibility of managing the scheme. The Nigerian Health Sector Market Study Report discloses that there was a mandate by the Nigerian President to the National Health Insurance Scheme (NHIS) to fast track the scale-up of coverage of health insurance from less than 5 percent in 2013 to 30 percent before the end of 2015. The report also reveals that there was a presidential summit on Universal Health Coverage (UHC) in March 2014 to give an ultimate political support to the UHC drive. The only result from the summit was the target of 30 percent health insurance coverage[279].

The objectives of the scheme[280] are to: ensure that every Nigerian has access to good health care services, protect Nigerians from the financial burden of medical bills, limit the rise in the cost of health care services, ensure efficiency in health care services, ensure equitable distribution of health care costs among different income groups; equitable patronage of all levels of health care, maintain high standard of health care delivery services within the scheme, improve and harness private sector participation in the provision of health care services, ensure adequate distribution of health facilities within the federation and ensure the availability of funds to the health sector for improved services.

Looking at these objectives, many Nigerians are perplexed about the situation of the Nigerian health system because with the National Health Insurance Scheme and other plans and policies on ground, many are

---

[278] Cfr. F. MONYE, «An Appraisal of the National Health Insurance Scheme of Nigeria», *Commonwealth Law Bulletin*, 32:3 415-427.

[279] Cfr. PHARM ACCESS FOUNDATION, Nigerian Health Sector, *Market Study Report…*, 19.

[280] Cfr. M. O. WELCOME, «The Nigerian health…».

deprived of the primary health services. In addition, many wonder why the rate of children under five who die in Nigeria every year is so high, why there is poor maternal health and very low life expectancy[281]. The instances of health insurance in Nigeria are very few. There are scanty free health care services provided for the citizens. The government provides for the government employees through a special health insurance scheme and the insurance by the private firms and the private health care providers[282]. The following affirmation of A. Awosusi, T. Folaranmi and R. Yates, gives a clear picture of Nigerians with regard to health insurance: "Less than 5% of Nigerians have health insurance coverage; most enrolees are in the formal sector with poor coverage in the informal sector"[283]. The number of people covered by insurance in Nigeria is very scanty.

The NHIS regulates health insurance in Nigeria and in the formal sector, it covers all federal government workers. For those in the informal sector, it introduced the Community-based health insurance (CBHIS) programmes, encouraging the various states of Nigeria to join the programme or set-up other health insurance scheme to cover their population. According to the Nigerian Health Sector, Market Study Report most states are reluctant to adhere to the scheme. Those in the formal sector are automatically covered. The informal sector accounts for over 70 percent of Nigerians, majority of which are not covered. Some are of the view that most citizens are not using the insurance because they are not compelled to, so they think it should be made compulsory for all in order to achieve the set targets[284].

2.2.3. National Health Bill

The National Health Bill emerged at the dawn of 2014. The National Health Bill is the first attempt in Nigeria to make available legislative clarification and funding sources to support the Primary Health Care

---

[281] Cfr. Ibid.,

[282] Cfr. R. J. VOGEL, *Financing Health Care in Sub-Saharan Africa*, Greenwood Press, Michigan 1993, 101-102.

[283] A. AWOSUSI – T. FOLARANMI – R. YATES, «Nigeria's new government and public financing for universal health coverage», *The Lancet Global Health*, 3(2015), e514-e515, in http://dx.doi.org/10.1016/S2214-109X(15)00088-1 [23-11-2017].

[284] Cfr. PHARM ACCESS FOUNDATION, Nigerian Health Sector, *Market Study Report...*, 19.

(PHC). It includes provisions for a Basic Health Care Provisions. At its origin, there was the hope that it would ensure notable increases of government financing for PHC. The major target of the National Health Bill is universal coverage with at least basic services. To realize its major objectives, the Bill strives to guarantee a Basic Health Care Provision Fund (BHCPF), which is to be funded thus: the consolidated fund of the federation, an amount not 1% of its value, grants by international donor partners; and funds from any other source[285]. It is proposed that: 50% of the fund shall be used for the provision of basic minimum package of health services to all citizens, in eligible PHC facilities through the NHIS, 25% of the fund shall be used to provide essential drugs for primary healthcare, 5% of the fund shall be used for the development of human resources for eligible PHC facilities; and 5% of the fund shall be used by the Federal Ministry of Health for National Health Emergency and Epidemic Response.

In Nigeria, it is the responsibility of the states to guide the registration and regulation of the public and private hospitals as well as monitoring the health facilities to ensure quality health care services. The federal level councils and boards have the duty of regulating the production and licensing of health workers[286]. The bill proposes that the distribution of funds for essential drugs for the primary health care and facility maintenance and human resource development be assigned to National Primary Health Care Development Agency. This role will be executed through State Primary Health Authorities. Additionally, the bill establishes that the state and Local Government Area should contribute 10% and 5% respectively of the total cost any state or local government block grant project[287]. The National Health Bill was a proposal waiting to be passed into law. When this was done in 2014, through a legislative process, it became the National Health Act of 2014, which will be the next object of our study.

---

[285] Cfr. Ibid., 21.

[286] Cfr. Ibid., 39.

[287] Cfr. B. S. C. UZOCHUKWU – M. D. UGHASORO – E. ETIABA – C. OKWUOSA – E. ENVULADU – O. E. ONWUJEKWE, «Health care financing in Nigeria: Implications for achieving universal health coverage», *Nigerian Journal of Clinical Practice*, 18(2015), 437-444.

2.2.4. National Health Act 2014

The National Health Act, 2014 is a bill for "An Act to provide a framework for the regulation, development and management of a national health system and set standards for rendering health services in the federation; and for related matters"[288]. The Nigerian President signed the National Health Act in Nigeria into law in 2014. The main purpose of the Act is serving as a framework for regulation, development and management of the National Health System and the role of health professionals. The Act was intended as a viable framework for arriving rapidly at the Universal Health Coverage (UHC) and meeting the Millennium Development Goals (MDGs). The National Health Act prepares the requisites for ascertaining adequate public resources for health by strengthening primary health care through the Basic Healthcare Provision Fund[289]. The provision of healthcare insurance for the groups that remained uncovered was one of the reasons why the National Health Act came into being. Some authors see at the core of the implementation of this Act, the counterpart funding from the state and local governments. For this, it was thought that resource mobilisation and accountability are important for the successful implementation of the Act[290]. This is in line with one of the reasons at the origin of the Act: improving funding of health care services at the rudimentary level to reach the unreached and the vulnerable.

O. Enabuele and J. E. Enabuele believe that NHA has all it takes to change significantly the nature of the Nigerian health care system by its impact on the practice by health professionals, health care quality, and health care outcomes[291]. The National Health Act is composed of seven parts and according to the above-mentioned authors; a proper implementation of these parts will bring good tides to the Nigerian health sector. The seven parts are divided thus[292]: 1. Responsibility for health and eligibility for health services and establishment of National Health System,

---

[288] National Assembly, *National Health Act, 2014: Explanatory Memorandum*, in http://www.nassnig.org/document/download/7990. [25-11-2017].

[289] Cfr. A. Awosusi – T. Folaranmi – R. Yates, «Nigeria's new government…».

[290] Cfr. Ibid.

[291] Cfr. O. Enabuele – J. E. Enabuele, «Nigeria's National Health Act: An assessment of health professionals' knowledge and perception», *Nigerian Medical Journal*, 57(2016), 260-265.

[292] Cfr. Ibid.

2. Health Establishment and Technologies, 3. Rights and Obligations of User and Healthcare Personnel, 4. National Health Research and Information System, 5. Human Resources for Health, 6. Control of Use of Blood Products, Tissue and Gametes in Humans, 7. Regulations and Miscellaneous Provisions. The National Health Act establishes how the Basic Health Provision Fund shall be financed[293].

2.2.5. National Strategic Health Development Plan

The Federal Ministry of Health describes the nature and some functions of the National Strategic Health Development Plan thus:

> The National Strategic Health Development Plan is the first of its kind in the history of the development of the Nigerian Health Care Delivery System which will serve as the overarching, all encompassing, reference document for actions in health by all stakeholders to ensure transparency, mutual accountability for results in the health sector[294].

The overarching goal of the National Strategic Health Development Plan is to improve the state of health of Nigerians by developing an efficient and sustainable health care system. In the preface of the National Strategic Health Development Plan, Professor C. O. Onyebuchi Chukwu, who was the Minister of health, affirmed that it "reflects shared aspirations to strengthen the national health system and to vastly improve the health status of Nigerians"[295]. Akin to the affirmation of the former Minister is the mission statement of NSHDP which reads: "To develop and implement appropriate policies and programmes as well as undertake other necessary actions that will strengthen the National Health System to be able to deliver effective, quality and affordable health"[296].

The first Presidential Summit on Health Care in Abuja, Nigeria was held under the theme "Accepting collective responsibility for improving our health in Nigeria"[297]. During the summit, the President, Vice-President,

---

[293] Cfr. National Assembly, National Health Act…

[294] Federal Ministry of Health: National Strategic Health…

[295] Ibid.

[296] Ibid.

[297] Ibid.

Executive Governors and Federal Capital Territory Minister of the Federal Republic of Nigeria, declared to have recognized the following characteristics of a good heath politics and policy in a healthy population that is economically productive, supported by a health care system that carters for all and sustains a life expectancy of not less 70 years by reducing to the barest minimum the burden of infectious and other debilitating diseases[298]. The Nigerian political leaders expressed their concern over the fact "that Nigeria is not on track towards achieving significant improvement in meeting the health expectation of its people[299]. The Summit also recognized that the challenges of health objectives in Nigeria are a result difficult to be achieved due to the weak health system, low levels of health care funding, inadequate financial protection for the poor, shortage and mal-distribution of the scarce health care resources, insufficiency in the standard of health care services delivery, inadequate and untimely availability of quality health commodities and weak partnership and coordination[300]. The principles of health are re-affirmed by the Nigerian leaders' health summit as a basic human right. The government, the political leaders agreed, has the responsibility of playing a leadership role in the improvement of the health status of the people. In this regard, the leaders pledged to be committed to the results oriented National strategic health plan and to the Primary Health Care (PHC) approach[301].

The federal Government of Nigeria, through the Federal Ministry of Health is convinced that a purposeful reform of the National Health Care Delivery System is necessary for strengthening the weak and fragile National Health Care Delivery System and improving performance of the country's entire Health System. For this, the government initiated a process that led the development of the National Strategic Health Development Plan (NSHDP) 2010-2015, which was developed in a highly participatory manner. The NSHDP was meant to serve as the overarching framework for health development in Nigeria. It drew inspirations from 36 States and the FCT Health Development Plans (SHDP). The strategic priority areas of NSHDP include: Leadership and Governance for Health; Health Service Delivery; Human Resources for Health; Financing for Health;

---

[298] Cfr. Ibid.

[299] Cfr. Ibid.

[300] Cfr. Ibid.

[301] Cfr. Ibid.

National Health Management Information System; Partnership for Health; Community Participation and Ownership; and Research for Health[302].

The final NSHDP which was approved by the National Council on Health (NCH) during its 53rd session in Asaba, Delta State, Nigeria in March 2010[303] includes that within the abovementioned areas, the Federal, State and Local Government Areas have the duty of developing and implementing strategic activities enacted for achieving the objectives of each priority area[304]. It also indicates in its implementation modalities that the three levels of government while implementing the plan are to collaborate with all stakeholders. The Medium-Term Sector Strategy (MTSS) is identified as an essential means for implementing the NSHDP through annual operational plans for all planning entities at the Federal, State and LGAs. It is established as the task of the Federal Ministry of Health to lead the implementation of NSHDP in the three levels of government.

The Steering committees of the State Health Development Planning level (SHDP) according to NSHDP was to be established at the Federal and State levels, with the responsibility of monitoring the implementation of the plan. At the Federal level, Permanent Secretary of the FMoH will head the committee; the Honourable Commissioner for Health will have the same duty at the State level, while it will be the duty of the Chairman of the Local Government Area or the Supervisory Councillor for Health (LHGA) to chair the committee at the Local Government level[305]. The vision of the National Strategic Health Development Plan is to reduce the morbidity and mortality rates due to communicable diseases to the barest minimum; reverse the increasing prevalence of non –communicable diseases; meet global targets on the elimination and eradication of diseases; significantly increase the life expectancy and quality of life of Nigerians[306]. The National Strategic Health Development Plan was estimated to cost Nigeria from 2010 to 2015, NGN3.997 trillion (USD 26.653 billion). The annual cost and investment requirement are NGN666.3 billion (USD 31.63)[307].

---

[302] Cfr. Ibid.

[303] Cfr. Ibid.

[304] Cfr. Ibid.

[305] Cfr. Ibid.

[306] Cfr. Ibid.

[307] Cfr. Ibid.

2.3. The Nature, Concept, Structure and Administration of the Nigerian Health System

2.3.1. Nature of Health Care System in Nigeria

– Public health care in Nigeria

"Public health establishment" means a health establishment that is owned or controlled by a government body"[308]. The public health care system in Nigeria is divided into three tiers. Each of these are linked to the three levels of government: federal, state and local government area[309]. The government provides public health care through national healthcare systems. The public health service has the unique responsibility to protect and improve the general health of the citizens and to see to the health needs of the entire population. In carrying out this delegated responsibility, the public health system involves its agencies, makes health and development programs carrying along everyone at the federal, state and local levels[310]. The public health care is believed to provide healthcare services that are mostly in favor of the poor. It is to guarantee the easiest way to achieve universal and equitable access to health care. The vulnerable, who cannot acquire their health needs on their own, put their hope on the public health system, which has the responsibility and the moral duty of taking care of them. In Nigeria, the basic health needs of the poor are hardly met and their hopes are continuously dashed by unimpressive performance of the public health system. Health funding is one of the major challenges of the public health system in Nigeria[311].

Misdistribution and mismanagement of health resources are among the major problems in the Nigerian health care system. Many citizens who can afford the cost of private health services consider the public health facilities in Nigeria as death traps. An already cited report in this regard discloses that "high burden of diseases and health system challenges that negatively impact quality of care have left a lot of Nigerians seeking care

---

[308] NATIONAL ASSEMBLY, National Health Act …,

[309] Cfr. President's Malaria Initiative, Nigeria, *Malaria Operational Plan FY 2017*, 14.

[310] Cfr. D. M. N. McDikkoh, *The Nigerian health…*, 90.

[311] Cfr. PHARM ACCESS FOUNDATION, NIGERIAN HEALTH SECTOR, *Market Study Report…*, 16.

outside Nigeria"[312]. Those who can afford to travel abroad for treatment do that, while the vulnerable who have no means of sponsoring themselves die without proper medical attention. The weak referral system according to A. J. Istifanus has succeeded in keeping facilities grossly under-utilized. He was alarmed that the public health system, which include, the tertiary and secondary health care institutions, "consume a disproportionate share of public health expenditure whereas most of the conditions that affect the majority of Nigerians can be managed at the primary health care"[313]. This represents an allocation inefficiency in Nigerian health care system that has led to situations where common conditions either were without treatments or received treatments at unnecessary high costs[314].

Other studies reveal that the public health facilities offer the most affordable options for the majority of Nigerians. It is cheaper, but the quality is far lower than what is obtainable from the private health facilities. This is where the problem lies. For example, "public health facilities are often characterized by inadequacy of supplies including medicines"[315]. Regarding the distribution of medicines, majority of Nigerians purchase through out-of-pocket payments. Since most African countries including Nigeria do not manufacture, but rather import medicines, they are usually expensive[316]. Nigerians prefer foreign drugs to made in Nigeria drugs. Such mentality is based on disappointment from the public health sector and various Nigerian made products. Often in Nigeria, drug dealers are not perturbed seeing people suffer and die because of the fake drugs they are buying and consuming. Most dealers are after making profits and do not care "whose ox is gored". Regarding this problem, the position of B. A. Ushie, D. B. Ugal and J. A. Ingwu is considerable:

---

[312]   Ibid.

[313]   A. J. Istifanus, «A Comparative Analysis…».

[314]   Cfr. Ibid.

[315]   B. A. Ushie – D. B. Ugal – J. A. Ingwu, «Overdependence on For-Profit Pharmacies: A Descriptive Survey of User Evaluation of Medicines Availability in Public Hospitals in Selected Nigerian States», *PLoS ONE* 11(2016), e0165707, in https://doi.org/10.1371/journal.pone.0165707 [30-7-2018].

[316]   Cfr. O. O. Odusanya, «Drug use indicators at a secondary health care facility in Lagos, Nigeria, Journal of Community Medicine & Primary Health Care», 16(2014), 21-24.

> There are serious limits to depending on private sector health
> care because the very reason for their existence is profit-making,
> meaning that while they can provide good services for those
> who can afford them, private sector health is unlikely to provide
> sustainable health services to the majority of Nigerians who live
> below the poverty line and are underserved[317].

In most Nigerian hospitals, the most prescribed medicines are often not found. This according to some "buttresses the notion that Nigerian hospitals are in a decayed state and nothing more than consulting clinics"[318]. This is evident is the following challenges identified by some Nigerian authors:

> Lack of access to affordable health care services, poor
> distribution of health facilities, shortage of drugs, poor attitude
> of health workers, the enormous cost of health services, which is
> sometimes out of the reach of the poor, poor infrastructure and
> poor health education strategy are some of the critical problems
> of health delivery in Nigeria[319].

It is not always easy to get care, especially medicine from the public health facilities because of the long procedure involved. This discourages those who can afford to pay more from going to the public health facilities. They resort to the private sector even though the cost is higher there[320].

---

[317] Cfr. B. A. Ushie – D. B. Ugal – J. A. Ingwu, «Overdependence on For-Profit Pharmacies: A Descriptive Survey of User Evaluation of Medicines Availability in Public Hospitals in Selected Nigerian States», *PLoS ONE* 11(2016), e0165707, in https://doi.org/10.1371/journal.pone.0165707 [30-7-2018].

[318] Ibid; Cfr. E. O. Innocent – O. A. Uche – I. B. Uche, Building a solid health care system in Nigeria: challenges and prospects, *Academic Journal of Interdisciplinary Studies*, 3(2014), 501.

[319] Ibid; Cfr. B. Uzochukwu – O. Onwujekwe, «Healthcare reform involving the introduction of user fees and drug revolving funds: influence on health workers' behaviour in southeast Nigeria», *Health Policy*, 75(2005), 1-8, in https://doi.org/10.1016/j.healthpol.2005.01.019 [1-8-2018]; Cfr. A. S. Jegede, «Problems and prospects of health care delivery in Nigeria: issues in political economy and social inequality», *Currents and Perspectives in Sociology*, Malthouse Press Limited, Ibadan 2002, 212-226.

[320] Cfr. C. B. Eke – R. C. Ibekwe – V. U. Muoneke – J. M. Chinawa – M. U. Ibekwe – O. M. Ukoha – B. C. Ibe, «End users' perception of quality of care

A steady availability of care is of paramount importance to the success of any health care system[321].

In synthesis, Nigeria's public health system challenges include: inadequate, inaccessible, and poor-quality service delivery, particularly at the periphery, where most primary health care facilities offer only a limited package of services due to limited availability of trained health workers; lack of necessary referral linkages between the different levels of health care; weak logistics system for commodities, with as many as six separate vertical commodities management systems with little or no coordination between them; poorly maintained infrastructure with many buildings and equipment in need of repair and/or maintenance; weak institutional capacity with inadequate supervision of health services; and limited availability of health workers, and poor deployment in the rural health facilities[322].

– Private health care system in Nigeria

"Private health establishment" means a health establishment that is not owned or controlled by an organ of the state"[323]. The private health care system serves a higher proportion of the population in Nigerian. It consists of primary, secondary, and tertiary health care facilities. There are also pharmacies, proprietary patent medicine vendors (PPMVs), traditional

---

of children attending children's outpatients clinic of University of Nigeria Teaching Hospital Ituku-Ozalla Enugu», *BMC Research Notes*, 7(2014), 800-805;Cfr. G. U. P. Iloh – J. N. Ofoedu – F. U. Odu – C. V. Ifedigbo – K. D. Iwuamanam, «Evaluation of patients' satisfactions with quality of care provided at the National Health Insurance Scheme clinic of a tertiary hospital in South-Eastern Nigeria», *Nigeria Journal of clinical practice*, 15(2013), 469-474.

[321] Cfr. O. E. Johnson – N. W. Adiakpan – M. C. Asuzu, «Drug availability and health facility usage in Bamako Initiative and a non-Bamako Initiative Local Government Areas of Akwa Ibom State, South-South Nigeria», *Journal of Community Medicine and Primary Health Care*, 27(2015), 73-82; Cfr. S. T. Adedokun – V. T. Adekanmbi – O. A. Utham – R. J. Lilford, «Contextual factors associated with health care service utilization for children with acute childhood illness in Nigeria», *PLoS ONE*, 12(2017), e0173578, in https://doi.org/10.1371/journal.pone.0173578 [3-8-2018].

[322] Cfr. President's Malaria Initiative…, 15.

[323] National Assembly, National Health Act…

medicine practitioners and other authorized and unregistered medicine and drug sellers[324]. "Services provided by the private sector are either subsidized (e.g. faith-based health facilities) or full-cost (e.g. privately-owned clinics and hospitals)"[325]. The public health system with its poor performance creates a big opportunity for private health facilities to gain more influence in the health care service provision in Nigeria. This is affirmed by the study commissioned by the Embassy of the Kingdom of the Netherlands.

According to the study report: "With mostly out-of-pocket expenditure, individual hospitals and their owners and not insurers, are the biggest decision makers in the choice of equipment, drugs and other procurement"[326]. As aforementioned, the performance of the public health sector in Nigeria does not encourage most people to trust it. Some Nigerians move abroad or to the Nigerian private facilities in a quest for quality health care services. "The private health sector's response to the increasing demand for quality services, increasing middle class and huge outbound medical tourism, is expansion of existing private hospitals and establishment of hospitals in Nigeria by Nigerian healthcare specialists in Diaspora…"[327]. It is obvious that the importance of the public health system in Nigeria is decreasing while the private health system is gaining more economic importance because of its quality services. According to a government source, about 76% of all secondary facilities and approximately 28% of primary health care facilities in Nigeria are private. The document adds that 42% of fever cases resort first to the private sector[328]. This as we have mentioned is because the private sector is easily accessible and offers quality health services. It is however generally accepted in Nigeria that quality of care in both the public and private health sectors needs substantial improvement[329].

---

[324] Cfr. President's Malaria Initiative…, 15.

[325] G. TIMOTHY – O. IRINOYE - U. YUNUSA - A. DALHATU - S. AHMED - A. SUBERU, «Balancing Demand and…».

[326] PHARM ACCESS FOUNDATION, Nigerian Health Sector, *Market Study Report…*, 12.

[327] Ibid., 18.

[328] Cfr. President's Malaria Initiative…, 15.

[329] Cfr. G. TIMOTHY - O. IRINOYE - U. YUNUSA - A. DALHATU - S. AHMED - A. SUBERU, «Balancing Demand and…».

2.3.2. Concept of Health System in Nigeria

The Nigerian health care system's administration is uniquely fashioned in accordance to its system of government to suit the health care exigencies in the geographical zones, considering the various cultures and traditions. Nigerian has a three-tier system of government. The federal government is responsible for the tertiary health care system; the state governments manage the secondary health system, and the local governments operates the primary health system. Since most of the population, about 55% live in the rural areas[330], the policies and plans that target the provision of health for all consider the community health, an aspect of the primary health system as an important means for the achievement of this goal.

This Nigerian way of conceiving the health care system is in line with the views of some authors who argued on the various concepts of health. According to the author S. Curtis[331], there is no single or unique concept accepted by all as the concept of health is open to differing interpretations. This, according the study by W. M. Gesler and R. A. Kearns[332] is because there are different cultures of health; different people have their models based on their cultural, religious, cosmological, moorings, which vary from place to place. Other authors[333] add that the different concepts of health could depend on class (social class), ethnicity, gender and other factors that represent the markers of social differences[334]. In the same vein, D. Gregory, R. Johnston, G. Pratt, M. Watts and S. Whatmore, sustain the argument in favour of widening the medical geography to include "a holistic focus on the great variability of the human condition, commonly at the scale of population within territories, but in principle also at that of individual people interacting with quite specific sites"[335]. Health care does not only

---

[330] Cfr. M. O. Welcome, «The Nigerian health…».

[331] Cfr. S. Curtis, *Health and Inequality: Geographical Perspectives*, Sage, London 2004, 2.

[332] Cfr. W. M. Gesler - R. A. Kearns, *Culture/Place/Health*, Routledge, London 2002, 30-32.

[333] N. D. Lewis - I. Dyck - S. McLafferty (eds.), *Geographies of women's health: place diversity and differences*, Routledge, London 2001, 15.

[334] Cfr. D. Gregory – R. Johnston – G. Pratt – M. J. Watts – S. Whatmore, (eds.), «Health and Health…».

[335] Ibid.

imply solely the provision of hospitals, clinics and other medical facilities, but also spaces, places, environments and landscapes[336].

The Nigerian government entrusted primary health to the local governments to ensure that health care services get to every citizen. Nevertheless, this noble objective of providing health for all starting from the grass roots, unfortunately remains a utopia in Nigeria. The rural areas, hence, the primary health care system is not accorded the consideration it merits. Funding at this level of the health care system is very poor. The situation affects the nature and performance of the entire health care system in Nigeria. Some authors commenting on the state of the Nigerian health care system write:

> The health system is in shambles, policy somersault and reversals tend to have under-mined several reforms in the sector over the years. Poor human resources and policy management have led to unprecedented brain drain in the health sector as health professionals in search for better conditions of service abroad often vote with their feet in droves. The Nigerian health system is in comatose, few hospitals with few drugs, inadequate and substandard technology and a lack of infrastructural support, including electricity, water and diagnostic laboratories resulting in misdiagnosis[337].

The considerations made by the above cited authors are not dissimilar to those of M. I. Olatubi, O. O. Oyediran, I. O. Adubi and O. C. Ogidan who present the deplorable condition of the Nigeria health system thus: "Primary Health Care (PHC), which forms the bedrock of the national health system, is in a prostrate state because of the poor political will, gross under funding, and lack of capacity at the LGA level, which is the main implementing body"[338]. The words are clear on the state of health system in Nigeria. The system is sick and needs the right ethical principles to bring it to an appreciable condition.

In poor communities, health care service is challenged by the problem of acceptability and out-of-pocket spending which represent about 70 percent

---

[336] Cfr. Ibid.

[337] G. Timothy – O. Irinoye – U. Yunusa – A. Dalhatu – S. Ahmed – A. Suberu, «Balancing Demand and...».

[338] M. I. Olatubi – O. O. Oyediran – I. O. Adubi – O. C. Ogidan, «Health Care Expenditure...».

of total private expenditure. The federal, state and local governments in Nigeria are thus invited "to live up to their responsibility of meeting the basic health care needs of Nigerians by equipping the health establishments with the requisite personnel/facilities as recommended by WHO and the 2004 Health Review Policy of the Federal Ministry of Health"[339]. Availability, accessibility and affordability are among the essential qualities of a just health care system. A health care service is available when it is there for the people. However, if it is available and not accessible to those in need of it or affordable for those for whom it is made, then its availability is useless. For a health care service, especially the basic health care service to be defined available in the real sense of the word, it must be accessible to all and affordable for all, especially the vulnerable. The status or nature of any health care system is often a reflection of the way it is being managed. We will now see the administration of the Nigerian health care system, in order to evaluate later how the Nigerian government responds to the problem of distribution of health care resources.

2.3.3. Structure and Administration of Health Care System in Nigeria

The health system administration in Nigeria depends largely on the political activities in the country. In the administration of the Nigerian health care system, it is the function of the federal government to handle the activities at the tertiary level; the university teaching hospitals and the federal medical centres. The state governments are to manage provisions at the secondary level, that is, the general hospitals and primary health care facilities. The primary health care provisions are under the jurisdiction of the local government areas. The federal government's role is mostly limited to coordinating the affairs of the university teaching hospitals and federal medical centres (tertiary healthcare) while the state government manages the various general hospitals (secondary healthcare) and the local government focus on dispensaries (primary healthcare), which are regulated by the federal government through the National Primary Health Care Development Agency (NPHCDA).

---

[339] S. I. EFE, «Health care problem and management in Nigeria», *Journal of Geography and Regional Planning*, 6(2013), 244-254, in https://doi.org/10.5897/jgrp2013.0366 [10-10-2016].

To understand better the Nigerian health care administration, it is important to understand the directives by the Nigerian Constitution on the allocation of revenues among the federal, state and local governments. As intimated above, Nigeria operates a federalist system of government. The system of governance was restructured with the Constitution of 1999, which distinguishes the functions and responsibilities of the three tiers of government; Federal, State and Local. According the prescription of the Constitution, the State government is responsible for the basic health care and education of the citizens. The State government is not alone in the responsibility as the Federal government also has a very significant role to play is such areas[340]. The 1999 Constitution specifies that revenues from oil, as well as from VAT, customs, and corporate income tax be divided between federal, state and local levels of government. This has to be done following strictly the formulae stipulated by the Revenue Mobilization Allocation and Fiscal Commission and endorsed by the National Assembly[341].

Oil revenue accounts for about 75% of all consolidated government revenue in Nigeria[342]. According to the current formulae, the modality for the distribution of the oil revenues is as follows: 13% should be given to the oil producing states (derivation principle) and then the remaining revenues should be divided between the Federal Government (53%), the State Governments (27%), and the Local Governments (20%). The allocation of revenue from customs, excise, and corporate income taxes are to be done following the same formula without the derivation principle. The division of revenues from the VAT goes thus: while 15% goes to the Federal Government, 50% is allocated to the State Governments, and 35% is given to the Local Governments[343]. The 1999 Constitution establishes that allocations to the Local Government should go "as stipulated in State Joint Local Government Account", under the authority of the State Government. This implies that it is within the powers of the State Government to decide the modality and what is to be allocated to the State and local government[344].

---

[340] Cfr. WORLD BANK, *Nigeria Economic Report*, n. 1, May 2013, 23-24.
[341] Cfr. Ibid., 24.
[342] Cfr. Ibid.
[343] Cfr. Ibid.
[344] Cfr. Ibid.

The brief exposition of the 1999 Constitution on the economic rapport between the three tiers of government in Nigeria, gives an insight on the administration of the Nigerian health system, which is styled following the three levels of government. Thinking in the same vein, R. Jeffrey aptly writes:

> The political economy of health care provides a necessary backdrop to an understanding of health policymaking [...] The political economy of health care is an attempt to specify the ways in which economic interests and political processes structure the provision of health services [...] the political process is seen to follow directly from economic determinants[345].

We will treat here the three levels of health care administration in Nigeria, paying more attention to the primary health care which is generally believed to be the most essential level among the three.

– Primary health care – Local Government

What is Primary Health care? Primary health care refers to the "first contact between a health professional and a patient with the professional who assumes responsibility on an ongoing basis for the patient's health needs"[346]. The nature of the primary Health care as the initial approach to a health worker to seek treatment or advice shows its importance. It is the foundation of most health care systems and it is practiced at the community level. "Primary health care services" means such health services as may be prescribed by the Minister to be primary health care services"[347]. The Local governments are constitutionally responsible for the provision of the Primary Health Care in Nigeria. The local government areas (LGAs) possess and fund the primary health care facilities. They are also responsible for management of health posts and clinics, health centres and comprehensive health centres that provide basic health care services[348]. The

---

[345] R. Jeffery, The Impact of Socioeconomic and Political Factors on the Provision of Health Care in India, in R. Akhtar (ed.) *Health Care Patterns and Planning in Developing Countries*, Greenwood Press, New York 1991, 99-114.

[346] D. M. N. McDikkoh, *The Nigerian health…*, 50.

[347] National Assembly, *National Health Act…*,

[348] Cfr. World Health Organization, Primary Care Systems Profiles &

importance of the primary health care system cannot be over emphasized. Primary health care facilities serve as the entry point, which introduces the community into the health care system. Primary health care facilities comprise of "health centres and clinics, dispensaries, and health posts, providing general preventive, curative, promotive, and pre-referral care to the population as the entry point of the health care system"[349]. In addition, the facilities "are typically staffed by nurses, community health workers, community health extension workers (CHEWs), and environmental health officers. LGAs are mandated by the Constitution to finance and manage primary health care"[350].

Being under the local government areas, the primary health care system is the least funded and worst organised among the three levels of government.

> This has over the years resulted in extensive dilapidation of primary healthcare infrastructure, lack of modern equipment, inadequate and poorly trained manpower and consequent absence or poor-quality services and loss of confidence in the system. Nigeria's poor health indices and lack of significant progress towards the millennium development goals (MDGs) has been directly attributed to the failure of the primary health care system as the highest burden diseases are mostly those that should have been managed at the primary care level[351].

The primary health system according to the Nigerian national health policy is the framework to achieve improved health for the population. For this policy, "a comprehensive health care system delivered through primary health centres should include maternal and child health care"[352]. During the first health summit in Abuja, Nigeria, the Nigerian political leaders pledged to commit themselves "to significantly improve the health status of Nigerians through the development of a strengthened and sustainable

---

Performance (PRIMASYS), in http://www.who.int/alliance-hpsr/projects/AHPSR-Nigeria-300916.pdf [11-12-2017].

[349] FEDERAL REPUBLIC OF NIGERIA, *National Human Resources for Health Strategic Plan 2008 to 2012*, 15.

[350] Ibid.

[351] PHARM ACCESS FOUNDATION, NIGERIAN HEALTH SECTOR, *Market Study Report...*, 20.

[352] FEDERAL REPUBLIC OF NIGERIA, *National Human Resources...*, 15.

primary health care delivery system"[353]. The improvement, strengthening, rendering more accessible basic health services, especially to the poor women and expansion of coverage of the maternal health care services are among the major aims of the Primary Health Care (PHC) in Nigeria[354].

–   Secondary health care – State Government

What is Secondary Health care? Secondary Health care is a second tier of the health system. Usually after the first contact at the primary health care system, some cases are referred to specialists at secondary health care facilities for treatment. Each of the 36 States in Nigerian is responsible for the secondary health system in its territory. The States through their Ministries of Health provide health care services through health care facilities. In addition, they offer technical assistance to the local government areas' Health Departments[355]. The major facilities in this phase are the general hospitals, which provide general medical, and laboratory services. They are also dispensers of specialized health services like surgery, paediatrics, obstetrics and gynaecology. Most of these cases are those that are referred from the primary health care that has no competence and equipment to handle them. This method of referring some problems demonstrates the synergy that exists between the primary and the secondary health care systems. Some of the health workers in the general hospitals include medical officers, nurses, midwives, laboratory and pharmacy specialists, and community health officers[356].

–   Tertiary health care – Federal Government

What is Tertiary Health care? Tertiary Health care refers to a third tier of the health system. At the tertiary level, cases referred from primary and

---

[353]   Federal Ministry of Health, *National Strategic Health Development Plan (NSHDP)*, 2010-2015, 11, in http://www.health.gov.ng/doc/NSHDP.pdf [25-11-2017].

[354]   Cfr. C. L. Ejembi – M. Alti-Mazu – O. Chirdan – H. O. Ezeh – S. Sheidu – T. Dahiru, «Utilization of maternal health services by rural Hausa women in Zaria environs, northern Nigeria: has primary health care made a difference?», *Journal of Community Medicine & Primary Health Care*, 16(2004), 47-54.

[355]   Cfr. World Health Organization, *Primary Care Systems…*

[356]   Cfr. Federal Republic of Nigeria, *National Human Resources…*, 15.

secondary levels are treated. Specialized medical personnel and equipment that are sophisticated and suit the cases they handle equip the tertiary health systems. In the urban settlements, the tertiary health care facilities provide extensive primary and first referral care to patients[357].

The federal government, through the Federal Ministry of Health is responsible for the stewardship of the affairs for health and the provision of the tertiary health care in Nigeria. The federal level carries out its duty through the network of tertiary, teaching and specialist hospitals. Several states are responsible for managing and funding the tertiary health care facilities within their state territories[358]. The Tertiary health care system is at the highest technical level of health care in Nigeria. Though the tertiary system occupies the highest level, according to many it is not as important as the primary level. The primary health care system, which is at the lowest level, is considered the most important because it assures basic health care for all. For this reason, S. I. Okafor affirms, "the Nigerian experience highlights the need for a review of the administrative arrangements for health care provision in the country"[359]. The tertiary health care facilities include specialist and teaching hospitals and federal medical centres (FMCs). While the primary health facilities refer patients to the secondary health facilities, the secondary health facilities refer patients to the tertiary health facilities for treatment. This evidences how the three levels work synergistically. The facilities at the tertiary level possess special expertise and full-fledged technological expertise that qualify them as resource centres for knowledge generation and diffusion. There is at least one tertiary facility in each of the 36 states[360].

2.4 Primary Health Care System in Nigeria

As we have intimated above, we are giving more attention to the Primary Health Care System because of the central position it occupies

---

[357] Cfr. T. M. AKANDE, «Referral system in Nigeria: study of a tertiary health facility», Annals of African Medicine, 3(2004), 130-133.

[358] Cfr. WORLD HEALTH ORGANIZATION, *Primary Care Systems…*,

[359] S. I. OKAFOR, «Spatial Aspects of Health Care Provision in Nigeria», in R. AKHTAR (ed.) *Health Care Patterns and Planning in Developing Countries*, Greenwood Press, New York 1991, 263-274.

[360] CFR. FEDERAL REPUBLIC OF NIGERIA, *National Human Resources…*, 15.

in the Health care system. It is the initial and as many believe the most important contact with the medical world during the battle with ill health. "Primary Health Care (PHC) is the foundation of the Nigeria National Health System"[361]. Over half of the Nigerian population live in rural areas. The 2013 National Demographic Health Survey (NDHS)[362] as cited by the Primary Care Systems Profiles & Performance (**PRIMASYS**), reveals that:

> Common preventable diseases such as malaria, diarrhoea and malnutrition are the major causes of morbidity and mortality in children; maternal mortality is 576/100,000; and under-five mortality rate 69/1000 live births. Antenatal care attendance and delivery by skilled health providers are 61% and 38% respectively; and only about a quarter of children are fully vaccinated[363].

This gives an insight of the state of primary health care service provision in Nigeria. It also reveals the general condition of the Nigerian Health care system and the quality of health of an average Nigerian. M. K.-Nimakoh, M. C.-Olah and T. V. McCann remark that the efforts at the global level to better the condition of women and children has never met the desired goal in sub-Sahara Africa, perhaps because of the conditions of primary health care[364].

An appropriate primary health care system is a necessary condition for realizing the Millennium Development Goals. Thus, it is widely believed that the primary aim of any health care system is to "efficiently provide evidence-based services that meet the clinical/medical needs"[365] of those in need of care. Quality health care services should be accessible, available, affordable and acceptable to the clients. This according to the aforementioned authors "is particularly important for vulnerable populations with specific needs,

---

361 WORLD HEALTH ORGANIZATION, *Primary Care Systems…*,

362 NATIONAL POPULATION COMMISSION, 2013, Nigeria Demographic and Health Survey in http://www.population.gov.ng/index.php/2013-nigeria-demographic-and-health-survey [11-12-2017].

363 WORLD HEALTH ORGANIZATION, *Primary Care Systems…*,

364 Cfr. M. K.-NIMAKOH – M. C.-OLAH – T. V. McCANN, «Access barriers to obstetric care at health facilities in sub-Sahara Africa–a systematic review», *Systematic Reviews*, 6(2017), 110, in https://doi.org/10.1186/s13643-017-0503-x [31-7-2018].

365 M. K.-NIMAKOH – M. C.-OLAH – T. V. McCANN, «Access barriers to…».

such as pregnant women and their infants"[366]. Regrettably, most facilities in many Nigerian hospitals and clinics are in various states of disrepair. In most states of Nigeria the primary health care facilities are in dilapidating conditions, with equipment and infrastructures being either missing or archaic[367]. For this reason, "health outcomes and utilization of health care in Nigeria have been found to be low"[368].

In the following part of the work, we will treat the evolution of Primary Healthcare in Nigeria, the structure of Primary Healthcare in Nigeria, the organizational structure of Primary Healthcare in Nigeria, the community health practice in Nigeria and the Ward Health System in Nigeria.

2.4.1. Structure of Primary health Care in Nigeria

The primary health care system in Nigeria is constitutionally under the jurisdiction of the last among the three tiers of government; the local government areas (LGAs). According to the Nigerian government, the reason for assigning the primary health system to the LGAs is that they are closer to the citizens than the federal and the state governments. This method has been strongly criticized by many Nigerian and foreign scholars owing to its unfruitfulness.

---

[366] Ibid.

[367] Cfr. I. S. ABDULRAHEEM – A. R. OLAPIPO – M. O. AMODU, «Primary health care services in Nigeria: Critical issues and strategies for enhancing the use by the rural communities», *Journal of Public Health and Epidemiology*, 4(2012) 5-13.

[368] A. OTOVWE – E. SARKI, «Utilization of Primary Health Care Services in Jaba Local Government Area of Kaduna State Nigeria», *Journal of Health Science*, 27(2017), 339-350, in https://dx.doi.org/10.4314/ejhs.v27i45 [31-7-2018]; O. B. TITUS – O. A. ADEBISOLA – A. O. ADENIJI, «Healthcare access and utilization among rural households in Nigeria», *Journal of Development and Agricultural Economy*, 7(2015), 195-203; V. Y. ADAM – N. S. AWUNOR, «Perceptions and factors affecting utilization of health services in rural community Southern Nigeria», *Journal of Medicine and Biomedical Research*, 13(2014), 117-124; F. A. AKESODE, «Factors affecting the use of primary health care clinics for children», *Journal of Epidemiology and Community Health*, 36(1982), 310-314); T. D. ODETOLA, «Health care utilization among rural women of child-bearing age: a Nigerian experience», *The Pan African Medical Journal*, 20(2015), 151, in https://doi.org/10.11604/pamj.2015.20.151.5845 [31-7-2018].

Primary health care is meant to be the corner stone of the Nigerian health system. Being closer to the people than the secondary and tertiary systems, it is considered as the means to drive health services to the grassroots. The major aim of the primary health system is to provide for the people at the rudimentary level, general health services that are preventive, promotional, curative and rehabilitative[369]. In carrying out this laudable duty, the local governments are to be assisted by the states and federal governments. The National Health Policy of 1988 and the National Primary Healthcare Development Agency (NPHCDA) established in 1992 were among the numerous attempts of the federal government to see that primary health care functions effectively. Despite the fact that these national health policies stand for the assistance of the states and federal governments, the LGAs' poor performances are often said to be due to lack of support from the state and federal levels of the government.

The LGAs under the primary health care programme are to plan, manage, monitor and evaluate the rendering of health care services. To make this administrative function feasible, every local government was divided into health districts of 10,000 to 30,000 people. Each district was entrusted to appoint a health committee for the smooth running of its primary health care. The villages or communities had a health committee of the neighbouring village or community with the responsibilities of controlling and managing the primary health care activities in their vicinity. The committees worked through the village heads or selected persons from the village in order to involve them in solving the health matters affecting their people[370]. In Nigeria, primary health care represented over 85 percent of the health care facilities in 2005[371].

2.4.2. The organizational structure of Primary Health care System in Nigeria

The organizational structure of the Nigerian Primary health care system is divided into 5 levels: The first level in an ascending order is made

---

[369] Cfr. S. A. ODUNBUNMI, *Primary Health Care in Nigeria: Structure and Performance*, LAMBERT Academic Publishing, Saarbrucken, Germany 2012, 37.

[370] Cfr. Ibid.

[371] Cfr. A. O AIGBIREMOLEM – I. ALENOGHENA – E. EBOREIME – C. ABEJEGAH, «Primary Health Care...».

up of Volunteers Health Workers (VHWs) and Traditional Birth Attendants (TBAs). The health workers at this level are trained informally. Community Health Extension Workers (CHEWs) form the second level. They receive formal training from Schools of Health Technology for 3 years and afterwards are awarded a diploma in community health care. At the third level are the Community Health Officers (CHOs). The CHOs are next to nurses in grade and are in charge of the primary health care centers in the absence of nurses. After receiving the training that qualifies one for the second level (CHEW), health workers undergo another one-year training in a teaching hospital to qualify as a CHO. Nurses/midwives are at the fourth level. These can head primary health care centers with the assistance of the medical officer of Health (MOH) in difficult cases. In the absence of the MOH in any local government, the most senior nurse substitutes as supervisor. The fifth and highest level is occupied by the MOH who is a medical doctor. The medical officer of health supervises a group of primary health care (PHC) centers found in each Local Government Area[372].

2.4.3. Community Health Practice in Nigeria

Regarding Community health practice, The Alma Ata Declaration (iv) states: "The people have a right and duty to participate individually and collectively in the planning and implementation of their health care"[373]. Community health practice implies "provision of health care services, through early diagnosis of disease, recognition of environmental and occupational hazards to good health and prevention of diseases in the community"[374]. Acceptance that the community is an important place for health care services

---

[372] Cfr. J. ABDULMALIK – L. KOLA – W. FADAHUNSI – K. ADEBAYO – M. T. YASAMY – E. MUSA – O. GUREJE, «Country Contextualization of the Mental Gap Action Programme Intervention Guide: A Case Study from Nigeria», *PLoS Medicine*, 10(2013), e1001501, in https://doi.org/10.1371/journal.pmed.1001501[23-11-2017]. (The organizational structure of the Nigerian Primary health care system is found in figure 2 in the cited work.)

[373] *Declaration of Alma-Ata, International Conference on Primary Health Care*, Alma-Ata, USSR, 6-12 September 1978 in http://www.who.int/publications/almaata_declaration_en.pdf [10-12-2017].

[374] A. S. IBAMA – D. A. DOTIMI – R. OBELE, «Community Health Practice in Nigeria – Prospects and challenges», *International Journal of Current Research*, 7 (2015), 11989-11992, in http://www.journalcra.com [23-11-2017].

commenced in the 1960s. In line with this trend, the primary health care in Nigeria came up as a product of the Basic Health Services in 1979[375]. Primary health care has the goal of Universal Health Coverage. For this reason, the basic essence of PHC is to ensure that the rudimentary health services are accessible and available to the vulnerable in rural areas.

Some afore-cited Nigerian authors[376], citing Alakija (2000), present the following perspectives for the definition of the Community health:

1. Part of medicine which is concerned with the health of the whole population and the prevention of diseases from which the population suffers.
2. It identifies the root causes of diseases and health problems not only from the individual but also from the family, the community and the environment.
3. The community resources are utilized principally in solving their problems. The resources from government and the private sector can also be used.
4. It aims at giving the highest level of health for all people in the community spanning physical, mental, moral, social and spiritual health.

The above description of the community health shows how the practice of community health is at the heart of the primary health care system. Community health through the application of simple scientific and cultural approved methods and skills, strives to ensure the prevention, promotion and treatment of health conditions in a specific community. Community health practice received notable attention in Nigeria starting from the period between 1975-1980, when through the Basic Health Service Scheme (BHSS), there was a systematic provision of health care at the community level by health workers who were majorly Community Health Practitioners. The Basic Health Service Scheme (BHSS) was instituted to facilitate the establishment of health centres in the communities to work with them, enabling the participation of the members of the community in reference[377].

---

[375] Cfr. Ibid.

[376] Cfr. Ibid.

[377] Cfr. Ibid.

This is akin to the Alma Ata Declaration definition of community participation as "the process by which individuals and families assume the responsibility for their own health and for those of the community and develop the capacity to contribute to their and the community's development"[378]. Community health is essential for a highly populated nation like Nigeria, if it wants to achieve the major objective of primary health care, which is that of touching the lives of every citizen and addressing the conditions that lead to the high mortality and morbidity rate that has become the emblem of the country. Community health adopts the approach of grass roots organization of the communities. This enables it to reach everyone especially the vulnerable who would have been ignored without such a rudimentary approach.

Community health practitioners in Nigeria comprise Community Health Officers, Community Health Supervisors (their training was stopped in 1990), Community Health Extension Workers (formerly known as Community Health Assistants but was changed in 1987), and Junior Community Health Extension Workers (formerly called Community Health Aides, the name was changed in 1987). According to the Health Reform Foundation in 2007, these Community Health Practitioners are the pillars of the Nigerian Primary Health Care system[379].

Community health practice in Nigeria has many challenges. Firstly, it has not been able to achieve the major goals behind its origin. Today in Nigeria there is no grassroot health care service for all because many citizens in the rural areas are gravely marginalized in terms of availability, accessibility and affordability of primary health care. Another issue is the lack of will of the government to fund primary health, causes this challenge according to many Nigerians and in particular, the community health programmes. Other obstacles of community health include uneven distribution of the insufficient community health workers, lack of adequate facilities and infrastructures, lack of organization on how to reach the unreached communities, unsatisfactory attitude of health workers and the insufficient knowledge of primary health care on the part of health professionals and those who make decisions on the issues in question[380].

Some authors ascertain that Nigeria's primary health care system has the potential to be effective based on the ratio of health worker/

---

[378] *Declaration of Alma-Ata…*

[379] Cfr. A. S. IBAMA – D. A. DOTIMI – R. OBELE, «Community Health Practice…».

[380] Cfr. Ibid.

population. They cited an example of the year 2006 where one centre alone (Community Health Extension Workers) had 117,568 (91/100,000 population) operating in the country. Therefore, they think that health care providers, in addition to mass media efforts, have to educate community members and their leaders to ensure a better knowledge of the community health practice. Mass education and mobilization according to them are the necessary conditions for establishing the Ward Health System (WHS). This implies a rapid improvement on Health information transfer and access to communication media[381].

2.4.4. Ward Health System (WHS)

Before adopting the Ward Health System (WHS), Nigeria, just like other countries in sub-Sahara Africa, operated the District Health System. With this model, "there was no clear demarcation of the "districts", as all LGAs carved themselves into what they perceived as districts. The entire LGA was considered then as the functional unit and there was no uniformity"[382]. Therefore, there was the need for a new system in order to achieve the set goals relative to health care services at the grass roots level. The federal government of Nigeria, in December 2000, introduced the Ward Health System[383]. This was done to re-vitalize the National Primary Health Development Agency (NPHCDA) enacted in 1992 and to respond to the recommendation of the World Health Organisation (WHO) of 1992 that "community mobilization would greatly be assisted if the boundaries of the health district are the same as the electoral ward (10,000 to 30,000 people) which elect a councillor to the LGA"[384 385]. This means replacing the District/village structure with the LGA-ward Community/village structure[386].

---

[381] Cfr. O. A. Abosede – P. C. Campbell – T. Olufunlayo – O. O. Sholeye, «Establishing a Sustainable Ward Health System in Nigeria: Are Key Implementers Well Informed?», *Journal of Community Medicine & Health Education*, 2(2012), 164. http://dx.doi.org/10.4172/2161-0711.1000164 [10-12-2017].

[382] Ibid.

[383] Cfr. S. A. Odunbunmi, *Primary Health Care...*, 40.

[384] World Health Organization (1992), *The Report of WHO Review*, 10.

[385] O. A. Abosede – P. C. Campbell – T. Olufunlayo – O. O. Sholeye, «Establishing a Sustainable...».

[386] Cfr. S. A. Odunbunmi, *Primary Health Care...*, 40.

The Federal Ministry of Health (FMOH) reacted immediately to the adoption of WHS by providing resources to construct 200 model Ward Health Centres in the wards without health facilities in the 6 health zones of the country. This move by the ministry was seen as another attempt by the government to establish standard national health centres in the country and part of the efforts to foster the development of primary health care services. The year after the adoption of the WHS, the President of Nigeria, through an Appropriation Bill, ordered the NPHCDA to facilitate the building of these 200 health centres, which would serve as pivots for implementing primary health care. The federal government with this renewed its commitment to the development of primary health care in the country[387]. The project of constructing 200 health centres across the country was accomplished in 2003. The health centres were as the apex of all PHC services in the respective wards. During the construction, it was envisaged that the communities would be actively involved. After the construction, the centres were handed over to the Ward Development Committees (WDC), which consist of the community members.

Sources on the reviews of the development of the National Primary Health Care System in Nigeria reveal many problems among which are the inadequate community mobilization and participation, lack of proper orientation of the health work force, and mal-distribution of resources. One of the major reasons for the failure in realizing the objectives of the Basic Health Services Scheme according to some authors is relative to the poor and ineffective participation of the people, that is, the community in the provision of the health care services. This led to the abandonment of projects and stealing of facilities by hoodlums. The Scheme thus was inefficient and as a result a failure[388].

The primary goal of the Ward Health Service (WHS) is to involve the people at the local or grass roots level in the provision of health care services and in making more effective and efficient primary health care services in their communities[389]. The following are the general objectives of the WHS[390]:

---

[387] Cfr. O. A. Abosede – P. C. Campbell – T. Olufunlayo – O. O. Sholeye, Establishing a Sustainable…,

[388] Cfr. Ibid.

[389] Cfr. S. A. Odunbunmi, *Primary Health Care…*, 41.

[390] Cfr. Ibid., 41-42.

- To improve knowledge, attitude and practice on health issues in communities.
- To promote local initiatives through participatory learning activities.
- To encourage self-reliance.
- To reduce maternal and infant mortality rate by 25% in the target wards within 2 years.
- To make essential drugs available in the target wards.
- To encourage collaboration between stakeholders.
- To encourage poverty-alleviation activities such as small – scale industry etc.

For improving the effectiveness of health service, the WHS was to[391]:

- Improve the supervisory role of the junior community health workers.
- Build local capacity at all levels.
- Promote active participation of the people to increase ownership and sustainability.
- Phase implementation of the WHS.
- Motivate local resource mobilization and optimal use of funds.
- Build on lessons learned and successes achieved in the target wards to develop other wards.
- Support poverty alleviation strategies through inter-sectoral collaboration.
- Promote information sharing with other stakeholders.
- Promote local initiative.

The programme structure of the Ward Health Service[392] includes the provision of primary health care facilities and services to a political defined ward constituency with an elected councillor. The referral ward health centre provides general services "to cover all PHC components as apex health facility"[393]. Each ward centre has health workers and personnel who carry out the function of supervising and coordinating the health care

---

[391] Cfr. S. A. ODUNBUNMI, *Primary Health Care…*, 42-43.
[392] Cfr. Ibid., 43.
[393] Ibid.

services administered with the particular ward. In urban areas, the wards are subdivided into sections, while those in rural areas are subdivided into groups of villages. A resident Junior Community Health Extension Worker (JCHEW) supervises each of these subdivisions[394].

The passage from "do-for" (where the government does and provides everything alone) as the only approach to health care provision to the "do-with" approach (an approach that involves the community members in health care provision) was a gigantic step towards the achievement of a formidable WHS. It is as a matter fact accepted that with the "do-with" approach, participation of the community members was very crucial to the implementation of WHS. With this approach, the community members were seen working hand in hand and supporting the development committees in their areas to tackle their health problems, thereby improving their quality of health[395].

O. A. Abosede, P. C. Campbell, T. Olufunlayo and O. O. Sholeye think that including training on the WHS in the medical and dental curricula is an essential strategy. According to them, having the training on the WHS as part of their primary health care curriculum would help the doctors and dentists who may be assigned to work in rural areas during the National Youth Service programme to be an important means for community education and mobilization. For these authors: "Re-orientation on the WHS ought to be part of their orientation programmed in camps"[396].

2.5. Health Workers in Nigeria

According to the World Health Organisation (WHO), (2006), Human Resources for Health are "those who promote and preserve health as well as those who diagnose and treat diseases. Also included within human resources are health management and support workers, those who help to make the health system function, but who do not provide health services directly"[397]. Human Resources could be described as the heartbeat or corner stone of health service delivery. This is verified in the services

---

[394]   Cfr. Ibid.

[395]   Cfr. O. A. ABOSEDE – P. C. CAMPBELL – T. OLUFUNLAYO – O. O. SHOLEYE, Establishing a Sustainable …

[396]   Ibid.

[397]   FEDERAL REPUBLIC OF NIGERIA, National Human Resources…, 12.

rendered by the health workers. If these services are of a standard quality, they can positively influence immunization coverage, increased outreach of primary care, maternal, neonatal and child health and other the delivery of most life-saving health services and vice versa. The above arguments explain the reason for the following affirmation that the health workforce determines health outputs and outcomes and the health systems performance[398].

2.5.1. The training of Medical Doctors and Nurses in Nigeria

The training of a medical doctor in Nigeria has its remote beginning from the high school years. A student who wants to become a physician starts by showing his interest in science subjects like chemistry, biology and physics. At end of secondary education, the student sits for the West African Examination Council (WAEC) or the General Certificate of Education (GCE) and must acquire credit or distinction in five subjects including the above mentioned. With this and the required grade for medical education in the Joint Admission and Matriculation Board (JAMB), the student can start medical education at University. The basic subjects for medical degree include anatomy, biochemistry, microbiology, physiology and immunology. After the rudimentary phase which lasts for two or three years, the student passes to the clinical phase, which may last for two of three years. Here students participate in lessons relative to internal medicine, surgery and their specialist areas like paediatrics, obstetrics, genecology and psychiatry. During the period of training, the student has the possibility of practical experience to enable them to acquire concrete knowledge of the medical profession, especially in the important aspect of doctor-patient relationship[399]. At the end of training, the medical school evaluates the scholastic activities of the student, after which the student is promoted and graduates if the school's judgement is positive.

Nursing is similar to the medical profession and this similarity is extended to the training of nurses. To be a nurse, one is required to possess both knowledge and skills. The curriculum of nursing in the strict sense ranges from biological, physical, social, medical, pharmaceutical to other nursing science. Nursing requires a broad knowledge and sense

---

[398] Cfr. Ibid.
[399] Cfr. D. M. N. McDikkoh, *The Nigerian health system's…*, 111.

of professionalism because, the term nurse by definition implies the occupation of one who is devoted to the care of the sick. This brings the nurse to intervene in almost all aspects of the patients' life[400]. Secondary education requirements of nursing in Nigeria are similar to that of the medical doctor. In Nigeria, after graduation, it is obligatory for the student to take a licensure examination to qualify as a Nigerian Registered Nurse (NRN)[401]. The nurse carries out diagnosis, orders laboratory test and interprets test results. It is also the duty of the nurse to order treatments and minor surgeries.

2.5.2. Dentists

The dentist in Nigeria, just like in other countries, is a health worker specialized in dental health problems. They treat problems specifically for the strengthening of teeth (orthodontics); take care of teeth and surrounding tissues affected by diseases (endodontics); substitute with artificial teeth, treat gums and bones affected by diseases and teeth decay problems in adult and children caused by sugar and inadequate mouth hygiene. Some oral diseases in Nigeria include malocclusion, traumatised teeth, dental fluorosis and oral tumours[402]. The dentist treats these and other dental public health issues. The dentist is an important figure in Nigeria because oral health is considered an essential aspect of the general health and contributes to the improvement of the quality of life[403].

2.5.3. Pharmacists

The pharmacist is a trained health worker who is responsible for the hospital's pharmaceutical store where drugs and medications are conserved. In some Nigerian hospitals, in the absence of trained pharmacists, pharmacy or dispensary attendants are placed in charge of this sector. There are also

---

[400] Cfr. Ibid., 113.

[401] Cfr. Ibid., 116.

[402] Cfr. E. S. AKPATA, «Oral health in Nigeria», *International Dental Journal*, 54 (2004), 361-366, in https://doi.org/10.1111/j.1875-595x.2004.tb00012.x [15-9-2017].

[403] O. B. BRAIMOH – E. D. ODAI, «A survey of dental students on global oral health issues in Nigeria», *Journal of International Society of Preventive & Community Dentistry*, 4(2014), 17-21.

qualified pharmacists who work in private pharmaceutical stores, where drugs and medicine can be purchased. The pharmacist's specific functions are procuring, storing and dispensing drugs and various chemical product for medicinal purpose. Pharmacists control the supply of drugs and make sure the right drugs are administered to patients. To be a qualified pharmacist in Nigeria, one has to meet the required standard of the profession being specialized in the study relevant to drugs and medicines.

2.5.4. Laboratory Technicians and Laboratory Technologists

A laboratory technician is a health worker trained to handle issues relative to laboratory instruments and test procedures. The difference between the laboratory technologist and laboratory technician lies in the fact that while the former is a physician who can diagnose and decode laboratory test results, the later cannot because they are not a physician. A laboratory technologist is a physician specialized in technical and pathological aspects of medication realities.

2.5.5. Environmental Health Workers

Environmental health is an important sector of public health though many in Nigeria consider it old-fashioned. Environmental health comprises of the aspects of human health, including human life conditioned by physical, biological, chemical and social factors. The environmental health worker ensures there is a proper monitoring of the environment to prevent diseases that may arise from unhealthy environment. Their services are geared towards maintenance of environmental integrity. The role of the environmental health worker in very important as it has to do with the control of all factors that may have direct or indirect effect on physical, social and mental well-being of man in his environment. In Nigeria today, there is a conspicuous indifferent attitude towards the environmental health workers by the government, who in the majority of its institutions makes no provision of office for them. When their work was appreciated in Nigeria, the environmental health officers, formerly known as "sanitary inspectors" were the major motivators who tirelessly moved from house-to-house to inspect the environment of the people. They played the role of educating people on the necessity of sanitation and hygiene. They diligently enforced environmental sanitation laws and regulations.

2.5.6. Private/Public Health Workers

Private health workers are all those who do not practice under the public health system. They work in their private health facilities following the laws and regulations established by the government to regulate their activities. In Nigeria, most doctors who own private hospital or work in private clinics work as both private and public health workers. In fact a good number of Nigerian physicians are officially in private practice despite the fact that much of their income comes directly from the public fund. Most health providers employed by faith-based and non-governmental organizations in many settings act in that mode. The government officially employs Public health workers and they are officially in public practice and get their income directly from the public purse[404].

2.5.7. Community Health Worker

The community health workers play vital roles in realizing the Universal Coverage of basic health services. Community health workers are paraprofessionals or lay individuals who with their well-grounded knowledge of the language, culture and traditions of a place and their job-related training help in providing culturally appropriated health services to the community assigned to them[405]. In the classification of community health workers in an ascending order,[406] the first category is those with little or no formal education but with some days or weeks of informal training. These are simply known as lay health workers. The second are those known as level 1 paraprofessionals, that is, community health workers with some form of secondary education, followed by informal training. The third category are the level 2 paraprofessionals, individuals who attended secondary education and later had a job-related formal training of a few months and in some cases exceeding one year. Simple lay health workers

---

[404] Cfr. *The World Health Report 2006*, Health Workers: A Global Profile.

[405] Cfr. A. OLANIRAN, H. SMITH, R. UNKELS – S. BAR-ZEEV – N. VAN DEN BROEK, «Who is a community health worker? – A systematic review of definitions», *Global Health Action*, 10(2017), in https://doi.org/10.1080/16549716.2017.127 2223 [16-5-2017].

[406] Cfr. Ibid.

provide their services gratuitively; level 1 and 2 paraprofessionals tend to receive income[407].

2.5.8. Informal Health Workers

Informal health workers fall under the private health practice. In Nigeria, many informal health workers provide health care in commercial settings like shops and markets. Though they are mostly without formal medical education, they act like professional doctors and nurses because they interrogate their clients, take medical histories and go ahead to diagnose and to prescribe drugs. In a situation where the formal health services are neither available nor accessible to citizens, as it is mostly the case in Nigeria, informal health workers are the primary and most important reference points for people in need of health services. Most of them are addressed as 'doctors' and 'nurses' by the poor and illiterate patients.

The activities of informal health workers are at times monitored and they are invited to follow the rules and regulations set by the ministry of health to guide their activities. Most of them do not follow these rules, thereby constituting threats to the life and health of many poor Nigerians. They sell fake and adulterated drugs and administer services like abortion causing the death of many teenagers. D. M. N. MacDikkoh describes this problem in the following statement:

> In societies where the rule of law exists, drugstores are manned and run by pharmacists and trained pharmacy technicians or attendants, even in rural areas. In Nigeria, however, this is not so as most drugstores and pharmacies are run by untrained personnel, the majority of which have never attended any formal training in the pharmaceutical discipline or, for that matter, any of the health professional training. Occasionally, you will find some who have never attended school of any kind and yet sell powerful medications that are complex and capable of altering human constitution, or even kill, under the supervision of people trained in that discipline[408].

---

[407] Cfr. Ibid.

[408] Cfr. D. M. N. McDikkoh, *The Nigerian health system's…*, 71.

Patent Medicine Vendors (PMVs) and Community Pharmacists (CPs) are the most common informal health workers. As we mentioned earlier, they handle complicated issues that are not within their competence. Most often they serve as short-cuts for some who do not want anyone to know what they are suffering. Most cases are sexual transmitted diseases. In their observations on how young people's sexual reproductive health care needs are met in Abuja, Nigeria, A. D. Okonkwo and U. P. Okonkwo note that the Community Pharmacists and the Patent Medicine Vendors provide young people with "a seamless and non-judgemental access to contraceptives, sexual health advice and post-sexual risk exposure care"[409]. The PMVs and CPs, colloquially called *"chemists"* in Nigeria, are not experts in these areas and so can easily mislead the young girls who go to them for reasons such as "teenage pregnancy and sexually transmitted infections (STIs) which young people putatively prevent and/or manage by patronizing Patent Medicine Vendors (PMV) and Community Pharmacists (CP)"[410].

The CPs are legally authorized to sell and dispense prescriptions. They can sell drugs following a presentation of formal prescriptions. Whereas the PMVs can only sell patent medicines that are considered safe by the Nigerian regulatory authorities. These medicines must be sold in their original manufacturer packages[411]. CPs and PMVs also sell house hold provisions to meet the needs and demands of their clients[412]. In Nigeria, though the PMVs and the CPs are only permitted to sell Over The Counter (OTC) drugs like anti malaria drugs, pain relieving tablets, cough syrups, they often stock OTC controlled drugs like antibiotics and steroids and engage in practices and procedures that are not covered by their license[413]. For this reason, authors like K. Peterson and O. Obileye

---

[409] A. D. OKONKWO – U. P. OKONKWO, «Patent medicine vendors, community pharmacists and STI management in Abuja, Nigeria», *African Health Sciences*, 10(2010), 253-265.

[410] Ibid.

[411] Cfr. R. ADISA – T. FAKEYE, «Assessment of the knowledge of community pharmacists regarding common phytopharmaceuticals sold in south-western Nigeria», *Tropical Journal of Pharmaceutical Research*,5(2006), 619-625.

[412] Cfr. F. O. OSHINAME – W. R. BRIEGER, «Primary care training for patent medicine vendors in rural Nigeria», *Social Science & Medicine*, 35(1992), 1477-1484.

[413] Cfr. M. U. ADIUKWU, «Sales practices of patent medicine sellers in Nigeria», *Health Policy Planning*, 11(1996), 202-205.

think that pharmacy practice in Nigeria is under-regulated. Such under-regulation is obvious in the afore-mentioned notice of the CPs and the PMVs, and in the fact that patent medicine practice in Nigeria favours fake medicines which lead illness and often to untimely death of victims[414]. As a result of this abuse, the National Agency for Food & Drugs Administration and Control (NAFDAC), often checks and sanctions the illegal sales of drugs in Nigeria[415].

The inefficiency of the primary health care system in Nigeria promotes the activities of the PMVs and CPs[416]. Some authors affirm that CPs and PMVs are highly involved more than any other sector in handling the preventive and therapeutic sexual reproductive health care needs of young people in Nigeria[417]. According to A. D. Okonkwo and U. P. Okonkwo: "Nigerian CPs and PMVs retail these products, and their (re)combination, to young people who need preventive and restorative sexual reproductive healthcare"[418].

---

[414] Cfr. K. Peterson – O. Obileye, «Access to drugs for HIV/AIDS and related opportunistic infections in Nigeria», *Policy Project/Nigeria* 2002, 1-45; Cfr. M. U. Adikwu – K. C. Okoye, «Patient factors militating against the laws governing prescriptions-only medicines in Nigeria», *Nigerian Journal of Pharmacy*, 23(1992), 7-11.

[415] Cfr. T. Edike – C. Obinwanne, National Agency for Food & Drug Administration and Control (NAFDAC), Destroys N14bn Fake Drugs, *Vanguard*, Nov. 7, 2006.

[416] Cfr. P. O. Erah, «The changing roles of pharmacy in hospital and community pharmacy practice in Nigeria», *Tropical Journal of pharmaceutical Research*, 2(2003), 196-196.

[417] Cfr. W. R. Brieger – P. E. Osamor – K. S. Salami – O. Oladepo – S. A. Otusanya, «Observations of patent medicine vendor and customer interaction in urban and rural areas of Oyo State, Nigeria», *Health Policy Planning*, 2004, 19(2004), 177-182; W. R. Brieger – L. A. Salako – R. E. Umeh – P. U. Agomo – B. M. Afolabi – A. K. Adeneye, «Promoting pre-packaged drugs for prompt and appropriate treatment of febrile illness in rural Nigerian Communities», *International Quarterly of Community Health Education*, 21(2002), 19-40.

[418] A. D. Okonkwo – U. P. Okonkwo, «Patent medicine vendors...», *African Health Sci...*; Cfr. W. R. Brieger – J. Ramakrishna – J. D. Adeniyi, Self-treatment in rural Nigeria, a community health education diagnosis, Hygiene International Journal of Health Education, 5(1986), 41-46.

2.5.9. The Key Regulators of Health Care Workers in Nigeria

A Federal government document reveals that Nigeria has a huge number of health workers. Only two countries in Africa, Egypt and South Africa, can be compared to Nigeria in terms of numerical capacity of workforce in the health sector. The document released in 2008 affirms that in Nigeria, "there are about 39,210 doctors and 124,629 nurses registered in the country, which translates into about 30 doctors and 100 nurses per 100,000 population"[419]. The problem lies in their regulation, organisation, distribution, remuneration and their attitude towards patients. These factors seriously affect the outcome of the services rendered by these health workers.

The following are the key regulators for the training and activities of health care workers in Nigeria[420]:

- Medical and Dental Council of Nigeria (MDCN) – 1. Regulate training including medical education 2. License doctors and dentists and enforce professional conduct.
- Pharmaceutical Council of Nigeria (PCN) – 1. Regulate training including continuing professional development2. License pharmacists to practice and enforce professional conduct 3. Inspect and license pharmacy premises.
- Nursing and Midwifery Council of Nigeria (NMCN) -1. Regulate training including continuing professional development 2. License nurses and midwives to practice and enforce professional conduct.
- Medical Laboratory Science Council of Nigeria (MLSCN) - 1. Regulate training including continuing professional development 2. License Laboratory Scientists, Technician and Assistants to practice and enforce professional conduct 3. Regulate the production, importation, sales and stocking of diagnostic laboratory reagents and chemicals 4. Inspect regulate and accredit Medical Laboratories (public and private).
- National Agency For Food and Drug Administration and Control (NAFDAC): The vision of NAFDAC is to safeguard the public health of the nation. Its mission is to safeguard the public health

---

[419] FEDERAL REPUBLIC OF NIGERIA, *National Human Resources…*, 16.
[420] Cfr. Nigerian Health Sector, *Market Study Report …*, 40.

by making sure that only the right quality food, drugs and other regulated products are manufactured, exported, imported, advertised, sold and used.

2.5.10. Human Resources for Health: The Experience of Health Work Force in Nigeria

The experience of health workers in Nigeria does not show that of a nation which understands the importance of health and that of a health work force. The results of a study on the health workforce in Nigeria reveals that "the Nigerian health system is relatively weak and there is yet a coordinated response across the country"[421]. The just cited authors identified some problems that must be addressed in this regard. According to them:

> A number of health workforce crises have been reported in recent times due to several months' salaries owed, poor welfare, lack of appropriate health facilities and emerging factions among health workers. Poor administration and response across different factions engaged in protracted supremacy challenge. These crises have consequently prevented optimal healthcare delivery to the Nigerian population[422].

The health workforce cannot be ignored if the Nigerian health system wants to continue to render its services to the nation. This is affirmed in the position that "the health workforce–all persons involved in activities primarily devoted to enhancing health–is an essential block of any functioning health system in any country, in the absence of which clinical and public health services cannot be delivered to the population"[423]. It has been reported that Nigeria faces serious challenges in "training, funding, employment, capacity building and efficient deployment of its

---

[421] D. Adeloye – R. A. David – A. A. Olaogun – A. Auta – A. Adesokan – M. Gadanya – J. K. Opele – O. Owagbemi – A. Iseolorunkanmi, «Health workforce and governance: the crisis in Nigeria», *Human Resources for Health*, 15(2017), 32. https://doi.org/10.1186/s12960-017-0205-4 [30-7-2018].

[422] Ibid.

[423] Ibid; Cfr. World Health Organization, *The World Health Report 2006– working together for health*, Geneva, World Health Organization, 2006.

workforce"[424], just like many other African countries. Crisis in this regard seems to be more severe in Nigeria: "According to the 2006 World health Report, 57 countries were in severe health workforce crisis [...] Nigeria, the most populous African country, possibly contributes even more to these crisis [...] Nigeria, has been adjudged a major factor in countries with severe health workforce crises"[425].

The above cited report observes that "based on our findings, it is evident that health workforce crises in Nigeria have continued to deteriorate due to some specific factors, mostly related to poor health leadership"[426]. The problem of leadership is a major constraint of development in Africa. Little wonder why the World Health Organization has always maintained the position that a "robust finance structure, well-remunerated and trained workforce, sufficient and highly maintained facilities" are qualities of a strong health system. It also sustains that the above mentioned characteristics could be guaranteed only with appropriate governance[427]. Such characteristics according to some authors are lacking in Nigeria. According to them, "the Nigerian health system is lacking full capacity in leadership and governance, with this reflecting in the health workforce crises and poor health service delivery in recent years"[428].

2.6. The Nigerian Health Care Financing System

Health is classified among the most important conditions of human life[429]. Any financial barrier is an obstacle to access to healthcare for the

---

[424] D. ADELOYE – R. A. DAVID – A. A. OLAOGUN – A. AUTA – A. ADESOKAN – M. GADANYA – J. K. OPELE – O. OWAGBEMI – A. ISEOLORUNKANMI, «Health workforce and...»; Cfr. WORLD HEALTH ORGANIZATION, Nigeria, in *Global Health Workforce Alliance*, Geneva, World Health Organization, 2016.

[425] Ibid.

[426] Ibid.

[427] Cfr. Ibid; Cfr. WORLD HEALTH ORGANIZATION, *World Health Report* 2010, Health *systems financing: the path to universal coverage*, Geneva, World Health Organization, 2010.

[428] Ibid.

[429] Cfr. A. O. LAWANSON – O. S. OPELOYERU, «Equity in healthcare financing», *Journal of Hospital Administration*, 5(2016), 53-59, in http://dx.doi.org/10.5430/jha.v5n5p53 [7-11-2017].

citizens in the low socio-economic bracket. This according to some authors calls for the effort to ensure that the entire population has access to quality health services without risking financial catastrophic outcome. This is the thrust of universal coverage. According to the Declaration of Alma Ata on Primary Health Assistance: "Primary Health Care is essential health care based on appropriate and acceptable methods and technology made universally accessible to individuals and families in the community"[430]. The Alma Ata Declaration acclaimed by some as the most important event in the International Health Politics, underlines the importance of primary health, indicating that it represents a valid strategy towards the realization of the project of providing health for all by the year 2000[431]. The project of providing health services to every Nigerian citizen is yet to be realized in 2019. The country's poor economic condition is a major factor responsible for this failure. It is evident that the current economic recession in Nigeria has a notable negative impact on Nigerian health sector. The effect of the recession is evident in the high cost of drugs, poor financing of the health sector, high cost of treatment, high disease morbidity and mortality and the continuous increase in out-of-pocket spending on health care[432].

2.6.1. Budgetary allocations to the health sector
by the Nigerian government

During the first Presidential health Summit held on 10th March 2014 in Abuja, the President and Vice-President together with the governors and other political leaders, pledged to commit themselves to significantly improve the health status of Nigerians by "increasing budget allocation at the Federal, State and LGAs from the present level by at least 25% each year towards achieving the Abuja Declaration target of 15%; committing to at least 90% release and 100% utilization by the end of the year"[433]. The World Health Organisation notes that the general expenditure by the Nigerian government

---

[430] I. D. Askew, «Planning and Implementing Community Participation in Health Programmes», in R. Akhtar (ed.) *Health Care Patterns and Planning in Developing Countries*, Greenwood Press, New York 1991, 3-19.

[431] Cfr. J. E. Eko, «Implication of Economic Recession on the Health Care Delivery System», *Nigeria Social Science*, 6 (2017), 14-18, in https://doi.org/10.11648/j.ss.20170601.13 [17-1-2018].

[432] Cfr. Ibid.

[433] Federal Ministry of Health, National Strategic Health…,

on health as a percentage of total government expenditure was very low at 3.3% in 2002, increasing consistently per year to 9.4% in 2007, and dropped to 6.7% in 2012[434][435]. The World Bank in an assessment in 2010 discloses that the dysfunctional state of the Nigerian health system is because it is grossly under-funded with a per capita expenditure of US$9.44[436]. In 2013, Nigerian allocated N279 billion to health an amount a bit higher than the N262 billion allocated in 2014. The state of the Nigerian budgetary allocation has not improved either recently as "a recent review of health-system financing for UHC in Nigeria shows high out-of-pocket expenses for health care, a very low budget for health at all levels of government, and poor health insurance penetration"[437].

Due to the poor performance of the Nigerian government in its budgetary allocation to health, private expenditure on health as a percentage of total health expenditure has remained high in the country, dropping slightly from 74.4% in 2002 to 68.9% in 2012. Out-of-pocket expenditure as a percentage of private expenditure on health has continued to increase, going above 90% since 2002, while it was 95.7% in 2012[438]. Despite the fact there are clear evidences that adequate public financing is key to the achievement of Universal Health Coverage (UHC), government expenditure on health in Nigeria has remained below standard. Nigeria's health expenditure is relatively low, even when compared with other African countries[439]. This analysis of the Nigerian health expenditure is a clear evidence of poor funding of public health. Many Nigerians are forced to spend high on health and this penalizes and threatens the health and lives of the vulnerable. Rwanda's exemplary health-system reforms according to A. Awosusi offer important lessons for Nigeria in this regard[440]. E. N. Anyika observes that there is the need to match structures,

---

[434] Cfr. WHO, Global Health Observatory Data Repository Nigeria, Statistics Summary (2002–present), in http://apps.who.int/gho/data/node.country. country-NGA [23-11-2017].

[435] Cfr. A. Awosusi – T. Folaranmi – R. Yates, «Nigeria's new government...».

[436] Cfr. A. O. Lawanson – O. S. Opeloyeru, «Equity in healthcare...».

[437] A. Awosusi – T. Folaranmi – R. Yates, «Nigeria's new government...».

[438] Cfr. Ibid.

[439] Cfr. B. O. Olakunde, «Public health care financing in Nigeria: Which way forward?», *Annals of Nigerian Medicine*, 6(2012), 4-10, in https://doi.org/10.4103/0331-3131.100199 [15-4-2017].

[440] Cfr. A. Awosusi – T. Folaranmi – R. Yates, «Nigeria's new government...».

systems and strategies with political and financial resources, and policy guidelines related to the health care system in Nigeria to achieve laudable health outcomes[441].

Some Nigerian authors rightly believe that good reproductive health care is a necessary condition for human capital development of any nation: "maximum productivity and output, good health is essential as is good maternal health for babies/offspring"[442]. Therefore they argue:

> For there to be effective, durable economic productivity in an area or nation; the health of the individuals in that particular location must first be optimal through provision of adequate health care services. Improvement in health care is a compulsory factor to be considered in the enhancement of the Human Capital Development in every single economy[443].

The just cited health/economic condition of the citizens and consequently of the nation, is achieved through appropriate government expenditure on health. Since government expenditure is a major source of financing health in many societies, the positive or negative health outcomes of the people are said to depend mostly on it. "In a nutshell, health investments have the capability to lead to improvement in a nation's maternal health and thus to resultant improvement in human capital"[444]. Correspondingly, R. K. Edeme affirms: "Public health expenditure is very important for decision makers to know the amount of government-funding on health care, the effectiveness of health care programs and the level of efficiency of this public health expenditure on achieving improvements in health outcomes"[445].

---

[441]   Cfr. E. N. ANYIKA, «Regulatory uncertainties in the pharmaceutical sector: perceptions among Nigerian pharmacists and policy implications for decision making», *Journal of Hospital Administration*, 5(2016), 48-55, in https://doi/10.5430/jha.v5n3p48 [28-7-2018].

[442]   R. N. OGU – B. C. E.-EMMANUEL, «Nigeria Government Expenditure, Economic Productivity and the prevention of Maternal Mortality: A Call to Action», *Journal of Economics, Management and Trade*, 21(2018), 1-9.

[443]   Ibid.

[444]   Ibid; J. O. YAQUB – T. V. OJAPINWA – R. O. YUSSUFF, «Public Health Expenditure and health outcome in Nigeria: the impact of governance», *European Scientific Journal*, 8(2012), e – ISSN 1857 – 7431.

[445]   R. K. EDEME, «Public health Expenditure and Health Outcome in Nigeria»,

2.6.2. Total Expenditure on Health as % GDP

The source of Health care system financing in Nigeria is a combination of tax revenue, out-of-pocket spending, funding from donors, and social and community health insurance. According to the Federal Ministry of Health:

> The National Health Accounts (NHA) for Nigeria over the period 2003 to 2005(CBN Report 2006) estimate that the Total Health Expenditure (THE) in Nigeria has grown from N6661.662 billion in 2003 to N976.69 billion in 2005. While the THE has grown in absolute terms by nearly a third during this period, THE as a share of Gross Domestic Product (GDP) has actually declined from 12.25% in 2003 to 8.56% in 2005. Federal government health expenditure was estimated to have grown three fold from N47.02billion in 2003 to N130.76billion in 2005, while the estimated expenditure for the same period by states grew from N48billion to N78.8billion and that of LGAs nearly doubled from N28.63billion to N44.64billion[446].

In his brief comparative analysis, B. O. Olakunde, observes that Nigeria's total health expenditure (THE) as percentage of the gross domestic product (GDP) between 1998 and 2000 was less than 5%, not meeting with the commitments in other developing countries like Kenya (5.3%), Zambia (6.2%), Tanzania (6.8%), Malawi (7.2%), and South Africa (7.5%)[447]. The document of the National Strategic Health Development Plan (HSHDP) reveals that the average share of the Total Government Expenditure on health increased from an average of about a fifth of the Total Health Expenditure (20.65%) between 1998 and 2002, to about a quarter of THE (24.1%) from 2003 to 2005[448]. In the same trend, B. O. Olakunde affirms: "The total government expenditure as proportion of THE was estimated as 18.69% in 2003, 26.40% in 2005. Remarkably, the federal budgetary component of health expenditure has increased

---

[446] *African Journal of Biomedical and Life Sciences*, 5(2017), 96-102, in https://doi.org/10.11648/j.ajbls.20170505.13 [21-8-2018].

[446] FEDERAL MINISTRY OF HEALTH, National Strategic Health...

[447] Cfr. B. O. OLAKUNDE, «Public health care...».

[448] Cfr. Federal Ministry of Health: National Strategic Health...

over the years. It increased from 1.7% in 1991 to 7.2% in 2007"[449]. Some other sources highlight the increment of the allocation to the health sector. According to one of these sources, "the total budget allocation to health at the federal level has increased by 67% from NGN154.6 billion in 2009 to NGN266.7 billion in 2011 and the federal budget allocation to health, accounts for 5.4% of the total federal budget and 0.7% of the national gross domestic product"[450].

Despite the above-mentioned increments, the Nigerian health sector is still not in a good state and the Nigeria health indicators are identified among the worst globally. Additionally, the Nigerian government has not been able to keep to the commitment of the African Union Countries in the Abuja declaration, to allocate at least a 15% ratio of the general budget to the health sector. Since the Abuja declaration in 2001, the government's budgetary allocation to the health sector has never surpassed 6%. In fact, a document of the Federal Ministry of Health, Nigeria, confirms this in the following declaration: "The poor performance of Nigeria's health system can therefore also be primarily attributed to poor financial resourcing of health services"[451]. The Primary Care Systems Profiles & Performance (PRIMASYS), a document produced in collaboration with WHO, affirms:

> With a gross domestic product (GDP) per capita of US$1091 and income inequity [...] Nigeria is still ranked among the poorest countries in the world, with about 70% of the population living below US$1 per day. Economic indicators show that as of 2013, total health expenditure as a proportion of GDP was 3.7%, and out-of-pocket payments represent over two thirds of health expenditure[452].

The Central Bank of Nigeria reveals that the proportion of the Federal Government's total expenditure on the social sector from 2001 to 2005 was between 12% and 19%. Some other sources also claim that absolute terms expenditure on health from 2001 to 2005, increased by more than 150%[453].

---

[449] B. O. OLAKUNDE, Public health care...

[450] B. S. C. UZOCHUKWU – M. D. UGHASORO – E. ETIABA – C. OKWUOSA – E. ENVULADU – O. E. ONWUJEKWE, «Health care financing...».

[451] FEDERAL MINISTRY OF HEALTH, National Strategic Health...

[452] WORLD HEALTH ORGANIZATION, Primary Care Systems...

[453] Cfr. FEDERAL MINISTRY OF HEALTH, National Strategic Health...

The claimed increase of government's expenditure on health does not reflect on the health care system and the life expectation of the population. For instance, some authors who carried out a study on the Universal Health Coverage in Nigerian report the hindrances caused by underfunding in some states in Nigeria. According to their report:

> In most states of the federation, the proportion of states' and LGAs budgets allocated to health remains below 15%. It is as low as 2% in Ondo and as high as 15% in Bauchi State. The per capita health expenditure of $10 is far below the $34 recommended by the macro-economic commission on health as required for provision of basic package of essential health care services[454].

Similarly, the Federal Ministry of Health reports that house hold out of pocket expenditure has remained the largest source of health expenditure in Nigeria. According to the Ministry of Health, the household out of pocket expenditure increased from N489.79 billion in 2003 to N656.55 billion in 2005[455]. The Nigerian health care system since its origin has been plagued by inadequate general government expenditure on health. This problem has been an obstacle towards achieving Universal Health Coverage. The general government health expenditure as a percentage of the total health expenditure increased from 32% in 2009 to 35% in 2000. The federal government expenditure touched 6% in 2012, but over the years the allocation to health has been equivalent to 3.2% of the total federal spending. The fact that total government allocation to the health sector remains below the 15% agreement of the African Union's Abuja declaration in 2001, remains a concern of the Nigerian health care system[456].

---

[454] B. S. C. Uzochukwu – M. D. Ughasoro – E. Etiaba – C. Okwuosa – E. Envuladu – O. E. Onwujekwe, «Health care financing…».

[455] Cfr. Federal Ministry of Health, Nationa Strategic Health…

[456] Cfr. B. S. C. Uzochukwu – M. D. Ughasoro – E. Etiaba – C. Okwuosa – E. Envuladu – O. E. Onwujekwe, «Health care financing…».

2.6.3. Health Expenditure Per Capita in Nigeria
at Average Exchange Rate (US$)[457]

The per capita total health expenditure in Nigeria at average exchange rate (US$) from 1999 to 2014 is as follows: 1999 – 16.26, 2000 – 17.22, 2001 – 18.28, 2002 – 17.89, 2003 – 38.50, 2004 – 44.94, 2005 – 53.09, 2006 – 61.01, 2007 – 81.37, 2008 – 88.52, 2009 – 74.36, 2010 – 80.34, 2011 – 93.23, 2012 – 90.39, 2013 – 110.37 and 2014 – 117.52.

Per capita government expenditure on health at average exchange rate (US$)[458] from 1999 to 2014 is thus: 1999 – 4.74, 2000 – 5.76, 2001 – 5.73, 2002 – 4.57, 2003 – 8.63, 2004 – 14.69, 2005 – 15.48, 2006 – 20.10, 2007 – 26.79, 2008 – 32.55, 2009 – 23.26, 2010 – 21.03, 2011 – 29.12, 2012 – 28.31, 2013 – 26.30 and 2014 – 29.55.

An overview of the total health expenditure per capita from 1999 to 2014 reveals that it touched the maximum after 19 years, by reaching the value of US$117.52 in 2014. Between 1999 and 2014, there was a continuous increase, which however was not stable. The total government expenditure per capita suggests that the Nigerian health care situation needs improvement especially in budget allocation. A general analysis demonstrates that the Nigerian government spends low on health, comparatively less than some other African countries[459].

2.6.4. The Abuja Declaration

Heads of states of the African Union countries converged in Abuja in April 2001 and pledged to allocate 15% their total annual budget to the health sector. This agreement is for the purpose of improving the health sector and to make better the health conditions of their citizens[460]. During the meeting, "they urged donor countries to "fulfil the yet to be met target of 0.7% of their annual *GNP* as official Development Assistance (ODA) to developing countries"[461]. The Alma Ata Declaration strongly affirms that health is a fundamental human right and it is the duty of the government

---

[457]   Cfr. WORLD HEALTH ORGANIZATION, *Global Health Observatory*...

[458]   Cfr. Ibid.

[459]   Cfr. Ibid.

[460]   Cfr. WORLD HEALTH ORGANIZATION, *Abuja Declaration: Ten Years On*, in http://www.who.int/healthsystems/publications/Abuja10.pdf [2-12-2017].

[461]   Ibid.

to provide conditions for the people to enjoy good health[462]. Observing the development of government's health care funding in Nigeria, one may doubt if the Nigerian government agreed with the concept of health as a right and that it is the responsibility the governments towards the people. B. S. Aregbeshola and S. M. Khan make clear their doubt thus:

> Health is rarely seen as a fundamental human right by policy makers in Nigeria; hence, the inability to implement the Abuja Declaration in which African heads of state pledge to set a target of earmarking at least 15% of their annual budget to improve the health sector. Increasing investment in health of the people has been a challenge for decision makers in spite of evidence showing the link between health and economic development[463].

The above-mentioned authors disclose that Nigeria is among the many African countries that fall short of the Abuja Declaration of 2001[464,465]. The 2016 health expenditure for the year was 4. 13% and in the 2017 budget, a total of N303.81 was allocated to the health sector from the grand total of N7. 298 trillion mapped out for expenditure for the year. The sum allocated to health is 4.16%. Comparing the 4.13% health allocation of 2016 to the 4.16% health allocation of 2017, there is an increment of 3%. But with the current inflation rate and devalued naira, it may be right to say that the 2017 allocation is less than that of the previous year. Since the Abuja declaration where the African leaders agreed to allocate at least 15% of the total annual budget to the health sector, Nigeria's allocation to the health sector has never surpassed 6% (5.7% in 2012).

As aforementioned, Nigeria has been oscillating between 3% and 6% with the national budget allocated to the health sector. With this, it is clear that the performance of the country is still poor and below the Abuja declaration's standard. The World Health Organisation in this regard emphasizes: "It is therefore important to consider ways to develop new sources of funds and examine more critically how to improve the efficiency of health spending, while always protecting the poor vulnerable"[466]. To

---

[462]   Cfr. B. S. AREGBESHOLA – S. M. KHAN, «Primary Health Care...».

[463]   Ibid.

[464]   Cfr. Ibid.

[465]   Cfr. WHO, *Abuja Declaration: Ten...*

[466]   Ibid.

sustain the vulnerable, it is necessary to strengthen the primary health care. This calls for the implementation of the Abuja Declaration.

2.6.5. National Health Financing Policy

The financing of the public health sector depends on funding from the federation account. In the sharing of funds for health among the three tiers of government, the federal level receives half of the total share, while a quarter is shared among the 36 states and the remaining quarter is distributed among the 774 local government areas. One of the reasons behind the decentralisation policy, which assigns primary health care to local government is that it is easier to have more efficient services when government is closer to the people. This could be true in a nation where the right and dignity of the human person is really taken into consideration and when allocations are being executed following the right principles of justice.

To tackle the problem of disjunction between finances and responsibility and between communities and the political administration of primary health care, the federal government of Nigeria adopted the National Primary Health Care Development Agency (NPHCDA), which should monitor the implementation of primary health care at local and state levels. Some health care experts who have noticed the technical, financial, managerial and political lacunae of local governments in the provision of adequate primary health care services have suggested the state governments or the federal government take over the responsibility, while the local governments assume the role of supervision. This suggestion is motivated by the aim of seeing that the basic life-saving health care services are available and accessible to all, especially to the most vulnerable.

> The National Health Act "sets the background to earmark adequate public resources to health towards strengthening primary health care through the Basic Healthcare Provision Fund. 50% of the fund will be managed by the National Health Insurance Scheme to ensure access to a minimum package of health services for all Nigerians and 45% by the National Primary Healthcare Development Agency for primary health-care facility upgrade and maintenance, provision of essential drugs, and deployment of human resources to primary health-care facilities. The Federal Ministry of Health will manage the

remaining 5% for national health emergency and response to epidemics[467].

According to some already cited authors "Policy documents on health in Nigeria emphasize the pursuit of equity in health and healthcare through improved access to quality healthcare by the poor and vulnerable"[468]. Equity implies "fair" distribution of available resources across the population. Equity is similar to equality but does not mean the same thing as equality. Both concepts cannot be used interchangeably. Equity helps us to address concretely the problem of each person. Equity in health fosters the principle of a preferential option for the poor and the vulnerable. There is no doubt about the fact that the health and financial policies in Nigeria declare the intention of improving the life of the poor and the vulnerable. The problem is that instead of improving, their lives deteriorate because of the lack of will to implement properly the policies on ground.

Large investment in health care is very important but alone it cannot make the Nigerian Health system appreciable. To really improve the health and quality of life of the population and to reduce morbidity and mortality rate of any country it is important to have the will to consider political, economic, educational, social and other health-enhancing interventions on aspects like infrastructure and environmental safety improvement. These can have notable effects on the effectiveness of the health care provision and the quality of health and life of the people.

Conclusion

The history of a systematic health care in Nigeria as this chapter reveals started with the contribution of the Christian (catholic) missionaries. With the activities of the colonial masters, there were also some affairs in the area of health care. This chapter disclosed the catholic missionaries delivered health care, placing the human person; the weak and the poor at the centre. On the contrary, the colonial masters delivered services that were gain oriented; for selfish interests. This is exactly why this dissertation is proposing the catholic principles for a person-centred health care delivery in Nigeria. From 1960 when Nigeria gained her independence, the idea

---

[467] A. Awosusi – T. Folaranmi – R. Yates, «Nigeria's new government…».
[468] A. O. Lawanson – O. S. Opeloyeru, «Equity in healthcare…».

was that of developing a health system that could provide basic health care for all following the catholic-western-hospital system.

With this, there was the first idea of adopting the Primary Health Care (PHC); a system in synergy with the catholic health care delivery. Thus, the Nigerian government adopted the Basic Health Service Scheme (BHSS) in1979. The trend continued in this line giving rise to the National Development Plan (1975 - 1979), inaugurated to make health care services accessible at the grassroots levels, the primary health care plan launched in 1987 by Professor Olikoye Ransome-Kuti, who was the Minister of Health in Nigeria, the National Primary Healthcare Development Agency (NPHCDA), launched in 1992 and the Ward Health System established in 2001. The Nigerian history from the political point of view, as we saw in the previous chapter, never allowed these plans to take root and to realize the goals for which they were established.

However, The Nigerian health system as our work has revealed continued to evolve and to increase its relentless efforts with: the National Health Policy, the National Health Insurance Scheme, the National Health Bill, the National Health Act 2014 and the National Strategic Health Development Plan. These served as the reformative measures for the health system as well as instruments for the improvement of the people's health. The National Health Policy for instance has the stance that it is a human right to have access to quality and affordable health care. For this, it is poised to achieve the goal of making basic health care available to all. In the same vein, the federal government instituted the National Health Insurance Scheme in May 1999 with the target of giving many Nigerians the possibility of receiving health care services.

Likewise, in 2014, the National Health Bill emerged as the first attempt in Nigeria to take a legislative stance and to fund the Primary Health Care (PHC). In order to further strengthen the health system, the National Health Act was signed into law in 2014 by the Nigerian President. It was meant to guide both the health system and health professionals in the bid to quickly achieve the Universal Health Coverage (UHC) and reach the Millennium Development Goals (MDGs). One of the major targets of the Act was to reduce the child and infant mortality rate in Nigeria. Another initiative is the National Strategic Health Development Plan which as we saw in this chapter had the mission of improving the health of Nigerians by establishing an efficient and sustainable health care system.

Theoretically, Nigeria has optimal health policies, plan, schemes, bills, etc., but lacks principles that can help to apply them justly. This is evident in the Nigerian health indicators and the causes of death and how the main pathologies in Nigeria are addressed. Surely, there have been some efforts of the Nigerian health system in some of these aspects, but the general results show that something is missing. This missing-link is what our dissertation will reveal in chapter four; the principles that can put the Nigerian Health System back on the right track.

The study of the nature, structure and administration of the Nigerian health system in this work showed it is divided into private and public health systems. The public health system is composed of three sectors following the model of three-tier system of government in Nigeria. While the public health system provides more affordable health services, the services made available by the private system are not easily affordable for the poor, who form the greater part of the Nigerian population. Both of them have the intention of making services accessible to all. Nigerians as we have seen in this chapter lament the poor quality of the services obtainable from the public sector, a phenomenon which constrains many to resort to the private sector for services.

The public health facilities are government entities. The activities of the public sector are directly linked to the political decisions. The administrative structure as this chapter has revealed is divided into three: the federal government controls the affairs of the tertiary level which comprises the university teaching hospitals and the federal medical centres. State governments control the affairs at the secondary level, which include: the general hospitals and primary health care facilities. Local government areas operate at the primary level.

The primary level is the lowest and it is controlled by the lowest of the levels of government in Nigeria. Consequently, it receives the lowest fund when the allocation to the health sector is shared. Our work has shown its contrariety to this form of allocation because the primary health system occupies the section of health that makes services reach the grassroots. All the initiatives like the MDGs, SDGs, UHC and the health policies and plans in Nigerian are geared towards making health care accessible to all especially at the primary level. For this, we retained that the administration of the health care system is not coherent to these initiatives.

We retain important the human resources; the health workers, which we defined in this chapter as the heartbeat or corner stone of health service delivery. We did not concentrate only on how there are trained, regulated and distributed, but also on how they are treated; their remuneration. The quality of this class of persons and how they are treated, obviously affects the health outputs and outcomes and the health systems.

One of the major characteristics of a good financing system is the capacity to realize a fair distribution of the burden of the health care services, thus protecting the people from heavy spending on health services, which may result in catastrophe for families. A sound financing system is also expected to reduce the barriers to health care services by ensuring a fair distribution of public expenditures[469]. The Nigerian government does not seem to have the above mentioned characteristics because while the health care needs of the population increase, the government expenditure on the health sector remains low. It is reported that "Nigeria, with an estimated population of over 180 million, and largest economy ($509 billion in 2014) in Africa, commits around 5% of GDP to healthcare financing"[470]. For this, the commonest way of obtaining health care services is out-of-pocket spending.

This has unfavourable effects on the pockets of many Nigerians who cry foul every day. Many Nigerian who feel disappointed from the performance of the Nigerian politics and the health system resort to traditional medicines. Our study has demonstrated that primary health care is the foundation of Nigerian health care and how the inadequate funding and support to this important level jeopardizes the entire health care system in Nigeria. The next chapters will search for a solution in the principles of justice which if chosen and applied rightly could lead to making the Nigerian Health care system more appreciable.

---

[469] Cfr. A. O. Lawanson – O. S. Opeloyeru, «Equity in healthcare…».
[470] Ibid.

Chapter 3

THE MORAL PRINCIPLES IN HEALTH CARE – THE SECULAR PERSPECTIVE

Introduction

This chapter studies how human health is maintained through a fair distribution of health care resources. It treats the problems relevant to the question: whether there is a right to health care. If this right exists, how does society respond to it? With what criteria of justice does society address the issue of distribution of health care resources? What moral principles, theories and approaches are applied to the distribution of health care resources? The problem of distribution of health care resources is an ethical issue that has been in existence for some time now and continues to give rise to interminable debates. Because of its nature, "different concepts of justice generate different ideas about fair distribution of healthcare resources"[471]. Most issues of health care allocation as we will see in this chapter focus on "the role of public financing in ensuring the ethically justified access to

---

[471]   C. Leget – R. Hoedemaekers, «Teaching medical students about fair distribution of healthcare resources», *Journal of Medical Ethics*, 33(2017), 737-741, in http://dx.doi.org/10.1136/jme.2006.017095 [22-12-2017].

and utilisation of health care by members of society"[472], especially the most vulnerable members. Since there are differing needs among the members of our society, what is the best way to distribute health care resources? To address this question, we will treat in this chapter, the various models pertinent to the health care allocation, studying the concept of 'distributive justice' and the various theories and approaches of distributive justice applied to the allocation of health care resources.

Because of the delicate nature of decision-making in ethical issues on what to do, it is recommended that "considered judgements" be adopted as decision-making guidelines. "A considered judgement implies that a degree of thinking and reasoning occurs before making a decision"[473]. Ethical principles and theories are good instruments for deliberations to reach decisions. They can also assist with their characteristics in confronting public and individual health situations to convince and motivate people to accept such decisions. This means, applying reflective equilibrium, which according to J. Summer entails the use of reason to select from among the ethical principles, theories, approaches and common morality and applying them to decision on present cases[474]. The principle of justice is very necessary though it is seen as a complex principle because it includes multiple ways of interpreting and understanding rights. More so, because there are unsettled discussions on the nature, that is, what is justice and how to arrive at it. "Justice Principles start from the idea that in the distribution of burdens and benefits, the allocation should be equal unless there is a material reason to discriminate"[475]. The principles of justice may be considered as the overriding principles of bioethics because they cut across broad ethical situations and, in most cases, other principles are applied in respect to justice. Regarding giving to each what is due to him or her, we can say that what is owed to individuals or what they deserve can be determined by the nature of the person, by the condition of the individual and by what the social institutions have determined. Because

---

[472] J. Hurley, «Ethics, economics, and public financing of health care», *Journal of Medical Ethics*, 27(2001), 234-239, in http://dx.doi.org/10.1136/jme.27.4.234 [22-12-2017].

[473] J. Summer, «Principle of Healthcare Ethics», in E. E. Morrison (ed.) *Health Care Ethics: Critical Issues for the 21ˢᵗ Century*, Jones and Bartlett Publishers, Sudbury MA 2009², 41-58.

[474] Cfr. Ibid.

[475] Ibid.

of the difficult tasks the principles of justice have to tackle, it is widely believed that understanding the various conceptions of rights and justice is very necessary in resource allocation at both the organizational level and at the government policy-making level[476].

In this chapter we will evaluate the moral principles, theories and approaches applied to health justice and later adopt what we retain positive in them and compatible with the Catholic principles, to apply them in chapter four to the concrete issues of health care in Nigeria mainly seen in chapters one and two. Suffice it to mention that one of the major goals of our work is to demonstrate that the catholic principles which we are treating in the next chapter are the best for the realization of a fair distribution of health care resources in Nigeria.

We will immediately study the concept of justice and afterwards see some proposed principles, theories and approaches to the allocation of health care resources. This will be followed by ethical evaluations of the right to health, equity in health and need principles and then conclusion.

3.1. The Concept of Justice

The *Penguin dictionary of Philosophy* defines Justice as "an attribute of *political systems, relations between individuals, actions,* and we can say of *persons* that they are just"[477]. We have two kinds of particular justice: Distributive justice, which operates at a society level and is concerned with the fair allocation of benefits and burdened, and Corrective or Commutative justice, which operates between two parties and strives to maintain or restore a balance[478]. Justice is ranked among the most important moral and political concepts. Globally, there have been many debates on the necessity of social justice to address the problems of inequalities in the right to health and access to and utilization of health care resources. Thus, T. L. Beauchamp and J. F. Childress affirm that "issues concerning the fairness of a distribution generate questions about principles of justice"[479].

---

[476] Cfr. Ibid.

[477] T. MAUTNER (ed.), *The Penguin Dictionary of Philosophy*, Penguin Books, London 1999, 288.

[478] Ibid.

[479] T. L. BEAUCHAMP – J. F. CHILDRESS, *Principles of Biomedical Ethics*, Oxford University Press, Inc., New York 2001⁵, 227.

Understanding the various nuances of rights and justice is very important in order to discuss the issue of health resource allocation. In explaining the concept of 'justice', many philosophers have been using terms like fairness and entitlement. With this, Justice has been variously defined to include fairness, equity and appropriate treatment regarding what is due or owed to persons. Injustice thus is verified where there is "a wrongful act or omission that denies people benefits to which they have a right or distributes burden unfairly"[480].

3.1.1. Distributive Justice

Distributive justice is the aspect of justice that "concerns the right way of allocating benefits and burdens"[481]. The authors T. L. Beauchamp and J. F. Childress define distributive justice thus:

> The term distributive justice refers to fair, equitable, and appropriate distribution determined by justified norms that structure the terms of social cooperation. Distributive justice refers broadly to the distribution of all rights and responsibilities in society, including, for example civil and political rights[482].

Accordingly, "the concept of distributive justice relates to determining what is fair when decision makers are determining how to divide burdens and benefits"[483]. At the heart of the distributive version of the principle of justice is the allocation of benefits and burdens. Distributive justice requires that the benefits and burdens available be identified and that the benefits be distributed equitably. The same is applicable to burdens, like the cost of providing the benefits.

The application of distributive principles is very important to achieve a just health care system. Some think that health care workers need not worry about the principles of distributive justice since determining the base package to be available and its distribution to people fall under the realm of social policy. But it has been revealed that at a practical level that the health professionals working in clinics encounter problems of distribution

---

[480] Ibid., 226.
[481] T. Mautner (ed.), *The Penguin Dictionary…*, 101.
[482] T. L. Beauchamp – J. F. Childress, *Principles of Biomedical…*, 228.
[483] J. Summer, «Principles of Healthcare…».

of health care resources, thus needing the principles of distributive justice. The application of the principle of distributive justice is necessary in cases such as, whether or not to charge standard or reduced prices to persons who do not have the capacity to pay, whether to charge higher prices to the rich in order to compensate the poor, when the request is on the higher side in respect to the available goods, as it is usually the case, whether a certain approach to treatment is cost worthy, especially when someone else, rather than the patient is to foot the bill, whether the poor and the vulnerable are to be granted their health needs knowing full well they will not be able to pay. In these cases, distributive justice becomes the central issue.

The fact that resource allocation is necessary at different levels (macro and micro) of health care helps us to understand and appreciate the concept of distributive justice in health care. Distributive justice is applied when the physician decides on the time to spend beside the patient's bed or to listen to each patient, the time the nurse should spend answering the call button for each patient etc. Is it fair to spend more time with one patient in dialogue or treatment giving less to the other? Decisions are not so easy when you stand face to face with those in need and you do not have all the necessary resources to address the problems of all of them. This accounts for the growing agreement among some authors "that equal access is the central issue for a just distribution of health care"[484]. These and more issues highlight the delicate nature of the problems where distributive justice are applied in health care resource distribution.

Importantly, "the principle of distributive justice demands decisions such as allocating and rationing health care made fairly within the political process"[485]. Distributive justice involves equal allocation, unless there is a material reason to discriminate. It includes determining what is fair in decision-making about how to divide burdens and benefits. Many ask if it is fair that some people or zones receive very little resources while others have them abundantly. Reacting to this question, there are people who think that in most cases some use very little resources because they are healthy, so do not need much resources. Others believe that in other cases,

---

[484] R. L. SHELTON, «Human rights and distributive justice in health care delivery», *Journal of medical ethics*, 4(1978), 165-171, in https://doi.org/10.1136/jme.4.4.165 [15-9-2017].

[485] G. P. SMITH, «Distributive Justice and Health Care», *Journal of Contemporary Health Law & Policy*, 18(2001-2002), 421-430.

those who use less are constrained to do so because they have limited or no access to the health care resources.

By considering these provocations and the subsequent reactions, it should be apparent that issues of health care distribution tend to or mirror general questions about distributive justice. The issue of distribution of health care resources however is not a simple one because the distribution of actual goods involves making decisions that have impacts on real people in real situations. Given that resources are limited, hard choices are inevitable. This accounts for multiple debates on the question of fair distribution of health care resources, especially on some particular issues such as cost, affordability, availability, accessibility, universality and quality.

It is commonly believed that "establishing fair procedure for the distribution of health care resources is a crucial goal for contemporary society to set and, hopefully, to achieve"[486]. To attain a fair procedure in the distribution of resources, there is the need to understand and solve the problems surrounding allocation, like the problem of discrimination. One of the reasons for discrimination in distribution is relative to material. This is classically described as material reason. The fundamental principle of distributive justice affirms equal share of burdens and benefits. Exceptions could be permitted if there are material reasons to discriminate. Among the material reasons is when the person deserves care or needs it. Regarding the concept "deserve", many believe that who does well deserves a prize and who commits a crime deserves punishment. Those who work hard are rewarded with promotion. There are some who believe that this mentality should be applied to decision-making processes in health care. The concept of "need" is considered differently from that of "deserve", in the sense that, the fact that a person "needs", serves as a material reason to discriminate. A person who needs could be one who is experiencing a situation of misfortune, physically or mentally disabled, a person or persons going through an unfavourable condition consequent to a past discrimination that was not in their favour and all those classified as vulnerable.

The questions to ask here are: Can there be modifications to application of the principles of justice? Is it possible to go beyond it without getting involved in actions that are not morally permissible? Some believe that 'need', 'charity' or 'compassion' can move one to go beyond the principle of justice by providing health care to a patient, even though justice does not

---

[486] Ibid.

permit it. Treatments can be given to patients with low level of probability for success in their particular health situations. For instance, treatments may be given free of charge in some cases where resources are surplus. Taking care of the need of the above-mentioned classes is the hallmark of a just society. For S. Capp, S. Savage and V. Clark, "distributive justice is an appropriate starting point for a consideration of what features could characterize a just health care system"[487].

The particular aspect of justice we are treating here is the distributive justice and its application to the distribution of health care resources. "Justice in health care, however, is more broadly concerned with equalising as far as possible the distribution of health care resources and opportunities for care and treatment"[488]. Justice to the individual precisely means "primarily non-discrimination on the basis of sex, religion, social standing, political affiliation, youth, old age, handicap or mental disorder, and equal opportunity in terms of access to resources, including preventative and treatment health services and benefits of research"[489]. The authors, T. L. Beauchamp and J. F. Childress note that many expect from valid principles of justice, to determine how social burdens, benefits, and positions ought to be allocated[490]. This refers in particular to the distributive justice. The just mentioned scholars rightly affirm that "issues concerning fairness of a distribution generate questions about principles of justice"[491]. In their view, "no single principle can address all the problems of justice"[492]. They affirm that "several principles of justice appear in the common morality and merit acceptance. One principle of justice is *formal*, the others *material*"[493].

— Formal Principle of Justice

"Common to all theories of justice is a minimal formal requirement traditionally attributed to Aristotle: Equals must be treated equally, and

---

[487] S. Capp – S. Savage –V. Clarke, «Exploring distributive justice in health care», *Australian Health Review*, 24 (2001), 40-44.

[488] I. E. Thompson, «Fundamental ethical principles in health care», *British Medical Journal (Clinical Research Ed.)*, 29(1987), 1461-1465.

[489] Ibid.

[490] T. L. Beauchamp – J. F. Childress, *Principles of Biomedical...*, 226.

[491] Ibid., 227.

[492] Ibid.

[493] Ibid.

134

unequals must be treated unequally"[494]. This principle of formal justice is described as being "formal" because it very plain in nature. It does not give detailed information regarding in what respects equals ought to be treated equally and it is silent on the criteria for determining "whether two or more individuals are in fact equals"[495]. T. L. Beauchamp and J. E. Childress maintain that the formal principle lacks substance because what it affirms does not stimulate any debate. This principle also described as principles of formal equality does not help us in terms determining how far should equality extend. The aforementioned ethical experts present a typical problem in this regard:

> Virtually all accounts of justice in health care hold that delivery programs and services designed to assist persons of a certain class, such as the poor or the elderly, should be made available to all members of that class. To deny benefits to some when others in the same class receive benefits is unjust. But is it also unjust to deny access to equally needy persons outside of the delineated class (e.g., workers with no health insurance)?"[496].

– Material Principles of Justice

The material principles of justice unlike the formal principle of justice "specify the relevant characteristics for equal treatment [...] identify the substantive properties for distribution"[497]. These principles are also called *material* because they are specific about the substantive features for distribution[498]. The principle of need is among the principles of material justice. According to the principle of need, a just distribution of social resources is done in accordance to needs. A situation of need arises when a person is without something, and this absence can lead to harm or seriously affect him or her. "We are not required to distribute all goods and services to satisfy all needs [...] our obligations are limited to *fundamental* needs"[499]. Fundamental needs are those needs whose absence can lead to serious

---

[494] Ibid.

[495] Ibid.

[496] Ibid.

[497] Ibid.

[498] Cfr. Ibid.

[499] Ibid., 228.

harm or damage of the person. The fact that not all needs can be satisfied is obvious, but the duty to satisfy the fundamental needs, like basic health needs and the need for health care is categorical. T. L. Beauchamp and J. F. Childress explain further explain:

> All public and institutional policies based on distributive justice ultimately derive from the acceptance (or rejection) of some material principles and some procedures for specifying, refining, or balancing them, and many disputes over the right policy or distribution spring from rival, or at least alternative, starting points with different material principles[500]

"Philosophers and others have proposed each of the following principles as a valid material principle of distributive justice"[501].

1. To each person an equal share
2. To each person according to need
3. To each person according to effort
4. To each person according to contribution
5. To each person according to merit
6. To each person according free-market exchanges[502]

According to the above-cited authors more than one of these principles can be accepted without difficulties. They affirm that some theories of justice accept all the six retaining them to be plausible. There is a valid moral position which affirms that "each of these material principles identifies a prima facie obligation whose weight cannot be assessed independently of particular context or spheres in which they are applicable"[503]. Some scholars accept the six principles because according to them, they can be combined to arrive at a just distribution of social resources. Others accept only a few of the six principles, because they believe that not all principles can lead to a fair distribution of resources. T. L. Beauchamp and J. F. Childress affirm that conflict among these principles can lead to a serious priority problem and will be an obstacle to the objective of any

---

[500] T. L. BEAUCHAMP – J. F. CHILDRESS, *Principles of Biomedical...*, 228.

[501] Ibid.

[502] Cfr. Ibid.

[503] Ibid.

moral system striving to establish a coherent framework of principles[504]. For example "if, by contrast, one were to accept only a principle of free-market distribution, then one would oppose a principle of need as a basis for public policy"[505]. This means that it is necessary to specify and balance the principles[506]. With this brief consideration of the concept of justice, we will proceed to treat the principles of distributive justice with some of the proposed theories and approaches of justice that are usually applied to the distribution of health care resources.

3.2. Some Proposed Principles, Theories and Approaches of Distributive Justice

One of the most important issues in health care is the problem of justice. The various ways of understanding justice give rise to different approaches to distribution of healthcare resources[507]. In this section, we are going to analyse some present principles, theories and approaches of distributive justice and later, as aforementioned, integrate their strong points to the Catholic principles we intend to apply to the Nigerian health system. There are notable similarities among the proposed models on how best to allocate health care resources. Nevertheless, they have notable divergences in their notions of health care allocation.

3.2.1. Procedural Justice

Procedural justice is essentially defined in terms of due process. Hence, procedural justice establishes rules that guarantee fair distribution of resources. Equality before the law is a form of procedural justice. This means receiving equal treatment as others. This theory of justice evokes the notion of fair procedures that represent the best means of reaching fair outcomes. This is because procedural justice helps to make and implement decisions following fair process. According to J. Summer:

---

[504] Cfr. Ibid., 229

[505] Ibid., 228.

[506] Cfr. Ibid. 229.

[507] C. LEGET – R. HOEDEMAEKERS, «Teaching medical students …».

> Procedural justice or due process means that when you get your turn, you receive the same treatment as everyone. One can apply this to the concept of health care. For example, if you are waiting to see your primary care physician, did others get to go ahead of you without any clear reason?[508]

Some authors believe that in procedural justice, it is more convincing when procedures are adopted in accordance with the principle of respect and dignity of the human person. Outcomes of such procedures are willingly accepted[509].

There are four pillars involved in the process of procedural justice: Consistency (fairness), Impartiality, Giving Voice and Transparency. Hence, procedural justice asks: "Were fair procedures in place, and were those procedures followed?"[510] To determine if a procedure is fair, some authors think that it must have the quality of consistency. This means that it must guarantee that like cases are treated similarly[511]. The process as well as those involved in the decision-making must be unbiased, hence impartial, with the intention of treating people fairly while taking into consideration the needs and viewpoints of interested parties[512].

In decision-making, those directly affected by the decisions should have the opportunity of expressing their views and they should be well represented. For a procedure to be fair, the processes that are implemented must be transparent. In a legal context of legal proceedings, procedural justice ensures fair trial and in the application of the law, it strives to guarantee impartiality, consistency and transparency. The four pillars of procedural justice expressed here include fairness, impartiality, giving voice and transparency. Some people believe that, procedural justice is not

---

[508] J. SUMMER, «Principles of Healthcare…».

[509] Cfr. M. DEUTSCH, «Justice and Conflict», in *The Handbook of Conflict Resolution: Theory and Practice,* M. DEUTSCH – P. T. COLEMAN (eds.), Jossey-Bass Inc. Publishers, San Francisco 2000, 45.

[510] J. SUMMER, «Principles of Healthcare…».

[511] Cfr. R. T. BUTTRAM – R. FOLGER – B. H. SHEPPARD, «Equity, Equality and Need: Three Faces of Social Justice», in *Conflict, Cooperation, and Justice: Essays Inspired by the Work of Morton Deutsch,* B. B. BUNKER – M. DEUTSCH (eds.), Jossey-Bass Inc. Publishers, San Francisco 1995, 272.

[512] Cfr. R. T. BUTTRAM – R. FOLGER – B. H. SHEPPARD, «Equity, Equality and…», 272.

enough, because they think that reaching fair outcomes is more important than implementing fair processes, others on the other hand believe that fair procedures are important since they could lead to fair outcomes[513].

As a principle of distributive justice, procedural justice implies fair procedures in setting rules to regulate the acquiring and transferring of goods. Being faithful to the right allocation rules according to many will certainly guarantee fairest distribution of health resources. The relationship between fair rules and mediation or negotiation processes is very important in reaching decisions that are acceptable to all parties. The critical dimensions of procedural justice show that there must be the clear perception that all parties have been heard; clear perception that people are treated with dignity and respect; the clear perception that the decision-making process is trustworthy; clarity on the process of decision-making; and a clear perception that the system players are concerned about the personal situation of the persons involved.

3.2.2. Libertarian Theories of Justice

Libertarianism is defined as "the view which, in opposition to determinism, asserts that it is possible for human agents to act freely, independently of necessitating causes"[514]. In the area of health care, the libertarian theory retains that any kind of health care service will be made available provided there is a demand from the self-paying or insured person. If the number of payers (those who have the ability to pay) is not sufficient, the service will not be provided even when it is the need of the community. Therefore, the need of the people is not relevant when there is no possibility of having sufficient payers for the services. This could be described as a clear commercialization of medicine or health care services. In this regard, it is always important to underline that health is a common good and not a commercial good. The commercialization of health is the dehumanization of medicine.

> The libertarian theory of justice is treasured by the free marketers
> who have great faith in the ability of the market to satisfy human
> wants. Any suggestion of an imposed equalisation process or

---

[513] Cfr. W. NELSON, «The Very Idea of Pure Procedural Justice», in *Ethics*, 90(1980), 502-511.

[514] T. MAUTNER (ed.), *The Penguin Dictionary ...*, 317.

> social intervention is anathema to libertarians as it represents
> a threat to individual liberty. An implicit characteristic of a
> health based on this theory of distribution is the need to have
> health insurance or an ability for services as required[515].

This is a theory that discriminates against the poor and the vulnerable. The uninsured have no hope of receiving health care where such principle is involved. The application of this policy in this manner makes health a commercial good controlled by a particular group of marketers. "Almost striking example of a health system based on libertarian value is found in the United States of America (U.S.A)"[516]. The libertarian principle practiced in the USA, favours the free market approach to the distributions of health care resources based on the material principle of ability to pay. The principle retains that a just society safeguards people's rights of property and liberty thereby putting them in the position to improve their circumstances and protect their rights to health. With this, health care is not considered as a service to be provided but acquired. "Libertarians generally support a health care system in which health care insurance is privately and voluntarily purchased [...] In this system, the state does not coercively take any one's personal property to benefit another [...] and society is not morally obligated to provide health care"[517]. Such a libertarian position raises moral questions concerning the hope of the poor and the vulnerable. It applies the rule and method that tend to abandon the disadvantaged to die in their indigent conditions.

According to the libertarian theory, only a person who demonstrates his or her ability to pay can be identified as being willing to receive health care services. "The theory's ideology assumes patients are the best judges of their own welfare with priorities that are self-determined and manifested through an ability pay"[518]. Hence, inability to pay means absence of treatment. The vulnerable who cannot afford to pay are not considered, therefore they are excluded and unjustly discriminated against. Further critique by S. Capp, S. Savage and V. Clark states that "the inability of this theory to accommodate the needs of the disadvantaged by a mandated redistribution of society's assets makes this a difficult concept to

---

[515] S. Capp – S. Savage –V. Clarke, «Exploring distributive justice...».

[516] Ibid.

[517] T. L. Beauchamp –J. F. Childress, *Principles of Biomedical...*, 232.

[518] S. Capp – S. Savage –V. Clarke, «Exploring distributive justice...».

embrace"[519]. Again, the authors affirm that such principle cannot lead to a fair allocation of health care resources. According to them, the "ability and needs of patients to access the health system are not necessarily congruent and the inevitable consequence is a distorted distribution of services"[520]. Services delivered following this theory cannot satisfy the requirements a just health care system because it favours only the groups of marketers and the rich and not all members of the society.

3.2.3. Utilitarian Theory of Justice

"Utilitarianism is an approach to morality that treats pleasure or desire-satisfaction as the sole element in human good and that regards the morality of actions as being entirely dependent on consequences or results for human (sentient) well-being"[521]. The issue of "purpose of life" has been at the centre of many philosophical and moral arguments for many years. Most philosophical theories agree that a just society is one that promotes the ultimate end of life. The proponents of utilitarianism believe that the ultimate human end consists in happiness, so a good society is one that maximizes the human happiness of its members. For utilitarianism, health is ethically good only if through it, man attains his desired happiness. "Among the various "goods" that contribute to the ultimate end, health is often accorded special ethical significance because it is necessary to achieving most intermediate and ultimate ends [...] and ill health represents a time of considerable vulnerability and dependency on others"[522].

For those who sustain utilitarianism, human well-being and happiness are the touchstones for all moral evaluations[523]. Contemporary utilitarianism has as the main object of its belief whatever satisfies people's desires or preferences or makes people happy[524]. However, the major ethical element in most contemporary utilitarianism is based on direct consequentialism. According to this approach (direct consequentialism), "the rightness and

---

[519] Ibid.

[520] Ibid.

[521] T. HONDERICH (ed.), *The Oxford Companion to Philosophy*, Oxford University Press Inc., New York 1995, 890.

[522] J. HURLEY, «Ethics, economics, and…».

[523] Cfr. T. HONDERICH (ed.), *The Oxford Companion…*, 890.

[524] Cfr. Ibid.

goodness of any action, motive, or political institution depends solely on the goodness of the overall state of affairs consequent upon it"[525]. With this, "most current direct (or act-) utilitarians want to say that an act is morally obligatory, if and only if, it produces a greater balance of pleasure over pain, or desire satisfaction, than any alternative action available to the agent"[526]. For act-utilitarianism therefore, an act can be defined morally right, or not wrong if and only if it produces a great balance of pleasure over pains as any alternative action at the disposition of the executor. From this utilitarian claim about rightness and obligation originates the various forms of the Principle of Utility[527]. A direct utilitarian view believes that an act moral evaluation is a form of instrumental evaluation because acts are right or obligatory not necessary because of their inherent character, their motives or their dependent on divine or social dictate, but rather, their being right or obligatory depends on how much overall human happiness or well-being they produce[528].

Not all utilitarian supporters agree with direct act consequentialism. The contrary group prefers 'rule-consequentialism' to 'act-consequentialism'. According to 'rule-consequentialism', "the rightness of an action depends on the consequences not of the action itself, but of various sets of rules"[529]. So while direct act-utilitarianism evaluates actions directly based on the consequences, rule-consequentialism evaluates them indirectly, that is, not based on their consequences but on a set of rules. For act-consequentialism, the 'end justifies the means'. If the end which is the attainment of the people's happiness and well-being is achieved, the action is right and obligatory. The moral evaluation solely depends on the end or result, the means has no significant relevance. So if most people are happy and healthy at the expense of the sad and sick few, the result, that is the happiness of the majority justifies the action.

Morally speaking, act-utilitarianism could be said to be discriminatory. It discriminates against the weak, the poor, the few in favour of the majority, the rich and the most powerful. Again, there is a widely accepted moral position, which affirms that a negative means cannot be justified

---

[525]   Ibid.

[526]   Ibid.

[527]   Cfr. Ibid.

[528]   Cfr. Ibid.

[529]   Ibid.

by a positive end. For example, if one steals in order to help the poor, the underlying motivation of one's action is morally acceptable but the means disqualifies the positive end. Therefore, the action of 'stealing' cannot be justified by one's good intention to help the poor. For clarity, it is generally believed that the end is not always that which comes at the end but, that which guides and motivates the action, thus, the end does not always justify the means.

Some critiques against the rule of utilitarianism claim that it does not give enough reasons why rules should be evaluated by their consequences but actions should not be. There is a conception that utilitarianism is "an impartial and impersonal view"[530]. The author, J. J. C. Smart distinguished between act-utilitarianism and rule-utilitarianism. According to him:

> Act-utilitarianism is the view that the rightness or wrongness of an action is to be judged by the consequences, good or bad, of the action itself. Rule-utilitarianism is the view that the rightness or wrongness of an action is to be judged by the goodness and badness on the consequences of a rule that everyone should perform the action in like circumstances[531].

In his objection to rule-utilitarianism, J. J. C. Smart argues that if rule-utilitarianism claims to advocate for human happiness, why then should it request abiding by a rule that obviously in a particular circumstance will not be most beneficial abiding by it. He therefore concludes that "to refuse to break a generally beneficial rule in those cases in which it is not beneficial to obey it seems irrational and to be a case of rule worship"[532]. Act-utilitarian doctrine teaches that if action "A" makes people happier than action "B", there is every reason to encourage the fulfilment of action "A" because it creates occasion for more benefits than "B". Thus, "A" in this case is preferred to "B". Despite what seems to be a positive impact of act-utilitarianism, "some good-hearted readers may reject the utilitarian position because of certain considerations relating to justice"[533].

---

[530]   T. Honderich (ed.), *The Oxford Companion ...*, 892.

[531]   J. J. C. Smart – B. Williams, *Utilitarianism for & Against*, Cambridge University Press, New York 1973, 9.

[532]   Ibid., 10.

[533]   Ibid., 31.

The negative utilitarianism upholds that it is necessary to minimize misery and pains. This according negative utilitarian approach is the "sole ultimate ethical principle"[534]. This position is in line with the proposal by Karl Popper that our concern should be that of maximizing happiness which comports minimizing suffering"[535]. The idea of minimizing suffering may convince many who agree that it is right to remove misery from their lives. In fact "people will be less ready to agree on what good they would like to see promoted than they will be to agree on what miseries should be avoided"[536].

The utilitarian theory of justice follows the trend of maximising public utility to attain the greatest benefit for society. With this mode of proceeding according to some authors, there will always be potential losers because "marginal groups who have little to offer to society but have a high propensity to consume health resources would be difficult groups to justify supporting"[537]. J. Hurley thinks that health care is ethically valuable since it contributes to health. For this reason, "it follows directly that the ethically justified distribution of access to and utilisation of needed health care is the one which generates the desired level and distribution of health"[538].

Health care resource allocation conducted in accordance to utilitarian theory therefore does not reflect an ethically justified distribution of access since it cuts off those who have little to offer to society. An ethically justified distribution is one that carries along each and every member of the society, providing their basic health care needs where it is possible. A critique describes the worst aspect of "utilitarianism result when professional judgements determine the social worth and liberty of the individual"[539]. According to the same critique, "the utilitarian view would support allocating funds to where the greater number receive care and not necessarily to the most deserving"[540]. Health care according to the utilitarian perspective should concentrate more on balancing such factors as public and private benefits, predicted cost saving, risk involved and necessary trade-offs.

---

[534] Ibid. 29.

[535] Ibid., 28.

[536] Ibid., 30.

[537] S. CAPP – S. SAVAGE –V. CLARKE, «Exploring distributive justice…».

[538] J. HURLEY, «Ethics, economics, and…».

[539] S. CAPP – S. SAVAGE –V. CLARKE, «Exploring distributive justice…».

[540] Ibid.

In contrast to the utilitarian view, G. P. Smith thinks that the major factor during the treatment of the patient should be his or her health condition. He adds that the course of treatment should always be guided "by the goal of humane, loving care which reduces human suffering, enhances the common good, as well as safeguards the dignity of the human spirit"[541]. In the same vein, R. Gillon highlights the typical features of a health care perspective that satisfies the standards of medical ethics: "Ethics and morals govern that everybody should have an equal opportunity to benefit from a public healthcare system. The chance of them benefiting, the quality of the benefit or the length of lifetime left to enjoy the benefit should not affect the allocation of resources"[542]. In line with the series of critiques, telling the hard truth on the utilitarian principles some renowned authors write: "Principles of utilitarian justice thus present serious problems [...] when carefully restricted in scope, they do have a legitimate role in forming health policies"[543].

3.2.4. Egalitarian Theories of Justice

Egalitarianism as defined by the *Penguin Dictionary of Philosophy* is "an outlook that opposes privilege and favours equality between individuals"[544]. In its application to health care, "egalitarian principles require that health care be distributed so as to reduce "inequality" (for example in terms of lifetime health)"[545]. To have distribution of health resources done in such a way that it reduces inequalities in health, the egalitarian theory confirms "fair innings" as a form of equalising principle. Fair innings indicates similar long and healthy life for everyone. This is considered as a strict principle of equalising lifetime health. Another equalising principle affirms "equalising people's opportunity for lifetime health, rather than achieved levels of health, to account for individuals' freedom of choice and autonomy in making choices that influenced health"[546].

---

[541] G. P. Smith, «Distributive Justice and...».

[542] R. Gillon, «Medical ethics: four principles plus attention to scope», *British Medical Journal*, 309(1994), 184 -188.

[543] T. L. Beauchamp – J. F. Childress, *Principles of Biomedical ...*, 231.

[544] T. Mautner (ed.), The Penguin Dictionary ..., 160.

[545] R. Cookson – P. Dolan, «Principles of justice in health care rationing», *Journal of Medical Ethics*, 26(2000), 323-329.

[546] R. Cookson – P. Dolan, «Principles of justice...».

The egalitarian theory of distributive justice affirms equal distribution of both social benefits and burdens. According to S. Capp, S. Savage and V. Clarke, there are two principles which give persuasive description of egalitarianism because of the emphasis on the concepts of equality, fairness and opportunity. Explaining the two principles, the authors affirm that the first principle states that "each person is to have an equal right to the most extensive total system of equal basic liberties compatible with a similar system of liberty"[547], while the second principle states that "social and economic inequalities are to be arranged so that they are both (a) to the greatest benefit of the least advantaged [...] (b) open to all under conditions of fair equality of opportunity"[548]. Justice literally means equality and fairness. Equitable distribution of health care resources means justice in health care. In the health care industry, it is believed that all individuals have equal rights to seek health care and to participate in the plan of care that concerns them.

The egalitarian theory sustains the non-discriminatory ideals of a just community. It considers the ability of the community to access a range of services and permits all individuals to have access to a decent minimum range of services. The theory advocates for a fair opportunity to access health care service. "However its application in the area of resource allocation is more problematic. The objectives of seeking a fair opportunity to access health care implies an ability of the system to provide such a service and this will not always be possible"[549]. For this, it is recommended that allocation policies be made explicit and the difficult allocation decisions which are inevitable be faced honestly. This has to be done always with the intention of improving the situation of the poorest, that is, the neediest and most vulnerable, in society. "Equality underpins distributive justice. An individual's right to healthcare resources should not be affected by who they are, including their age, sex, quality of life, socioeconomic status and race. The rich and poor should be treated as equals in terms of healthcare provisions"[550].

---

[547] S. CAPP – S. SAVAGE –V. CLARKE, «Exploring distributive justice...».

[548] Ibid.

[549] Ibid.

[550] J. HARRIS, «The rationing debate: Maximising the health of the whole community. The case against: what the principle objective of NHS should be», *British Medical Journal*, 314(1997), 669-672, in https://doi.org/10.1136/bmj.314.7081.669 [23-7-2017].

The position of J. Harris aptly represents the true sense of justice in health care. Justice in health care implies respecting one's right to health and ensuring one's access to basic health care irrespective of one's social or economic background. A person who cannot by himself afford the basic health care he/she needs because of his/her age, health conditions, economic or social status and location of his/her residence should neither be ignored nor abandoned. "In an ideal world, sufficient health care would be provided to all who need it. However, this is not always possible and healthcare resources should then be distributed in relation to their need within a society that has equal access to healthcare"[551]. It is right to distribute according to needs of the society and it is wrong to withhold or withdraw health based solely on economic decisions. Every human person should be treated with equality and respect. This implies not quantifying a person's life monetarily. Money is important in health care, but health care is not all about money.

R. M. Veatch prefers an egalitarian view to the utilitarian approach in health care. Veatch believes that in the egalitarian view, there is the basic premise that everyone is entitled to an equal claim in health care. He upholds the principle that affirms as a requisite of justice that every human being should receive the resources needed to be healthy[552]. In a similar argument on the right to health care, D. Mechanic retains that right to health care implies a duty on the government to assure each person quality health services. It also means according to him, that in the case of rationing, the process is imposed because it is inevitable to do so. The rules for rationing should be applied fairly with seriousness and without discrimination. This for him does not mean that everyone has the exact right to the same services, just as public education does not mean giving in every instance identical opportunity to children who differ in their capacities and needs"[553]. D. Mechanic therefore accepts that discrimination has to be based on justified reasons.

The egalitarian principle strives to address the problem of inequality between the urban and rural areas and to reduce the gap between the rich and the poor with regard to distribution and access to health care goods and services. The vulnerable with the egalitarian principle have hope of

---

[551]   R. GILLON, «Medical ethics: four…».

[552]   Cfr. R. L. SHELTON, «Human rights and…».

[553]   Ibid.

being considered because the principle does not welcome discrimination against them in the distribution of the health resources. The egalitarian principle largely assures the vulnerable of their right to health and access to and utilization of health care, where the resources and services are possible.

3.2.5. Rawls' Theory of Justice

John Rawls (1921-2002) was an American political philosopher in the liberal tradition. His work of political philosophy and ethics, *A Theory of Justice* is considered by many as an important approach to distributive justice. Defining the main idea of his theory of justice, Rawls states:

> The guiding idea is that the principles of justice for the basic structure of society are the object of the original argument. They are the principles that free and rational persons concerned to further their own interest would accept in an initial position of equality as defining the fundamental terms of their association. These principles are to regulate all further agreements; they specify the kinds of social cooperation that can be entered into and the forms of government that can be established. This way of regarding the principles of justice, I shall call "justice as fairness"[554].

In his theory of justice, the philosopher John Rawls elaborates his idea of justice as fairness. Rawls' theory of "justice as fairness" was meant to be "a substantial alternative to utilitarianism"[555]. According to Rawls, "in justice as fairness the original position of equality corresponds to the state of nature in the traditional theory of the social contract"[556]. He proposes the idea of choosing fundamental principles, which are in favor of everyone and do not offer advantages to any particular social group. To arrive at this choice, J. Rawls thinks of a veil of ignorance:

> The principles of justice are chosen behind a veil ignorance. This ensures that no one is advantaged or disadvantaged in the choice of principles by the outcome of natural chance or

---

[554] J. RAWLS, *A Theory of Justice* (Revised edition), The Belknap Press of Harvard University Press Cambridge, Massachusetts 1999, 10.

[555] T. MAUTNER (ed.), The Penguin Dictionary ..., 471.

[556] J. RAWLS, *A Theory of Justice* ..., 11.

the contingency of social circumstance. Since all are similarly situated and no one is able to design principles to favor his particular condition, the principles of justice are the result of a fair agreement or bargain[557].

Rawls' veil of ignorance entails a situation where no one knows their place in the society, the class to which they belong or their social status and no one knows their fortune in the distribution of natural assets, abilities, strength, etc. This according to him could be a solution to the problem of political injustice, because the veil of ignorance would permit individuals to select principles based solely on the basic general considerations. Explaining further, the author writes: "The original position is, one might say, the appropriate initial status quo, and thus the fundamental agreement reached in it are fair"[558]. The appropriate initial status quo Rawls believes would guarantee a fair agreement that will favor every citizen and not only special groups[559]. In addition, this for him "explains the propriety of the name "justice as fairness"[560]. Justice as fairness "conveys the idea that the principles of justice are agreed to in an initial situation that is fair"[561].

Rawls thinks that the original position will make egoism impossible, as a group that has the responsibility of making the choice of principles will not be able to decide in their own favor to the disadvantage of others, since they do not know their place in society, their class or social status, etc. Since no one knows the group to which he or she belongs, it will be difficult to choose principles, supporting for example the older generation or principles that will benefit the younger generation. For Rawls therefore, ignorance leads to the kind of justice, which he names "justice as fairness". According to Rawls' theory, the two principles individuals in the original position can choose are those of equality, then social and economic inequalities. The former implies the assignment of basic rights and duties, while the latter retains that inequalities of wealth and authority could be permitted only if they ensure benefits for everyone especially for the least advantaged

---

[557] Ibid.

[558] Ibid.

[559] Cfr. M. Gronebaum, *John Rawls' Theory of Justice: Justice as fairness*, Grin, Norderstedt Germany 2013, I-II.

[560] J. Rawls, *A Theory of Justice*, 11.

[561] Ibid.

citizens[562]. This view of accepting inequality only based on preferential option for the less privileged is in line with the ethical principles, which our thesis upholds. Discrimination could be permitted if and only if it is done for the benefit of the vulnerable and or those with emergencies.

Rawls is of the view that the principles permissible by interested parties should be the basis for the appropriate division of advantages. The parties that are involved must be all equal. The above mentioned two principles that determine the choice of individuals in the original position, according to Rawls, are "the heart of justice" that must be chosen by the equal parties in the original position to constitute 'justice as fairness'[563]. Rawls' theory of justice upholds that, with the initial position each is convinced that everyone is equally rational and similarly situated because no one is aware of his or her position. Consequently, the same basic rights for all is for the advantage of everyone and is accessible to all citizens. With this, Rawls concludes that, injustice arises from inequity that does not benefit every citizen.

Some authors perceive Rawls' idea of Justice as fairness as a project that looks out for everyone. It ensures that no one is left behind, especially the less privileged members of society. Justice as fairness implies helping the least advantaged without suppressing their liberty. Since justice as fairness requests benefit for everyone, it implies that any decision made in justice and in fairness must have first, considered all possible consequences that may arise for each person from such decisions. The two principles of justice as fairness some authors agree promote respect for one another and enhance the effectiveness of social cooperation[564].

The Utilitarian concept of justice is in broad contrasts with the theory of Rawls. While J. Rawls preaches that everyone should be carried along, the utilitarianism view advocates for the marginalization of some for the happiness of others. For utilitarianism, what makes most happy should be promoted even when it makes the minority sad or puts them in an unjust condition like slavery[565]. "Utilitarianism tries to maximize advantages for the most but not for all"[566]. In contrast to this, J. Rawls aptly remarks that

---

[562]   Cfr. M. GRONEBAUM, *John Rawls' Theory...*, III.

[563]   Ibid.

[564]   Cfr. Ibid., IV.

[565]   Cfr. Ibid., V.

[566]   Ibid.

"each person possesses an inviolability founded on justice that even the welfare of society cannot override"[567]. This inviolability "does not allow that the sacrifices imposed on a few are outweighed by the larger sum of advantages enjoyed by many"[568].

The article by R. L. Shelton mentions the observations of R. Green on John Rawls' theory according to which the object of inquiry of Rawls' theory of justice is not health care but social justice. The observation further remarks that certain implications of Rawls' theory of justice could be applied in health care especially the following three points:

1. Parties in the contract theory perspective would opt for a principle of equal access to health care to the most extensive health services society allows.
2. The theory seems to rule out direct income-based distributions of health care.
3. Basic preventive and therapeutic services have priority over expensive, high quality care and costly, esoteric research. Basic services should be rapidly brought within reach of every member of the society[569].

3.3. Critical Appraisal of the above treated Principles, Theories and Approaches of Justice

3.3.1. A General Assessment

The study of principle, theories and approaches of justice in this chapter shows how if strictly applied, some of them can help to improve the allocation of health care resources and the performance of the health care systems of many countries. No country can boast of a perfect health care system, but some principle, theories and approaches of justice can help health care systems to provide satisfactory answers to people, by redressing the salient issues in health care such as, right to health and access to care, dignity of the vulnerable, equalities and inequalities, cost, quality, affordability, availability, universality, etc. Part of the proposed

---

[567] J. RAWLS, *A Theory of Justice*..., 3.
[568] Ibid.
[569] Cfr. R. L. SHELTON, «Human rights and...».

theories and approaches meet with the standard for fair distribution of health resources, others do not. All the treated theories and approaches have their strong points and their limits.

The four pillars involved in the process of procedural justice guarantee the respect for the interest of all especially the weak members of the society. Thus, the principle of procedural justice ensures fairness because it provides clear regulations that help to avoid theft and arbitrariness in decision-making and in health care allocation. However, the principle is abstract and does not really address concrete health care problems. The libertarian theory does a good job of considering the health care resources available and strives to ensure their distribution. Nevertheless, its application manifests some shortcomings because it considers health as a commercial good and not a common good. In the application of this theory, the poor and vulnerable are not properly considered and they are unjustly discriminated against, because their inability to pay means absence of treatment for them. This way of considering health, as a commercial good is not ethically acceptable because health is a human and common good. The *commercialization* of health and health care can only lead to its *dehumanization*. The utilitarian theory approves maximizing utility by denying access to health care for some of the sickest and most vulnerable members of society. For utilitarianism, what makes most people happy should be promoted even when it makes the others in the minority sad or puts them in an unjust condition like slavery[570]. "Utilitarianism tries to maximize advantages for most but not for all"[571]. This theory is unjustly discriminatory especially against the poorest and the most vulnerable.

Distinctively, the egalitarian theory stands for the non-discriminatory ideals of a just distribution of health resources. It advocates for a fair opportunity in access and utilization of health care resources. For the egalitarians, individuals particularly the weakest and the poorest should have access to a decent minimum range of health care services. Egalitarian principles demand that law, polices, practices and the actions of the state and individuals be guided by impartial standards. Thus the principle advocates that all citizens should be treated impartially. Most of the views typical to the egalitarian theory are found in Rawls' theory of justice as fairness.

---

[570] Cfr. M. GRONEBAUM, *John Rawls' Theory…*, V.

[571] Ibid.

Rawls does not explicitly deal with health care questions; hence, we cannot appeal directly to his theory for solutions. We can only apply his theory using it to interpret certain concrete situations of health care resource allocations. Rawls stands for equality and non-discrimination. Unlike the utilitarian views, Rawls theory opines that everyone should be carried along in the distribution of health resources. Hence, J. Rawls aptly remarks each person possesses an inviolability which is founded on justice and such inviolability cannot be overridden by the comfort of society[572]. This inviolability does not permit sacrificing the interest of a few in favour a larger number of persons.[573]. Discrimination for Rawls can only be permitted if it is done in favour of the vulnerable. Rawls' idea of Justice as fairness is a project that looks for everyone. Rawls' idea of "original position" is very interesting and can largely bring about justice and fairness in the allocation of resources. Nevertheless, it is also limited in some aspects. The creation or actualization of the "original position" will be difficult in an existing state. For example, how will it be possible to guarantee equality of income for different standards of work? This makes some authors to think that "Rawls' theory of justice as fairness is very abstract"[574]. Another question concerns how the members of the parties will be elected and who will elect them?[575] For these and many other reasons, M. Groenebaum thinks, "one has to admit that, no matter how well Rawls' concept is grounded, it only is a hypothetical one, the actual realization would require further consideration and would probably be rather challenging"[576]. Rawls also admits that what he proposes is a "hypothetical situation of equal liberty". Yet, one of the major limits of Rawls' theory of justice is that his original state is hypothetical and cannot be easily realized concretely.

Further problems are identified in the fact that the idea of justice as fairness raises issues concerning which principles of justice would be chosen in the original position[577]. Regarding the principle of utility, Rawls argues that "In the absence of strong and lasting benevolent impulses, a rational

---

[572] Cfr. J. RAWLS, *A Theory of Justice…*, 3.

[573] Cfr. Ibid.

[574] M. GRONEBAUM, *John Rawls' Theory…*, V.

[575] Cfr. Ibid.

[576] Ibid.

[577] Cfr. J. RAWLS, *A Theory of Justice…*, 12-13.

man would not accept a basic structure merely because it maximized the algebraic sum of advantages irrespective of its permanent effects on his own basic rights and interest"[578]. With this argument, the philosopher affirms the incompatibility of the principle of utility "with the conception of social cooperation among equals for mutual advantage"[579]. The author identifies the problem of choice of principle as a very difficult one.

No one of these principles, theories and approaches seems to provide a very satisfactory criterion for a just health care system and shows the capability of resolving the problems arising from the distribution of health care resources. However, some of them possess some characteristics that can be applied together with the Catholic principles to guarantee ethical health care system in Nigeria. We continue our evaluation of the principles, theories and approaches using the health capability approach.

3.3.2. Consideration in the Light of Health Capability Approach

The scholar J. P. Ruger proposes *Health Capability* approach for the distribution of health care resources. Explaining his motivations for the model, he writes:

> Approaches provide different justifications that underlie health care and public health. Some models assert consumer rationality in health behaviours and willingness to forgo care beyond the individual's means. Other approaches focus on fair process, equality of opportunity, utilitarianism, or equal distribution of goods. Libertarians emphasize autonomy. However, none of these approaches captures a fundamental reality in the health ethics realm: people seek both good health *and* the ability to pursue it. Existing models cannot effectively address these twin goals because they typically favor either a consequentialist (outcome-oriented) or a proceduralist (procedure-oriented) perspective. The approach I develop captures both these intuitions in a concept I call health capability[580].

---

[578]   Ibid. 13.

[579]   Ibid.

[580]   J. P. RUGER, «Health Capability: Conceptualization and Operationalization», *American Journal of Public of Health*, 100(2010), 41-49.

In a further distinction between his Health Capability approach and other theories and approaches, J. P. Ruger remarks:

> Unlike other approaches, the health capability paradigm purports that the fundamental societal obligation is to ensure conditions for all to be able to be healthy, not to ensure equal welfare, or happiness, or employment opportunities. An unlike libertarianism, it does not support individuals opting out of social guarantees[581].

The foregoing reveals that the two global desires of good health and ability to pursue it have remained unfulfilled by the already proposed theories and approaches of the distributive justice. The just mentioned author claims that his approach is one that understands these two goals and the means to their attainment. Describing his model J. P. Ruger writes: "Health capability includes, but is broader than, health functioning and health itself; it is the ability to be healthy. A working model of health capability involves a number of different theoretical constructs at the individual and social level"[582]. Additionally, the author explains that individual health capability is dependent on how one's external environment enhances or detracts from an individual. The individual health capabilities are socially dependent but "the health capability paradigm rests on the notion that the individual is the unit of analysis for evaluating health policy and institutions"[583]. J. P. Ruger makes clear that health capability incorporates health outcomes and health agency. The concept: 'health agency' according to him refers to the ability of individuals to realize health goals they value and act as agents of their own health. Health functioning for him "is the outcome of the action to maintain or improve health. It is comprehensive, inclusive of mental and physical health functioning and more"[584]. Furthermore, he asserts that conceptually health capability is a means to understand "conditions that facilitate and barriers that impede health and ability to make health choices. It offers a more accurate evaluation of the aim and success of social policies and change"[585]. The model of health capability J.

---

[581]   Ibid.

[582]   Ibid.

[583]   Ibid.

[584]   Ibid.

[585]   Ibid.

P. Ruger reveals, strives to strike a balance between what the individual desires and what is offered to him; between paternalism and autonomy by respecting the consequences individuals encounter and their health agency[586]. This discloses that:

> Health capability allows the assessment of a wider range of injustices, beyond distribution of resources or liberties, to include attributes and conditions affecting individuals' freedom: self management, decision-making ability, skills, knowledge and competence, and social norms and relations, as well as structures within which resources distribution takes place[587].

This model of health capability strives to strike a balance between what the individual desires and what is offered to him; between paternalism and autonomy, thus defending the individual's right to health. For this reason, the aforementioned author thinks it is important "to conceptualize, operationalize and gather information on health capability from individuals rather than institutions"[588]. This explains why the notion that underlines the necessity to understand and measure the impact of the irreducibly social goods on the individual. The said understanding and measuring, that is the evaluation, has to be based on each individual circumstances, rather than evaluating the goodness or badness from the societal perspective. With this idea, J. P. Ruger unravels that in considering the irreducibly social goods – the good provided for entire groups of people rather than for individuals – the individual must be the criteria for the evaluation of the positive or negative impact of irreducibly social goods. Accordingly, he states: "The very existence of irreducibly social goods must therefore be evaluated and justified by their impact on individual health capability"[589]. This very argument is relevant to the evaluation of "the extent to which external characteristics such as social goods and structures enhance or impede one's health functioning and health agency"[590].

The above argument highlights that the government or society's duty is not and should not be limited to the provision of health care, but rather,

---

[586] Ibid.

[587] Ibid.

[588] Ibid.

[589] Ibid.

[590] Ibid.

extended to other social good. This is because the impact – good or bad – of the social good can help to ameliorate or worsen the health situation of the individual members of the society. Hence, it is clear that in various cases the individual health capability is consequent upon his or her external environment. Describing the health capability elements that are internal and external to the individual, the above-cited author writes:

> Internal factors include health status and health functioning; the ability to acquire accurate health-related knowledge and obtain health-related resources and to use both to prevent the onset and exacerbation of morbidity; the ability to link knowledge of potential health benefits and harms of behaviours and interventions to health outcomes; health-seeking skills, beliefs, and self-efficacy; values of health and health goals; self governance and self management to achieve health outcomes; the ability to make balanced decisions; motivation to achieve desirable health outcomes; and positive expectations about achieving outcomes. At the societal level, one's health capability includes external contextual influences: social norms; social network and social capital related to health outcomes; decisional power or latitude in familial and social contexts; group influences; material and social circumstances; economic, political, and social security; access to and utilization of health-related goods and services; the extent to which the public health and health care systems create an environment in which individuals can improve their health[591].

The above remark provides a list of the internal factors of health capability – strictly relevant to the individual's health – and the external factors – related to the societal level – demonstrating the link between the individual health capability and the social influences to highlight as aforementioned, how the former depends majorly on the latter. What is done at the societal level in the distribution of health care resources has inevitable consequences on the health situations of individual members of the society. Thus, the person has to be considered while decisions are being made on how to distribute the available goods in every society. The good of all is very important and it could only be achieved when the good of each is taken into consideration. This explains why "health capability

---

[591] Ibid.

is incarnate and measured at individual level"[592]. The Health Capability approach as J. P. Ruger remarks gears towards helping the individuals to be personally responsible for their health through health agency, that is, through the "individuals' ability to achieve health goals they value and act as agents of their own health"[593]. This is opposed to justifying health, health care, or public health equality of opportunity. For this author, the approach "holds that health functioning and health agency are ultimate ends of justice, not equality of opportunity"[594].

The internal perspective of health capability accentuates "self-management, self-governance, and confidence in one's ability to achieve health goals. Furthermore, it entails the ability to take responsibility for acquiring the information, knowledge, and skills necessary for good health"[595]. This remark is important because it evidences that right to health is accompanied by the fact that every individual (who is capable) has the duty of stewardship of his or her life and health. This entails the endeavour to be informed and to avoid every behaviour that puts one's health at risk, maintaining and improving one's health. Recognizing the capacity and the responsibility of the individual towards himself or herself health in terms of health care means respecting his dignity and his opportunity to participate in the distribution of health care resources.

This position however should not be understood as the absolutizing of the individual well-being, which compromises the communal well-being. It is also important to note that discarding the equality of opportunity approach is not advisable because a sane cooperation with it can help the health capability approach to achieve its goal of individual well-being. Therefore, making the individual experience the sole criterion and measure for the evaluation of outcome of the health care services as proposed by the conceptual model of health capacity is important and praise worthy position. However, thinking that everything should be based on the ability of the individual, making him the sole 'master' of his life and health, we think will not favour the individual. The equal opportunity to access and utilization of health care resources that is sustained by the egalitarian theory is a valid move to ensure the elimination of various inequalities

---

[592] Ibid.

[593] Ibid.

[594] Ibid.

[595] Ibid.

in health and to protect the weak, disadvantaged, poor and vulnerable. The health capability approach may risk not considering these classes of individuals by rejecting the equal opportunity to access and utilization of health care.

From the considerations made so far, we understand that while capacity has to do with the ability to produce, receive or contain, capability refers to "aptitude, a condition "capable of being converted or turned to use"[596]. Health capability is not limited to the individual skills, but includes also "a set of situations or conditions that enable optimal health"[597]. With this distinction, it is important to note that those who are not capable of being responsible for their health, because of their vulnerable conditions, should not be left to their own devices. In the same vein, individuals without the ability to pay should not be denied of the opportunity to enjoy health care, because health is a human and common good.

3.4. Ethical Evaluations of the Right to Health, Equity in Health and Need Principles (A Material Reason for Discrimination)

The principles, theories and approaches of justice treated above legitimate the claim that right to health is crucial to the justice. Whether individuals have right to health and how the society responds to this right is an important issue for our dissertation. The allocation of health care resources represents the most prominent way in which society confronts the issue of right to health and the maintenance of the health of the people. Thus health care allocation is essential for respecting peoples' right to health and ensuring their access to and utilization of health care. "Healthcare allocation is a controversial topic. It is not easy to apply principles of justice to the question of how to share out resources when there are not enough to satisfy every possible request. Nevertheless, decisions need to be made and it is imperative that we make decisions justly"[598].

The issue of distribution of resources is very controversial especially when it comes to trying to make a balance between needs that are on the higher side and insufficient available resources. In such situation, how

---

[596] Ibid.

[597] Ibid.

[598] P. GATELY – A. BECK – D. A. JONES, *Healthcare Allocation & Justice, Applying Catholic Social Teaching*, Incorporated Catholic Truth Society, London 2011, 5.

do we maintain equity? It is obviously a delicate task. Nevertheless, we cannot refrain from the noble responsibility of making just decisions on the distribution of health resources. In fact, some above-cited authors consider it "imperative" to make just decisions applying substantive ethical principles to the difficult problems in this regard, like the difficult decisions on "who gets what", in a situation where it is impossible for everyone to have everything. This makes particular reference to the issue of right to health, equity in health and the material reason for discrimination in the distribution of health care resources, that is, the need principles.

3.4.1. Right to Health and Access to Care

Among the entitlements essential to human fulfilment, the right to enjoy the highest attainable standard of physical and mental health is widely acclaimed to be the most fundamental. The right to health is fundamental because without good health, it will be difficult to exercise other civil and political rights. Good health is necessary for individuals and communities to reach their fulfilment. This underlies the claim that health is a necessary condition for well-functioning societies and human well-being.

The notion of the right to health in the sphere of the international law was first used in the 1948 Universal Declaration of Human Rights proclaimed unanimously by the UN General Assembly as a common standard for all humanity[599].

> The right to health is one of a set of internationally agreed human rights standards, and is inseparable or 'indivisible' from these other rights. This means achieving the right to health is both central to, and dependent upon, the realization of other human rights, to food, housing, work, education, information and participation[600].

It is generally accepted that 'Health' is a fundamental human right. Right to health is among the norms that are internationally recognized and

---

[599] Cfr. UNIVERSAL DECLARATION OF HUMAN RIGHTS, *United Nations General Assembly Resolution 217 A (III)*, United Nations, New York, NY 1948.

[600] UNITED NATIONS HUMAN RIGHTS, *Office of the High Commissioner: Special Rapporteur on the right to health* in http://www.who.int/mediacentre/factssheets/fs323/en/ [02-01-2018].

should be applied equally to all people everywhere in the world. Everyone is invested with this right but it is not always possible to exercise it because of the difficulty in receiving all that one needs in health care. In some cases, most people could have received what 'belongs' to them in terms of health care, but do not get it because of the lack of will of those in charge of disbursing the resources.

One of the major problems here is that "the debate about the right to health care has been characterized more by political rhetoric than careful analysis"[601]. The just cited authors note that the primary question regarding right to health and access to care relates to "whether the government should be involved in health care allocation and distribution, rather than leaving these matters to the market place"[602]. The question raised here is vital to the concept we are evaluating because in most countries people's right to health is violated and their access to care denied because of lack of clarity about where the government should intervene and what should be provided by the government and what should be acquired from the market. This is obvious in the fact that in most societies, the rule of ability to pay is allowed to determine the distribution of health care services. Where this rule serves as the only principle of distributive justice, the distribution of health resources cannot satisfy the ethical standards of a just society.

T. L. Beauchamp and J. F. Childress explain that "a right to health care can be general or specific"[603]. According to them, a specific moral and legal rights to health care contrast sharply with a general right[604]. Explaining this, they cite an example on how it is generally accepted as a moral obligation based on fairness to provide health care to military veterans. Similarly, it is supported that health care be provided and compensation be given to persons who sustain injuries during research undertaken on behalf of society[605]. In support of the general moral right to health care are two arguments: (1) an argument from collective social protection and (2) an argument from fair-opportunity"[606]. Right to health as entitlement "includes the right to a system of health protection that

---

[601] T. L. BEAUCHAMP – J. F. CHILDRESS, *Principles of Biomedical...*, 241.

[602] Ibid.

[603] Ibid. 242.

[604] Cfr. Ibid.

[605] Ibid.

[606] Ibid.

gives everyone an equal opportunity to enjoy the highest attainable level of health"[607]. An example of right to health as entitlement is the access to care especially basic care of every citizen. Prominent among the problems about the right to health care is how to specify entitlements and limits of the rights. Regarding this T. L. Beauchamp and J. F. Childress present two views that are widely accepted: "a right of *equal access* to health care and a right to a *decent minimum* of health care"[608]. These views are proposed by the egalitarians.

Among the various meanings of access to care is that "one is not legitimately prevented from obtaining health care"[609]. This interpretation of access to care implies that having a right of access does not mean the obligation on the part of others to provide or equitably distribute health care. Thus, to have access depends on one's free choice and one's ability to pay.

> More commonly, however, a right of access to health care refers to a right to obtain specified goods and services to which every entitled person has an equal claim. Here values of equality and solidarity are prominent. An inclusive understanding of this right requires that everyone has equal access to every treatment that is available to anyone[610].

The system based on freedom of choice and ability to pay is preferred by the libertarians, while the system that sustains giving to everyone equal access to the available treatments is of the egalitarian principles and it is expressed in Rawls' theory of justice as fairness. The exponents of right to decent minimum of health care sustain the provision of primary health for all. For them, basic health care should be universal and accessible.

> The decent-minimum approach entails acceptance of a two-tiered system of health care: enforced social coverage for basic and catastrophic health needs (tier 1), together with voluntary private coverage for other health needs and desires (tier 2). The first tier distributes health care based on need, and meets needs by universal access to basic services. This tier would presumably

---

[607] UNITED NATIONS HUMAN RIGHTS, *Office of the…*

[608] T. L. BEAUCHAMP – J. F. CHILDRESS, *Principles of Biomedical…*, 244.

[609] Ibid.

[610] Ibid.

cover at least public health protections and preventive care, primary care, and acute care, as well as special social services for those with disabilities[611].

Right to health and access to care implies giving everyone the opportunity to enjoy at least the primary health care service. Guaranteeing the basic health care services for the population is a hallmark of a just health care system. Health is a common good, and ensuring that each person enjoys the common good is the reason for the existence of the state. A certain view understands rights in relation to the common good and to human flourishing. Hence, it is affirmed that there is a right to healthcare, and like all human rights, the right to health care is rooted in the dignity of the human person. It includes a right of access to a substantial level of healthcare in the context of the resources of the society. In line with the foregoing, C. Petrini opines that "humans have a right to the resources necessary for health"[612]. This view captures accurately the connection between right to health, access to care and the principle of the common good and it demonstrates why it is important to consider this connection in the distribution of health care resources. Right to health is respected when the dignity of the human person is at the centre of the decision, polices, programmes and practices relevant to the distribution of health care and other resources.

3.4.2. Right to Health as a Primary or Basic Right (Does Everyone Has a Right to Healthcare?)

"The first right of the human person, the right to life, entails a right to the means for the proper development of life, such as adequate health care"[613]. The inseparability of right to health from the right to life legitimates

---

[611] Ibid.

[612] C. PETRINI, «Theoretical Models and Operational Frameworks in Public Health Ethics», *International Journal of Environmental Research and Public Health*, 7(2010), 189-202, in https://doi.org/10.3390/ijerph7010189 [17-8-2018].

[613] UNITED STATES CONFERENCE OF CATHOLIC BISHOPS, «Ethical and Religious Directives for Catholic Health Services (2009⁵)», in E. J. FURTON – P. J. CATALDO – A. S. MORACZEWSKI (eds.), *Catholic Health Care Ethics. A Manual for Practitioners*, The National Catholic Bioethics Center, Philadelphia 2009², 389-400.

the fundamentality of the right to health. Threatening somebody's health is as good as threatening his or her life. Right to health is a basic right that cannot be denied anyone. Thus, everyone has the right to heath care. The World Health Organization, by affirming health as one of the fundamental rights of every human being and by stating clearly the responsibility of the governments for the health of their people, made an important step towards codifying the right to health as international law[614].

The fundamental right to life and the right to health can be considered as two sides of the same coin. The right to health care is a companion to the fundamental right to life, and rights to the other necessities, such as among them food, clothing, and shelter[615]. This affirmation shows that everyone has right to health because the denial to this right implies denial of other fundamental rights, like rights to life, food, shelter and clothing. This underscores the fundamentality and universality of the right to health by associating human rights with the principle of the dignity of the human person.

3.4.3. Does Right to Health Imply the Duty of the Government to Provide Health Care for Everyone?

Right to health is a basic right and every human person possesses this right. The question many ask concerns whether the government should provide everything to everyone in terms of health care services. There are many debates on this issue, but the widely accepted view is the one that underlines the duty of the government to provide basic health care services to every citizen especially to vulnerable members of society. Some authors affirming this view write:

> The right to health, i.e. the right to highest attainable standard of health, makes governments responsible for the prevention, treatment and control of diseases and the creation of conditions

---

[614] Cfr. A. S. Christopher – D. Caruso, «American Medical Association (AMA) », *Journal of Ethics*, 17(2015), 958-965, in https://doi.org/10.1001/journalofethics.2015.17.10.msoc1-1510 [02-01-2018].

[615] Cfr. J. F. Naumann – R. W. Finn, «Principles of Catholic Social Teaching and Health Care Reform», in https://www.catholiceducation.org/en/religion-and-philosophy/social-justice/principles-of-catholic-social-teaching-and-health-care-reform.html [20-07-2017].

to ensure access to health facilities, goods and services required
to be healthy. Because all human rights – economic, social,
cultural, civil and political – are considered interdependent
and indivisible, governments are accountable for progressively
correcting conditions that may impede the realization of
the "right to health", as well as related rights to education,
information, privacy, decent living and working conditions,
participation, and freedom from discrimination. Systematic
attention to this range of rights by the health sector can provide
a coherent framework for a focus on conditions that may limit
people's ability to achieve optimal health and to receive health
services[616].

The above citation is clear on the responsibility of government towards
citizens regarding their right to health and access to care. The duty of the
state in this sense is not limited to the health care provision but is extended
to other important factors like health facilities and other health needs
where absence can thwart the government's effort to protect the right to
health of the population and to guarantee their access to care. Health
care is of special moral importance and meeting health needs is connected
with other goals of justice. "The principle of solidarity makes it clear that
ensuring healthcare provision is part of what the state is for"[617]. The State
has the duty of providing health care, particularly basic health care, to
every citizen where it is possible.

Basic health care provided to a citizen by the state should not be
considered as charity or favor done to this person but fulfilling the duty
of the State. We can understand this better with the definition of justice
as "giving each their due". In this case, the State has given the citizen
what belongs to him in justice. Some views that seem divergent to this
argument state: "The right of every individual to access health care does not
necessarily suppose an obligation on the part of the government to provide
it"[618]. The authors here are not necessarily saying that the State should
neglect its duty because the right to basic health cannot be ignored. What
they are pointing out is that the government cannot provide everything
to everyone, but there is the necessity on the part of the government to

---

[616]   P. BRAVEMAN – S. GRUSKIN, «Poverty, equity, human…».

[617]   P. GATELY – A. BECK – D. A. JONES, *Healthcare Allocation &…*, 35.

[618]   J. F. NAUMANN – R. W. FINN, «Principles of Catholic…».

guarantee a universal basic health care coverage. This concept has been embraced by almost all the countries of the world and by various trends of moral thoughts and beliefs. Referring to the Catholic teaching regarding this question, J. F. Naumann and R. W. Finn state:

> The teaching of the Universal Church has never been to suggest a government socialization of medical services. Rather, the Church has asserted the rights of every individual to have access to those things most necessary for sustaining and caring for human life, while at the same time insisting on the personal responsibility of each individual to care properly for his or her own health[619].

This affirmation obviously reminds each person of our duty towards ourselves and towards other. However, it should be reiterated that those who cannot acquire health care themselves should not be denied their rights to health. It is also important to emphasize the duty of the government to ensure that the vulnerable are not abandoned to die owing to negligence and indifferent attitude to their vulnerable conditions. The government has the duty to do whatever is possible and ethically acceptable to enable "persons who through no fault of their own are unable to work, to have means to acquire health care"[620]. This is a way of safeguarding their rights to health.

Some are convinced that the approach of not providing all health care needs awakes some sense of responsibility that will help to avoid unnecessary increase in cost of health care for everyone and abusive tendencies. For example, if an individual knows he or she has a personal financial obligation to pay even a portion of the cost of his or her medical care, the individual will be more responsible and prudent. Therefore, placing responsibility at the lowest level could be very useful. In a similar argument P. Gately, A. Beck and D. A. Jones write: "There seems no reason to require that to be fair a system must be free at the point of delivery [...] Furthermore, there is good reason to believe that charging can influence behavior and so reduce waste"[621]. The authors however agree with our thesis that the approach of financial obligation to pay cannot be applied to every person and to all situations. According to them: "Prenatal and neo-natal care are particularly

---

[619] Ibid.

[620] Ibid.

[621] P. Gately – A. Beck – D. A. Jones, *Healthcare Allocation &...*, 47.

crucial and should be given priority [...] Because of the unique vulnerability of the unborn and newly born child, such services ought to be provided regardless of ability to pay"[622]. The vulnerable cannot be abandoned, knowing full well that if the state and others do not provide for them, they cannot by themselves take care of their health and health care needs.

Government must not provide everything for everyone and must not interfere where people can provide for themselves, except for the decent minimum health care. The principle of subsidiarity, with principles of solidarity and common good reminds the state that one of the major reasons for its existence is the provision of basic health to the population. The right to health care does not imply that the state should deliver health care, but it reveals the duty of the state to provide basic health care especially to its vulnerable members. In the United Kingdom, for example, the state is the primary provider of education and health care[623]. However, the government is not the only provider of health care in all countries where there are private health care providers and other non-governmental and non-profit health care providers.

3.4.4. Is the Right to Health Absolute?

Distributive justice includes the aspects of rights to health and access to care. Treating the issue of right to health and access to care in relation to distributive justice, it is necessary to ask and give answer to the question: Is health a right or a purchased commodity? To say that something is a right or to claim something to be a right means that there is the legal basis, which stipulates that as a right or a moral claim, such right, is backed up by ethical principles and theories. A right in this sense is supported either by a legal reason or by a moral principle. There are rights that are classified as positive rights and they are called "social goods", which may or may not be provided by the society. According to M. E. Mahoney, these were named rights in order to create around them a higher sense of legitimacy to the public[624]. The positive rights are identified as legal rights. Calling them legal rights means there is someone whose responsibility it is to fulfil them.

---

[622] J. F. NAUMANN – R. W. FINN, «Principles of Catholic…».

[623] Cfr. P. GATELY – A. BECK – D. A. JONES, Ibid. 46.

[624] Cfr. M. E. MAHONEY, «Medical Rights and Public Welfare», *Proceeding of the American Philosophical Society*, 135(1991), 22-29.

The positive rights are also described as entitlements. These rights or entitlements are not always accomplished. For example, one may have right to certain health care, if the health care in question is not provided by anyone, that means the rights lose value. That particular service is not available, because it is not provided by anyone. From this example, it is understood that having certain rights does not imply that one must be able to exercise them always. This indicates that right to health care cannot be considered as an absolute right because being absolute means that it is stable and could always be exercised. This argument does not mean that people should be denied of their right to health with the excuse that rights to health is not absolute. Where it is possible, people's health needs and health care needs must be met because right to health is basic and universal. Everyone has a right to health, which must be respected by providing health care services where it is possible.

There are rights known as substance rights. These can be legal and sometimes not legal. The substance rights include health care, food, clean environment and other elements classified as basic need to maintain life[625]. In countries that show interest to respect for the rights and dignity of their citizens, substance rights can become legal rights, for instance one can get health care even when one does not have the capacity to pay. Whereas in the developing countries and countries where the libertarian principles are applied, these rights can hardly become legal rights because capacity to pay and out-of-pocket spending are the major source of health care funding.

We agree that it is contradictory to violate the right to health while promoting the right to life. The right to health, just like the right to life belongs to all men in an equal manner. In the same vein, pursuit of one's happiness will be difficult when one is denied of one's right to health. Health is an essential element for self-realization. With this, it becomes clear that right to basic health care belongs to all men and that basic health services must be provided to all by who has the responsibility to do so. This implies that where the possibility is ascertained, everyone is entitled to basic health care services. In a similar argument, J. Summer thinks that "an ideal right is a statement of a right that is meant to be motivational, a goal to seek. The WHO definition of health and its subsequent claim that everyone has a right to the highest attainable health care falls into this category"[626].

---

[625] Cfr. J. SUMMER, «Principle of Healthcare…».
[626] Ibid.

The government of every state with their health sectors therefore has the duty to aim for the highest attainable health care, as this would help to arrive at a performance in health care provision that does not fall below standard. It is generally accepted that there is no ideal health system in the world. The argument by J. Summer explains that the ideal right to health contained in the definition of the World Health Organisation is not easily attainable. No government can give every health care service to everyone, but the primary health care services where it is possible, should be made available to everyone. Health is a right that cannot be ignored without violating the fundamental right to life. P. F. Omonzejele indicates that "there are no rights without limitations; hence it then becomes relevant to know the minimum healthcare a member of a given society is entitled to, but such entitlement must not be evaluated on the basis of one's ability to pay for basic healthcare"[627]. When a person is denied the access to minimum or basic health care because of his or her economic, health and other conditions, we have a grave moral issue that connotes injustice.

3.4.5. What Kind of Health Care should be available to All?

The questions many ask about the distribution of health care services are: Are people entitled to a certain level of health care? If so, how do we distinguish between what should be available to all and what should not be? The truth of the fact as A. Fisher rightly mentioned in his lecture is that "not everyone can have every possible healthcare service"[628]. From what we have considered in the previous parts of this chapter, we have seen that it is widely accepted that the minimum decent health care should be available for all. That is to say that the primary health care must be universally available where there is the possibility.

In assuring the availability of certain health care services, it is important to consider as A. Fisher notes that "everything we choose to do in medicine we forego doing other things"[629]. This awakes our consciousness to knowing where to focus our attention. What we want to do in medicine, the service

---

[627] P. F. Omonzejele, «The Right to Healthcare in African Countries: Nigeria in View-A Moral Appraisal», *Etno Med*, 4(2010), 37-42.

[628] A. Fisher, «The ethics of health care (Lecture delivered to the annual symposium of the Guild of Catholic Doctors on April 24, 1993)», *Catholic Medical Quarterly*, 44(1993), 13-20.

[629] Ibid.

we want make available, is it worth doing, seeing the fact that it deprives opportunities in other sectors? Is it very essential? Does it fall under the logic of desire or is it a necessary need. Must all the medical needs of everyone be satisfied? These and more questions help in making decisions on what kind of health care services should be available to all. Meanwhile we retain that providing basic health care is very important knowing full well that what is primary in one country may be extraordinary in another.

3.4.6. QALY (Quality Adjusted Life Year) - What Is the Cash Value of Life?

In this part of the work apart from some objections that come from the secular perspective, we will see others of the Catholic origin, because QALYs dwells on the issues of life and dignity of the human person, which are at the heart of the Christian anthropology. One of the ethical questions in healthcare economics concerns the methods economists apply in measuring health benefits and the cost effectiveness of medical treatment. There is an interpretation of utilitarianism developed by Health economics, which is not based on market assessment of value but on the assessments of quality of life (QALY). Presenting this interpretation, P. Anand writes: "It has been argued by health economics that treatments should be offered so as to maximise the total number of QALYs produced by the total population"[630]. According to P. Anan, this "social choice rule" also called "health maximisation", sounds very interesting until its implications are properly scrutinized[631].

Most of the questions asked about the methods of the economists are relative to their being fair or unfair, just or unjust. "The QALY assumes that health improvement is equally valued between individuals"[632]. Some believe such assumption, that is, that health improvement is equally valued between individual in the QALY, is fair. Others believe it is not fair, since it does not leave any space "for alternative views over equity to be explicitly considered in societal decision making"[633].The QALY as a

---

[630] P. ANAND, «Capabilities and health…».

[631] Ibid.

[632] M. O. SOARES, «Is the QALY blind, deaf and dumb to equity? NICE's considerations over equity», *British Medical Bulletin*, 101(2012), 17-31.

[633] Ibid.

measure of individual health is a measure aimed to combine "the product of the years lived (QALYs), weighted by the quality in which that time is lived"[634]. Seen in this way, QALY may imply "that an individual would exchange time lived with quality–where a year lived in full quality of life is equivalent to more than 1 year lived at a lower quality"[635]. In terms of societal decision-making (on resource allocation), "QALY is aggregated across individuals"[636]. Such aggregation has to be done by averaging the total QALYs across individuals. This implies that, "a QALY gained by one individual is assumed to be equal to a QALY gained by another"[637].

Economists assign a utility value to life based on the health states. The value "between 0 (representing death) and 1 (representing good / best health), called the health-related Quality of Life value"[638]. Following this process, some health states are considered worse than death and are tagged with negative value. "In other words, the quality of life of an individual may be so poor that they are deemed to be better off dead"[639].With this method, some healthcare economists established a unified measure for morbidity and mortality. This move is to enable them to "combine the resulting clinical effectiveness of an intervention with its cost, so as to assess its cost effectiveness"[640]. This measure unifies life expectancy with quality of life based on actual health state of an individual. Such adjustment of the life expectancy of the individual is referred to as QALY. According to A. J. Culyer, "The most widely used measure of health gain is the Quality Adjusted Life Year (QALY)"[641]. O. J. Wouters, H. Naci and N. J. Samani addressing some issues of health economics write: "Economic considerations are increasingly common as health systems are under mounting pressure to maximise value for money. The quality-adjusted life year (QALY)–an outcome measure that expresses the duration and quality of life–is the main pillar of cost-effectiveness analysis"[642].

---

[634] Ibid.

[635] Ibid.

[636] Ibid.

[637] Ibid.

[638] P. Gately – A. Beck – D. A. Jones, *Healthcare Allocation &...*, 13.

[639] Cfr. Ibid.

[640] Ibid. 14.

[641] A. J. Culyer, «Economics and Ethics...».

[642] O. J. Wouters – H. Naci – N. J. Samani, *QALYs in cost-effectiveness analysis: an overview for cardiologists*, in http://dx.doi.org/10.1136/heartjnl-2015-308255

An example of the combination of life expectancy and quality of life considered as the actual health of an individual, shows that the QALY status of a stroke patient with life expectancy of 15 years is 9 years QALYs. This means that his or her 15 years life expectancy as a stroke patient is equivalent to 9 years in good health condition[643]. In the assessment of clinical effectiveness, for the healthcare economists to know the health benefits gained, "the expected QALY status after the medical interventions (allowing for probabilities of the various outcomes that can occur) is compared to the QALYs status immediately before, so as to determine the increase in the number of QALYs"[644]. To have an idea of its value for money, the figure–result of the above comparison or the health gains– is "divided into the cost figure for the intervention, we arrive at the cost effectiveness ratio for the intervention"[645]. This ratio represents the cost for the acquisition of an additional QALY. If the figure is low, that means the amount of gaining an extra QALY is low and this makes the intervention to be economically interesting[646].

Apart from its direct reference to the people's health situations, QALYs make indirect references to age. Highlighting QALYs' indirect reference to age criterion, P. Anad notes:

> Health maximisation is not directly age related in that QALYs are maximised whoever produces them, old or young. However, it is accepted that age enters indirectly, and significantly, in that young people will tend, *ceteris paribus*, to produce more QALYs. If ageism involves the inappropriate use of (old) age as a criterion for exclusion, then an important ethical question is whether the indirect age relatedness of health maximisation is ageist[647].

If justice to the individual defined in terms of primarily non-discrimination on the basis of old age, health situation and equal opportunity of access to resources, including treatment health services and

---

[3-1-2018].

[643] Cfr. P. GATELY – A. BECK – D. A. JONES, Ibid.

[644] Ibid.

[645] P. GATELY – A. BECK – D. A. JONES, *Healthcare Allocation &…*, 13.

[646] Cfr. Ibid.

[647] P. ANAND, «Capabilities and health…».

benefits of research[648], QALYs therefore violate the rules of justice. QALYs constantly give rise to moral questions because of their discriminatory nature and application that agrees with the exclusion of a class people, either because of their age or health conditions. For example:

> Suppose we can treat one of two people, both of whom if treated would fully recover but otherwise die. If these patients were equal in all material respects except age, then QALY maximisation would advocate treating the younger person because that person has greater amount of life left and generate more QALYs. A case for this so called fair innings argument which holds that older people, because of the length of life they have enjoyed compared with younger people, should yield priority to those who are younger[649].

Furthermore, the above-cited author retains that "the fair innings argument only supports some of the age discriminations that QALY maximisation makes"[650]. He notes that this specifically "applies to comparison where the age differences between those in need are substantial and where, therefore, one party might be said to have had a fair innings and another not"[651]. Following this trend, when making comparison between two patients of 35 years old and 50 years old, QALY maximisation would prioritise the younger patient based on his or her greater life expectancy. This according to P. Anand could be described as a form of ageism[652]. An evaluation of QALYs and related models by W. Thomas shows how the value of human life cannot be determined monetarily because it goes far beyond that. According to him "Valuation of life in terms of hard cash may be essential in establishing damages and compensation in a court of law, but in a doctor's surgery or in a hospital all that counts is life, irrespective of whatever market price may be attached to it"[653]. This according to P. F. Omonzejele implies that "the status, worthiness and input value of human

---

[648] Cfr. I. E. Thompson, «Fundamental ethical principles in health care», *British Medical Journal* (Clinical Research Ed.), 29(1987), 1461-1465.

[649] P. Anand, «Capabilities and health…».

[650] Ibid.

[651] Ibid.

[652] Cfr. Ibid.

[653] W. Thomas (ed.), *A Dictionary of Medical Ethics and Practice*, John Wright & Sons Ltd, Bristol 1977, 171.

life is of no consequence in the provision of health care"[654]. For these reasons, many authors have disagreed with QALYs. These objections will be treated subsequently.

3.4.7. Ethical Evaluations and Objections to the QALY

Some exponents of QALY uphold it because they claim it is objective. A critical examination rather shows QALY has some obvious limits that warrant some objections that have been raised against it. Some authors indicate QALY's shortcomings in the following statement: "QALY lacks integrity and is never truly objective"[655]. This position contrasts that of the proponents of QALY who retain its objectivity arguing that when a QALY is gained in one disease it is equivalent to a QALY gained in another. The supporters claim that the weight given to the gain of a QALY is the same and does not change based on "how many QALYs are currently enjoyed, how many are in prospect, the age, sex or ethnicity of beneficiaries or deservingness [...] it is also independent of any deprivation suffered outside health"[656].

Contrarily, there exist objections to quality of life measures as being contentious and as a misrepresentation of what the name suggests since they do not promote "cultural, ethnic, social and religious factors and the goods generally require for human flourishing"[657]. With the way the method of QALY proceeds, it is believed that the values inherent in QALY and the values the individuals place on their health and lives will not always tally[658]. The method of concentrating on a single health outcome is considered not enough as it offers a myopic view of the whole situation. There are other important health outcomes concerning the necessity of "access to health and social care after leaving hospital, social support and cognitive ability"[659]. Therefore, the calculation as it is done to determine the quality of life may result inaccurate because most important factors are not taken into consideration. A similar view maintains that QALYs are partial in their consideration. According to this view, "QALYs fail

---

[654] P. F. OMONZEJELE, «The Right to Healthcare...».

[655] Cfr. P. GATELY – A. BECK – D. A. JONES, *Healthcare Allocation &...*, 18.

[656] Ibid., 17-18.

[657] Ibid. 18.

[658] Ibid.

[659] Ibid., 18-19.

to take into account any benefits other than those relating to clinical effectiveness"[660].

The discriminatory characters of QALYs stand as clear motives for objections to them: "QALY status is clearly heavily dependent on age"[661]. This being the case, it is obvious that with QALYs, there must be discrimination against the elderly:

> Because heterogeneity in health is known to increase with age, it maintains that a focus on QALY status, based on age-determined life expectancies derived from mortality tables, can seriously misrepresent the prospects of those in old age who are in good health. Additionally, decisions can be made to exclude the elderly from clinical trial even though the elderly take the most medication[662].

The idea of excluding persons based on ethnicity, age, sex, economic, social, and geographical and other health conditions in health care programs connotes injustice. It violates the rights to health of every human being, which are inseparable from other rights. Similarly, the discriminatory treatment to those with disability and comorbidity problems in the name of QALYs gives more reasons to object to QALYs. Individuals with the above-mentioned health conditions could produce a lower QALY gain than those with a greater pre-treatment QALY status, despite the fact that they have the same life expectancy and they can all benefit in an equal manner from a particular treatment[663]. QALYs indicate the quality of life as the only or most important factor, neglecting the respect for the dignity of the human person that is relevant in every situation, irrespective of his health condition, and the important factors of the sacredness of every human life. If the quality of life as it is interpreted by QALYs, becomes the only measure, there will be a dehumanization of medicine and the health systems.

Besides, the use of QALYs will be an obstacle to reducing health inequalities associated with age and disability. A. Fisher and L. Gormally believe that QALY tends towards policies that give lowest priority to the

---

[660] Ibid., 19.

[661] Ibid.

[662] Ibid.

[663] Cfr. Ibid.

terminally ill, dying, elderly, and chronically sick or incapacitated, severely handicapped, and permanently unconscious and can easily permit their elimination even[664]. Additionally, it has been argued that with QALY, people with lower productivity such as children and elderly are considered to have health and health gains undervalued in comparison to people with higher productivity. In this way, the lower productive class is discriminated against[665]. It is also argued that when QALY is applied, there could be a case of discrimination when interventions that benefit fewer patients are deterred over interventions that benefit more patients[666].

The value of human life does not derive from a person's social or economic status but simply from his or her existence and his or her being created in the image of God. This means that beyond being young or old, healthy or sick and his presumed quality of life cannot determine the value of his life. The only thing that matters is his being in relationship with God[667]. This truth about the human life holds from conception to natural death. An ethical evaluation of QALY reveals many limits that disqualify it, especially based on its approach, which does not adequately respect the right to life, the right to health, and the dignity of vulnerable persons. There is the need for a change inspired by the fundamental principles and values inherent to the main features of an ethical health-care system that we will treat subsequently. Such features are enshrined in the catholic principles we will study in chapter four.

3.4.8. Equity in Health

"Equity means social justice or fairness; it is an ethical concept, grounded in principles of distributive justice"[668]. A common and plausible claim regarding right to health is that which confirms the right everyone has to a decent-minimum health care. This right according to the principle of equity should be given to each person according to what will be useful to him or her. Equity in health has been described "as the absence of

---

[664] Cfr. Ibid., 23.

[665] Cfr. M. O. Soares, «Is the QALY …».

[666] Cfr. Ibid.

[667] Cfr. M. P. Faggioni, *La Vita Nelle Nostre Mani. Manuale di Bioetica teologica*, Edizione Camilliane, Torino 2006², 42-43.

[668] P. Braveman – S. Gruskin, «Defining equity in health», *Journal of Epidemiology and Community Health*, 57(2003), 254-258.

socially unjust or unfair health disparities"[669]. Thus, the term equity in health refers to fairness in the distribution of health among individuals. Health inequities according to M. Whitehead, is defined as the differences in health that are unnecessary, avoidable, unfair and unjust[670]. Explaining further on the concept, "equity in health", P. Brave and S. Gruskin write:

> For the purpose of operationalization and measurement, equity in health can be defined as the absence of systematic disparities in health (or in the major social determinants of health) between social groups who have different levels of underlying social advantage/disadvantage – that is, different positions in a social hierarchy. Inequities in health systematically put groups of people who are already socially disadvantaged (for example, by virtue of being poor, female, and/or members of a disenfranchised racial, ethnic, or religious group) at further disadvantage with respect to their health; health is essential to wellbeing and to overcoming other effects of social disadvantage[671].

Health inequity penalizes the vulnerable who are already disadvantaged by the various forms of discrimination that have put them in such vulnerable conditions. Most of them are deprived of the key social determinants of health like, houses, drinking water and sanitation and health care. This means that certain people are treated without equity and unjustly. Often when a treatment is said to be unjust, we mean to say that it is morally wrong. In some cases, the term injustice is taken to signify unfairness or unfair treatment. A further description of the concept "equity" will be necessary for a better understanding of the various forms of unfairness or inequities in health. P. Braveman and S. Gruskin in a bulletin of the World Health Organization describes the concept "equity" thus:

> Equity is an ethical concept grounded in the principle of distributive justice. Equity in health reflects a concern to reduce unequal opportunities to be healthy associated with membership in less privileged social groups, such as poor

---

669 Ibid.

670 Cfr. M. WHITEHEAD, «The Concepts and principles of equity in health», *International Journal of Health Services*, 22(1992), 429-445, in <u>https://doi.org/10.2190/986l-lhq6-2vte-yrrn</u> [28-5-2018].

671 P. BRAVEMAN – S. GRUSKIN, «Poverty, equity, human…».

> people; disenfranchised racial, ethnic or religious groups; women: and rural residents. In operational terms, pursuing equity in health means eliminating health disparities that are systematically associated with underlying social disadvantage or marginalization. An equity framework systematically focuses attention on socially disadvantaged, marginalized, or disenfranchised groups within and between countries, including but not limited to the poor[672].

We can say that the principle of equity applied to the allocation of health care resources requests fairness in distribution. This means making every effort to see that all health inequalities are eliminated and no member of the society especially the vulnerable is denied his/her rights to health. One of the ways of eliminating inequalities in the distribution of health care resources according to Pope Francis is by remembering always that the rich and the poor have equal dignity[673].

Regarding how to go about the elimination process of health inequities, which reflect the absence of equity in society, some aforementioned authors write:

> Practical experience suggests that eliminating systematic health disparities between social groups requires correcting their fundamental causes, at least to some extent, as well as cushioning their health-damaging effects. Furthermore, a commitment to equalizing opportunities to be healthy inherently requires identification of the determinants as well as manifestations of health disparities. Concern for health equity thus implies a value–based commitment to tackle poverty and health, with or without conclusive evidence of aggregate utilitarian gains[674].

The authors, P. Bravemen and S.Gruskin, in this citation demonstrate that the problem of health disparities or health inequities have their roots in other problems. So, the problems should be traced to their roots, in order to achieve their proper eradication. For example, a budgetary allocation

---

[672] Ibid.

[673] Cfr. FRANCIS, «*LaudatoSì* Lettera Enciclica Sulla Cura della Casa Comune», n. 94, Paoline Editoriale Libri, Milano 2015, 72-73.

[674] P. BRAVEMAN – S. GRUSKIN, «Poverty, equity, human…».

done without considering the right principles of justice or based on the wrong principles and polices can lead to health disparities in a country.

Furthermore, Rice and Smith addressed the issue of inequality in relation to price. For them when we mention prices, we are not simply talking about money but also related to time costs, distances from the locations of health care facilities and many other factors which render the effective price higher than the financial price and cause substantial differences in the opportunities confronting different people in the same country[675]. This captures the image of a health care system like that of Nigeria where budgetary allocation to the health sector is always insufficient and the members of the society who live in the rural areas are serious penalized because the hospitals are situated far from their homes and they have to spend more time and money on transportation to have access to health care services. They are constrained to live in such situation when others in the urban areas have the health care services at their 'beck and call'. Whereas equity demands that those who need more be given according to their needs. The infrastructural problems are among the root causes of the health and other types of inequalities in many developing countries.

Efforts should be made in these areas in order to secure an equitable distribution of health care resources. Health is internationally included among the basic human rights. This means that inequity in health represents an infringement of human rights to health. Thus rights to health and equity in health are compatible in the efforts to eliminate health inequalities. In accordance to this argument, P. Braveman and S. Gruskin argue:

> Both equity and human rights principles dictate striving for equal opportunity for health for groups of people who have historically suffered discrimination or social marginalization. Achieving equal opportunity for health entails not only buffering the health-damaging effects of poverty and marginalization: it requires reducing disparities between populations in the underlying conditions – such as education, living standards, and environmental exposures – necessary to be healthy. Thus, both human rights and equity perspectives require that health institutions deal with poverty and health not only by providing care to improve the health of the poor but also by helping to

---

[675] Cfr. A. J. CULYER, «Economics and Ethics in Health Care», *Journal of Medical Ethics*, 27(2001), 217-222. https://doi.org/10.1136/jme.27.4.217 [15-10-2016].

alter the conditions that create, exacerbate, and perpetuate poverty and marginalization[676].

To reduce health inequities, health and other human rights must be guaranteed. As we have mentioned earlier, the violation of these rights in most countries is the cause of health inequalities. For instance, in most developing countries, poverty is among the major causes of health inequities. With the high rate of poverty, many live in unhealthy conditions and environments. At the root of poverty is corruption among the political leaders. Other factors apart from poverty are lack of education and discrimination of women and children. The complex nature of health inequity is epitomized in the following affirmation:

> A health disparity between more and less advantaged population groups constitutes an inequity not because we know the proximate cause of that disparity and judge them unjust them to be unjust, but rather because the disparity is strongly associated with unjust social structures; those structures systematically put disadvantaged groups at generally increased risk of ill health and also generally compound the social and economic consequences of ill health[677].

For some authors, "explicit adoption of equity and human rights approaches can ensure systematic attention to social disadvantage, vulnerability and discrimination in health policies and programmes"[678]. Equity in health and rights to health are important for a fair distribution of resources because they strive to ensure equal opportunity for health and the elimination of all kinds of health inequities and discriminations. Equity is a theory that looks out for everyone. If properly applied, we will be sure of a fair distribution of resources, because equity in health refers to fairness in the distribution of health across individuals. Nevertheless, some criticisms have been leveled against the Equity theory based on its assumptions and practical application. The homogenous perception of fairness (equity) will be difficult to be established since there are varieties in the ways people perceive equity or fairness. People differ in the models they use to make equity judgments.

---

[676]   P. BRAVEMAN – S. GRUSKIN, «Poverty, equity, human…»
[677]   Ibid.
[678]   Ibid.

3.4.9. Need Principles (A Material Reason to Discriminate in the Distribution of Health Care Resources)

The distribution of burdens and benefits equally is fundamental in distributive justice. But an exception can be condoned when there is a material reason for discrimination. One of the material reasons is that of "need". The concept of need is often employed to identify those health care services that a health care system should ensure is available for all citizens. Allocation according to some authors should be done in accordance to need because, "need is a central category for allocation"[679]. R. Cookson and P. Dolan explain that "need principles require that health care be distributed in proportion to "need" (for example, in terms of immediate ill health)"[680]. They believe that, "the distribution of health care according to need is perhaps the most widely discussed rationing principle in both academic and non-academic debates"[681]. The need principles advocate that the need of the people should be considered in the distribution of resources and not necessarily their ability to pay. Some think that in the distribution of health resources, "it is not access to or utilisation of health care services as such that is ethically justified, but access to or utilisation of needed health care services"[682].

Defining 'need' is difficult and this makes it difficult to identify what are needs in health care. In this vein, it is difficult to ascertain individual patients' health care needs in order to fashion services accordingly. It has been argued also that the wide variation in the description of 'need' has direct impact on the policies, strategies, plans and services geared towards meeting the people's health care needs. In their presentation of the definition of "need in terms of the degree of ill health" or "narrow definition of need as immediate threat to life" and the broader definition of need as ill health which would include immediate pain and suffering "as well as immediate threat to life", R. Cookson and P. Dolan, explain that these need principles or definitions "are both sometimes called the "Rule of Rescue"[683]. The concept of "Rule of Rescue" according to them implies

---

[679]   P. GATELY – A. BECK – D. A. JONES, *Healthcare Allocation &...*, 59.

[680]   R. COOKSON – P. DOLAN, «Principles of justice...».

[681]   Ibid.

[682]   J. HURLEY, «Ethics, economics, and...».

[683]   R. COOKSON – P. DOLAN, «Principles of Justice...».

the duty of the state and society towards those facing imminent threats to life and health[684].

According to some economists, the definition of "need" in terms of ill health is inadequate. For them, such definition does not help to understand how much benefit the health care could bring. So they assert that "need" should be defined or considered firstly in terms of the capacity of the individual to gain health from treatment. Going by this, a maximising principle would only consider focusing on allocation to patients in proportion to their capacity to benefit from treatment. This implies excluding those who have least capacity of gaining from treatment. "A (proportionate) need principle, by contrast, will always imply giving some health care to those with lesser needs (i.e., in proportion to those needs)"[685]. Among the clinicians of the British Medical Association, it is widely accepted that discrimination in health is permissible only on the grounds of clinical need[686]. On this account, they accept the principles of distribution according to clinical need. Need according to some cited authors is defined "in terms of the degree of ill health"[687]. The definition of need as ill health, described in terms of "Rule of Rescue", which implies the duty of society to do all it can to rescue those whose life or health are being threatened attracts some critiques. According to one of these critiques, this way of conceiving the need principles could create some problems. For example, in carrying out the moral duty of ensuring rescue for all in need (which is not always easy and possible), the rescue of one may lead to the denial of rescue for others[688]. This affirms the position that whatever decision we take in healthcare denies someone something elsewhere.

For the maximising principles, justice is done when health care is distributed in order to achieve the best possible consequences. Maximising principles some authors think, are utilitarian oriented. The likely consequences of actions are crucial in the maximising principles. Though the maximising principles are said to be utilitarian oriented, the same authors affirm they are not identical to the utilitarian principles. The difference between them lies in the fact that while the maximising principles

---

[684]   Cfr. Ibid.

[685]   Ibid.

[686]   Cfr. Ibid.

[687]   Ibid.

[688]   Cfr. Ibid.

lay emphasis on total population health, the utilitarian principles are concerned with maximising happiness which is not exclusively determined by good health, as other elements are included[689]. The implication of maximising principle depends essentially on the estimated health gain one is expected to make.

Some economists propose the idea of need as the individual's capacity to gain health from treatment[690]. This economists' approach in essence defines needs in terms of ability to benefit from health care provision[691]. Going by this definition of need, people who do not have the ability to benefit or have less capacity to benefit from health care provision will not be considered while the policies are made for health care services. In this sense, a maximising principle concentrates on investing more resources on one with the possibility of gaining most, avoiding another whose situation demonstrates the possibility of gaining least. According to the economists who do not agree with this mode of reasoning, it would not be fair to define need exclusively in terms of capacity to benefit because it would lead to discrimination of those who need expensive treatments. For instance, if there are two individuals who have the same capacity to benefit, and the treatment of one is more expensive than the other is, applying this concept of need means treating the one whose cost of treatment is less, despite the fact that they have the same need[692]. This means preferring economic gain to the health, life and dignity of certain individuals. The cost of treatment here is the measure and health is seen as a commercial rather than a common good. There are other considerations given based on abilities. For example, between the young and the elderly. Most prefer acting in favour of the young who have more life ahead of them to acting for the elderly who have little future abilities.

Theories based on discrimination against the sick, poor and the vulnerable, cannot be ethically justified. Where the consideration for economic gain outweighs the value for life and the dignity of the person, they cannot be ethically permissible as principles for the distribution of

---

[689] Cfr. Ibid.

[690] Cfr. Ibid.

[691] Cfr. A. STEVENS – S. GILLAM, «Needs assessment from theory to practice», *Bio Medical Journal*, 316(1998), 1448-1452, in https://doi.org/10.1136/bmj.316.7142.1448 [7-2-2017].

[692] Cfr. R. COOKSON – P. DOLAN, «Principles of Justice...».

health care resource allocation. R. Cookson and P. Dolan agree with economists' position that identifying need with capacity to benefit implies a bias against people who need expensive treatments. It may happen that "if two people, A and B, have the same need (capacity to benefit), but treating A is more expensive than treating B, then distributing expenditure according to capacity to benefit might mean that B gets treated but A does not, even though they have the same needs"[693]. Placing the cost of treatment first and above the health and life of the sick and the poor is a utilitarian method that is not ethically accepted. This calls for deliberations on applying the rights principles in order to make right decisions. Many ethicists have expressed their disapprobation on this because reduced potential and ability leads to discrimination against the vulnerable members of the society. The instances presented above highlight the difficulties encountered in the decision-making processes for the distribution of health care resources. The ethical principles must always be the guide.

There is a typical morality in health care, which permits discrimination for or against persons based on their need. A classic example is presented in the case of giving urgent attention to persons with emergencies. In a case of emergency, the long-time of waiting of those who came earlier does not count. Some cases of emergency like accidents or natural disasters are described as cases of need based on misfortune. In the same vein, there are other morally permissible discrimination based on the catholic principle that favour the disadvantaged, the poor and the vulnerable.

3.5. Main Features of an Ethical Health Care System

The main features of an ethical health-care system are those qualities that aid in pursuing a rights-based approach, health policy, strategies and programs that are formed particularly to improve the exercise of the people's right to health, access to care and utilization of health care resources. The human rights-based approach in this could be said to be is all-embracing[694]. The United Nations (UN) describes this approach as a means of realizing a fair distribution of health care resources. According to a UN document: "A human rights-based approach to health provides a

---

[693] Ibid.

[694] Cfr. UNITED NATIONS HUMAN RIGHTS, *Office of the…*

set of clear principles for setting and evaluating health policy and service delivery, targeting discriminatory practices and unjust power relations that are at the heart of inequitable health outcomes"[695].

The following are some of the core principles and standards of a rights-based approach we will treat in this section: Universality, Availability, Accessibility, Acceptability, Quality, Equality, and Non-discrimination. These qualities constitute the main features of an ethical health-care system. An ethical health care system is one that carries everyone along especially the poorest, weak, disadvantaged and respects their dignity as human persons. These features are considered necessary for the realization of such objectives.

3.5.1. Universality

"Human rights are universal and inalienable"[696]. Health as we have seen previously in this chapter is among the globally recognized fundamental rights. The right to health care is applied equally, to all people, everywhere, without distinction. This implies that no one should be deprived of this fundamental right because its deprivation can adversely affect other rights. For example, the denial of one's right to basic health care quickly affects the fundamental and inalienable right to life. Universality is a core component of the right to health because it ensures the primary health care for all which is a project embraced by many countries of the world. Without universality, it will be difficult to talk of an ethically accepted health care resource allocation.

3.5.2. Availability

To say that health care service is universal means it is available to all. Availability therefore "refers to the need for a sufficient quantity of functioning public health and health care facilities, goods and services, as well as programmes for all"[697]. In most countries, the availability of health care service is incomplete, that means the provision of services is not universal. This creates moral problems of inequality and other forms of

---

[695] Ibid.

[696] Ibid.

[697] Ibid.

injustice. An already cited document of the United Nations indicates how availability can be ascertained. According to this document, "availability can be measured through the analysis of disaggregated data to different and multiple stratifiers including by age, sex, location and socio-economic status and qualitative surveys to understand coverage gaps and health workforce coverage"[698]. The basic health care resources can be considered available when they are within the reach and utilizable by all, especially the weakest and the poorest classes.

3.5.3. Accessibility

Accessibility, Universality and Availability as core elements of human rights-based approach are intrinsically connected. Accessibility "requires that health facilities, goods, and services must be accessible to everyone"[699]. The four major overlapping aspects of accessibility are:

- Non-discrimination
- Physical accessibility
- Economic accessibility (affordability)
- Information accessibility[700]

Accessibility requires a proper analysis of the various barriers (physical, economic, social and others) which are present among people of different nations and individuals of the same nation. These barriers often penalize the poor and the disadvantaged. For this, accessibility calls "for the establishment or application of clear norms and standards in both law and policy to address these barriers, as well as robust monitoring systems of health-related information and whether this information is reaching all populations"[701].

3.5.4. Acceptability

Acceptability reveals the concrete and human face of medicine because it requires that policies, laws, programs, facilities, mode of rendering health

---

[698] Ibid.

[699] Ibid.

[700] Cfr. Ibid.

[701] UNITED NATIONS HUMAN RIGHTS, *Office of the...*

care services and the distribution of health care resources, should respect medical ethics and must be people-centered. This implies having a system that is based on the needs of the entire population and not a particular social group. Services here are provided for the people and the people are involved in most decisions in accordance to medical ethics and particularly with the ethics of community health care[702].

3.5.5. Quality

The quality of resources and services made available to the population must be of the required standard, that is, scientifically and medically tested and approved. "Quality is a key component of Universal Health Coverage, and includes the experience as well as the perception of health care. Quality health services should be:

- Safe – avoiding injuries to people for whom the care is intended;
- Effective – providing evidence-based healthcare services to those who need them
- People-centered – providing care that responds to individual preferences, needs and values;
- Timely – reducing waiting times and sometimes-harmful delays.
- Equitable – providing care that does not vary in quality on account of gender, ethnicity, geographic location, and socio-economic status;
- Integrated – providing care that makes available the full range of health services throughout the life course;
- Efficient – maximizing the benefit of available resources and avoiding waste"[703].

Quality applies to the quality of goods, facilities and services. Respecting the recommendations of these components of the human rights-based approach in the distribution of health care resources makes the services rendered more effective and efficient. They are very necessary for the attainment of an ethical health care.

---

[702] Cfr. Ibid.

[703] Ibid.

3.5.6. Equality and Non-discrimination

The principle of non-discrimination seeks to guarantee that in exercising human rights, no one is discriminated against because of his or her race, color, sex, religion, age, health status, place of residence, and economic and social conditions. The same principle prohibits discrimination and inequalities in access to health, as well as in means and entitlements for achieving this access. This is extended to other forms of actions that impair the equal enjoyment and exercise of the right to health[704].

The principle of equality and non-discrimination protects the interest of the disadvantaged against discrimination in the policies, programs and practices inherent to the distribution and provision of health care services. Furthermore, "non-discrimination and equality are key measures required to address the social determinants affecting the enjoyment of the right to health. Functioning national health information systems and availability of disaggregated data are essential to be able to identify the most vulnerable groups and diverse needs"[705]. There is no doubt that if this principle is properly applied, together with other ethically accepted principles of distributive justice and the features of an ethical health care system, it will guarantee a fair distribution of health resources, which is the main purpose of applying distributive justice to health care. Equality alone is not enough.

Conclusion

In this chapter, we have studied some major issues concerning how the human health is sustained through the distribution of health care resources. We have done this by considering properly some questions preannounced in the introductory part of this chapter: whether there is a right to health care. If this right exists, how does society respond to it? With what criteria of justice does society address the issue of distribution of health care resources? What moral principles, theories and approaches are applied to the distribution of health care resources?

To be able answer these questions correctly, out study in this chapter has demonstrated that a correct knowledge of the concept of justice is

---

[704]   Cfr. Ibid.

[705]   UNITED NATIONS HUMAN RIGHTS, *Office of the...*

essential. This justifies our analysis of the different interpretations of justice observing how these interpretations influence people's ideas and methods of allocating health care resources. The examinations done in this chapter reveal that many authors define justice in terms of fairness, equity and as giving attention to what is due or owed to persons. For them, there is injustice where these conditions are missing and where people are denied of their rights. This interests us because the main issue we are considering in this dissertation falls under distributive justice: the distribution of health care resources. How can the health care resources be distributed respecting the dignity of the human person; every human person?

As the present chapter has permitted to be seen, the issue of distribution of health care resources is an ethical question which has not ceased to provoke discussions at the political, economic, social and religious levels. We have thus surveyed many theories and approaches applied to the problem of health care resource allocation. All the theories and approaches viewed here addressed the questions regarding how best to distribute health care resources in a society where there are different needs among the its members. How can public financing satisfy the quest for fair access to and utilisation of health by the societal members. The models we attentively looked at are: Procedural Justice, Libertarian theories of justice, Utilitarian theory of justice, Egalitarian theories of justice and Rawls' theory of justice.

The study of the just mentioned principle, theories and approaches of justice in this chapter has revealed that their proper application can help to obtain to a certain point, an appreciable distribution of health care resources. We have also seen that not all of them stand for the notion of fairness or justice sustained by this dissertation. The various principles, theories and approaches of justice we have observed, despite their differences, converge on the importance of protecting the interest of justice. Nevertheless, they are all with shortcomings. There is therefore the need for an all-embracing set of principles, namely, the Catholic principles, which do not have the limits identified in the theories and approaches treated in this chapter. For this reason, we will treat the Catholic principles in the next Chapter applying it to the Nigerian Health care system. This is the major objective of our dissertation. We will also incorporate what we found good in the principles, theories and approaches considered in this chapter in our proposal of the Catholic principles in the next chapter.

The present chapter has evaluated some important issues of right to health taking into consideration questions like: Whether right to health as a primary or basic right means everyone has a right to healthcare? Does right to health imply the duty of the government to provide healthcare for everyone? Is the right to health absolute? What kind of health care should be available to all? Another important issue is that of QALY (Quality Adjusted Life Year). Regarding this, there is a question in reference to what is the cash value of life? Such questions as we have seen cannot be answered without an ethical assessment of the responses given by health, legal, political, economic, theological and philosophical experts.

In this section, an appraisal of the need principles as the material reason for discrimination and the questions proper to equity in health was very important to drive our point home. It is obvious from what we have seen so far in this work that we cannot meet all the health and health care needs of every individual with the limited resources available. In spite of this, we must be accountable for the reasonableness of the decisions we make about the distribution of health care resources. The third chapter of our dissertation has been able to address the issue of right to health, presenting the various models with which society approaches the quest for the respect of the right to health and access to and utilization of health care resources. A major problem that cuts across the themes the various theories and approaches confronted is that of inequalities. Why do some have more, while others have little or nothing to enjoy in health, which is a human and common good. This problem emerges from the misdistribution of health and other common goods. One of the remedies to the health inequalities and the injustice in health is the imperative of health care resource redistribution – from the rich to the poor, the vulnerable and the disadvantaged, from the healthy to the sickest – returning to the poor, the vulnerable and the sick what has been taken from them entails acting in conformity with justice. Making accessible and affordable the basic survival needs and universal health care is another way to tackle the problem of health inequalities and achieving a distributional fairness. The present dissertation affirms that basic health care is a right that should be accorded to every human person, without distinction.

The main features of an ethical health-care system evaluated in this chapter are close in intention to the Catholic principles we are proposing particularly in the fourth and final chapter, for a fair distribution of health care resources in Nigeria. The features include: Universality, Availability, Accessibility, Acceptability, Quality, Equality, and Non-discrimination. These are characteristics of an ethical health-care system; such that does not ignore anyone especially, the poorest, weak, disadvantaged and recognizes the dignity of every human persons. An ethical health-care system can be achieved in Nigeria through the application of Catholic principles which as we will see contain the just mention features of an ethical health-care system and all the positive points of the principles, theories and approaches treated in chapter three. Proving this, is one of the major objectives of the next chapter of this dissertation.

Chapter 4

DISTRIBUTION OF HEALTH CARE RESOURCES IN NIGERIA - APPLYING THE CATHOLIC PRINCIPLES OF DISTRIBUTIVE JUSTICE

Introduction

In chapter three of this dissertation, we examined the secular perspective of the moral principles in health care. We were able to study the principles, theories and approaches of distributive justice according to the secular line and we saw how these were applied to the distribution of health care resources in general. The ethical evaluation of the application of these secular principles, theories and approaches of distributive justice revealed how alone, they cannot guarantee a just health care system in Nigeria. This is because apart from their positive attributes, they exhibits weak points which make them incapable of offering a health care system that carries everyone along; a just and fair health care system. Some sources used in the foregoing chapter agree that when there is conflict among some principles, they can hardly be combined to achieve a coherent moral system able to offer justice and fairness. For example, the principle of free-market distribution is incompatible with the principle of need in the distribution of health care resources. This calls for a critical analysis of the principles to specify their characteristics. This was done in chapter three. In the fourth chapter, there is the intention of harmonizing the positive traits of the secular principles, theories and approaches studied in chapter three with the Catholic principles, in the bid to propose a better way of achieving a fair health care system in Nigeria. Suffice is it to mention that this chapter is dedicated majorly to the application of Catholic principles of distributive justice to the Nigerian health system in order to establish an appreciable health system in the country. We will also consider some main features of an ethical health care system, which are similar to the object of our study in the present chapter; the Catholic principles of distributive justice. These features will be used where they fit in directly.

The Catholic principles are global because they have everything positive in the secular principles, theories and approaches seen in chapter three, without containing any of the weak characteristics related to them. Therefore, we proffer the solution of applying the Catholic principles of distributive justice to the distribution of health care resources in the Nigerian Health Care System. The Catholic principles we are presenting in chapter four are: principle of dignity/integrity of the human person, principle of common good and solidarity, principle of preferential option for the most vulnerable, principle of subsidiarity. These principles will be applied in the examination of the major Nigerian health and health related matters we treated in chapters one and two, thus showing how the problems regarding health care resource allocation in Nigeria could be resolved by the use of the same principles.

We intend to study the problem of distribution of health care resources in Nigeria, following the Catholic concept of justice. The Catholic notion of justice retains that the dignity of the human person is a paramount theme. Justice according to the Catholic Doctrine is a human virtue[706]; one of the cardinal virtues. The Catechism of the Catholic Church defines justice, as "the moral virtue that consists in the constant and firm will to give their due to God and neighbour"[707]. When the duty of justice is fulfilled towards God, the Church describes it as "virtue of religion"[708]. Fulfilling the duty

---

[706] Cfr. The Catechism of the Catholic Church, n. 1804, Pauline's Publications-Africa, Nairobi, Kenya 1995, 439.

[707] Ibid., n. 1807, 439-440.

[708] Ibid, n. 1807.

of justice towards men means "to respect the rights of each and to establish in human relationships the harmony that promotes equity with regards to persons and to the common"[709]. The Church's Magisterium defines common good as "the sum total of social conditions which allow people, either as groups or as individuals, to reach their fulfillment more fully and more easily"[710]. Common good therefore implies the availability of the conditions that aid the members of the society to achieve their aims in life.

Common good means public good, shared and enjoyed by many persons, thus its distribution has to be done in fairness. This implies that no one should be denied the opportunity of enjoying or having his or her own share of the common good. In this regard, a Catholic author D. M. Gallagher affirms that "health care itself is clearly a common good of society, an essential element of the general common good"[711]. As a result, distributive justice demands the fair distribution of the common good to all members of the society. At all levels, efforts should be made to guarantee a just and fair distribution of health facilities[712]. The Catholic social teaching in the same vein affirms that to be faithful to the principle of common good, the state "should make accessible to each what is needed to lead a truly human life: food, clothing, health, work, education and culture, suitable information, the right to establish a family, and so on"[713].

The Church's social Magisterium gives greater importance to *social justice*, "which represents a real development in *general justice*, the justice that regulates social relationships according to the criterion of observance of the law"[714]. Such concept of justice is "related to social question which [...] concerns the social, political and economic aspects and, above all, the structural dimension of problems and their solutions"[715]. The Catholic understanding of justice is very important in the context of our study because it promotes the value, rights and dignity of every human person,

---

[709] Ibid.

[710] Ibid., n. 1906, 457.

[711] D. M. GALLAGHER, «The Common Good», in E. J. FURTON – P. J. CATALDO – A. S. MORACZEWSKI (eds.), *Catholic Health Care Ethics. A Manual for Practitioners*, The National Catholic Bioethics Center, Philadelphia 2009, 29-31².

[712] Cfr. PONTIFICIO CONSIGLIO PER GLI OPERATORI SANITARI, *Nuova Carta degli Operatori Sanitari*, Libreria Editrice Vaticana, Città del Vaticano 2016, 114.

[713] THE CATECHISM OF..., n. 1908, 457.

[714] PONTIFICAL COUNCIL FOR JUSTICE AND PEACE, *Compendium of the...*, 116.

[715] Ibid., n. 201, 116-117.

especially women and children. We will give more attention to women and children because we consider them as the most vulnerable in the Nigerian health care context, where they are often classified as the least and treated as such in the distribution health care and other resources. In addition, there is a cultural way of thinking in the African context that do not place women at the same level with men. This connotes injustice. In reaction to the above-mentioned issues, this Chapter applies the Catholic principles of distributive justice to the social, political and economic matters concerning the distribution of health care resources in Nigeria. This implies that our main preoccupation here will be that of a moral vision of the social realities of Nigeria considered in the first two chapters of this dissertation.

4.1. Catholic Principles of Distributive Justice

The Catholic principles of distributive justice could be recommended for any health care system to guarantee justice and fairness. The Catholic Social Doctrine on health care needs, especially those of the poor and the weak, is inspired by the mainstream Catholic anthropological and theological visions of social justice, which is person-centered.

Distributive justice in Health care is based on four fundamental principles:

1.   The principle of dignity/integrity of the human person
2.   The principle of common good and solidarity
3.   The principle of preferential option for the most vulnerable
4.   The principle of subsidiarity

"Catholic teaching offers a great deal of help for people working in health care who have responsibilities for allocation of resources"[716]. The Catholic Church in her teaching has developed an extensive theory of human rights that is based on the Christian doctrines that reveal the link between the dignity of the human person and the creation of man in God's image and likeness. Consequently, she teaches that all human beings are equal because all are created in the image of God [Genesis 1.26]. The Church also teaches the sacredness of life and of blood [Genesis Chapter 9].

---

[716]   P. GATELY – A. BECK – D. A. JONES, *Healthcare Allocation &…*, 29.

The right to life is inseparably related to the right to health care. For this, the Catholic social teaching invites each person to be his brother's keeper. The Universal Church understands health care in terms of 'care ethics' and this is applied in her teaching that "the right to healthcare cannot be detached from the notion of stewardship and the duty to care responsibly for our health"[717].

In addition, being our brother's keeper in the Catholic belief is a divine injunction. Taking care of the sick and the vulnerable is a concrete way of responding to this divine injunction. The main aim of this dissertation is the application of the above Catholic principles of distributive justice that represent the cornerstone of the Catholic social teaching to the distribution of heath care resources in the Nigerian health system, as a response to the right to health and health care of the Nigerian citizens. Here we are going study the principles and subsequently directly apply them to the concrete issues of health care resource allocation in Nigeria we considered in the first two chapters of this doctoral dissertation.

4.1.1. The Principle of Dignity/Integrity of the Human Person

Christian ethics is person-centered. This is obvious in the official documents of the Catholic Church that define the human person as a unified totality of body and soul. The Catholic Church thus sees and enjoins that the person be always considered as a psychophysical unity[718]. The principle of the dignity of the human person is a fundamental principle in the Catholic teaching. This principle in the Catholic health ethics concerns respecting the human dignity of every patient when making decisions on health and in giving health care services. The Catholic social teaching and the Personalist bioethics "are part of a broader moral framework". They share certain characteristics[719]. According to Catholic social doctrine:

> Men and women, in the concrete circumstances of history, represent the heart and soul of Catholic social thought[202]. The whole of the Church's social doctrine, in fact, develops

---

[717]   Ibid. 31.

[718]   Cfr. M. P. FAGGIONI, *La Vita nelle nostre Mani, Manuale di Bioetica Teologica*, Edizioni Camilliane, Torino 2004², 48-49.

[719]   J. B. HEHIR, «Policy Arguments in a Public Church: Catholic Social Ethics and Bioethics», *The Journal of Medicine and Philosophy*, 17(1992), 347-364.

> from the principle that affirms the inviolable dignity of the
> human person. In her manifold expressions of this knowledge,
> the Church has striven above all to defend human dignity in
> the face of every attempt to redimension or distort its image;
> moreover she has often denounced the many violations of
> human dignity[720].

In the same line, the Personalist bioethics affirms that "the human person is the reference point and standard for distinguishing licit from licit"[721]. Catholic social teaching conceives the human person as the origin of a moral vision for society. Similarly, the reflections of personalist bioethics are aimed at covering the whole existence of man[722]. Both Catholic social teaching and Personalist bioethics see the person as being social and they admit that people should come together to seek the common good. This implies that the category of "relationship" is the first constitutive essence of the person[723]. All the fundamental tenets of Personalist bioethics are contained in the person-centred Catholic social teaching.

The Catholic social doctrine sustains the safeguarding of the dignity of the human person from conception to death. Accordingly, some Catholic authors affirm that "our dignity as human persons is not negotiable"[724]. In faithfulness to the Catholic beliefs, the Papal Encyclical *"Pacem in Terris"* gives a list of the human rights:

> Man has a right to live. He has a right to bodily integrity and
> to the means necessary for the proper development of life,
> particularly food, clothing, shelter, medical care, rest, and
> finally, the necessary social services. In consequence, he has
> the right to be looked after in the event of ill-health, disability
> and old age[725].

---

[720] Cfr. PONTIFICAL COUNCIL FOR JUSTICE AND PEACE, Compendium of the...,
n. 107.

[721] E. SGRECCIA, *Personalist Bioethics – Foundations and Applications*, J. A. DI
Camillo – M. J. Miller (trans.), The National Catholic Bioethics Center,
Philadelphia 2012, 58.

[722] Cfr. R. FRATTALLONE, *Persona*, in S. LEONE – S. PRIVITERA (eds.), *Nuovo
Dizionario di Bioetica*, Città Nuova, Firenze 2004,856-863.

[723] Cfr. Ibid.

[724] P. GATELY – A. BECK – D. A. JONES, *Healthcare Allocation &...*, 29.

[725] JOHN XXIII, «*Pacem in Terris*, Encyclical Letter of on Establishing Universal

The same solemnity accorded to the dignity of the human person determines our reaction to the needs of every human being, his spiritual, social, economic and health care needs.

Answering the question concerning the basis for human equality among individuals, the Catechism of the Catholic Church states: "Created in the image of the one God and equally endowed with rational souls, all men have the same nature and the same origin [...] all therefore enjoy an equal dignity"[726]. Hence, the dignity of every human person does not depend on a person's economic or health condition, age, gender and social stratification. Each person is created in the image and likeness of God and is endowed with the dignity of the human person, which should be simply recognized, respected and safeguarded. In fact, according to the Catholic reflection "every human being has intrinsic, equal and inalienable dignity or worth, deserving uncompromising reverence and respect"[727]. For this, the Church affirms that some social inequalities are contrary to justice and to the dignity of the human person[728].

The Encyclical Letter *Pacem in Terris* continuing on human rights affirms: "The possession of rights involves the duty of implementing those rights, for they are expression of a man's personal dignity"[729]. Right to health care is a fundamental right that accompanies the fundamental and inalienable right to life. Failure to implement the right to health has the consequence of violating the dignity of the human person. The evaluation of the lackadaisical attitudes often noticed in some health care systems demonstrate how "poor care is always a failure to acknowledge the dignity of the patient as a person"[730]. In contrast to the aforementioned attitudes,

---

Peace», in Truth, Justice, Charity, and Liberty, n. 11, (1963), in C. CARLEN (ed.), *The Papal Encyclicals 1958-1981*, The Pierian Press, United States of America 1981,107-129.

[726] THE CATECHISM OF ..., n. 1934, 461.

[727] P. GATELY – A. BECK – D. A. JONES, *Healthcare Allocation &...*, 30.

[728] Cfr. THE CATECHISM OF..., n. 1938, 462; Cfr. CONCILIO VATICANO II, *Gaudium et Spes*, Costituzione Pastorale Sulla Chiesa nel Mondo Contemporaneo, n. 29, § 3, Testo ufficiale e traduzione italiana, Libreria Editrice Vaticana, Città del Vaticano 1998, 899-900.

[729] JOHN XXIII, «*Pacem in Terris*, Encyclical Letter of on Establishing Universal Peace», in Truth, Justice, Charity, and Liberty, n. 44, (1963), in C. CARLEN (ed.), *The Papal Encyclicals...*

[730] P. GATELY – A. BECK – D. A. JONES, *Healthcare Allocation &...*, 30.

the Church gives clues on the assessment of societal actions in reference to social justice: "Society ensures social justice when it respects the dignity and rights of the person as the proper end of the society itself"[731]. A society can be recognized as one that pursues social justice when it strives to respect the dignity of every human person and provides the conditions that permit every individual to obtain what is his or her due. The fundamental right to health regards the value of justice according to which there cannot be any distinction between persons owing to the objective situations of life[732].

The principle of the dignity of the human person together with the principle of respect for human life is the "driving force for care, and constitutive ground of human justice"[733]. In the social teaching of the Catholic Church, as already mentioned, the right to health care and the fundamental right to life are like two sides of the same coin. One cannot be preferred at the expense of the other. The state and the members of the society have the moral obligation to defend the lives of its members. The statement of the National Association of Pro-Life Nurses on health care Legislation aptly captures our assertion: "those lives and all lives are vulnerable and to be respected and cared for the best of our abilities. Care must be provided for any human being in need of care regardless of disability or level of function or dependence on others"[734]. Life is a gift from God; our responsibility is that of stewardship. Hence, any form of mistreating our own life/health or that of others is morally wrong. W. E. May, commenting on the unchangeable teaching of the Catholic Church on human life writes: "God the Lord of life has entrusted to men the noble mission of safeguarding life, and men must carry it out in a manner worthy of themselves. Life must be protected with the utmost care"[735].

According to the teaching of Pope John XXIII, each state must "have as its special aim the recognition, respect, safeguarding and promotion of the rights of the human person"[736]. To achieve an appreciable distribution

---

[731] Cfr. THE CATECHISM OF…, nn. 1929-1930, 460.

[732] Cfr. PONTIFICIO CONSIGLIO PER GLI OPERATORI SANITARI, *Nuova Carta degli…*, 114.

[733] J. F. NAUMANN – R. W. FINN, «*Principles of Catholic…*».

[734] *The statement of National Association of Pro-Life Nurses on health care Legislation* in www.nursesforlife.org/napnstatement.pdf [27-07-2017].

[735] W. E. MAY, *Catholic Bioethics and the human life*, Our Sunday Visitor Inc., Huntington, Indiana 2000, 152.

[736] JOHN XXIII, «*Pacem in Terris*, Encyclical Letter of on Establishing Universal

of health care resources, there is the need to respect the right to health, thus the dignity of every human person, especially that of the poor and the most vulnerable. When the right to health is not respected, there is no way the state can respect the right to life. "In 1994 Richard D. Lamm, former governor of Colorado wrote that health care system must change its model from the "individual patient" to the "population as a whole" and from "governed professionally" to "governed managerially"[737] in order to increase the access to and lower cost of health care. This is an erroneous interpretation of health as a common good. Perhaps, it is apparent why in 1984 Lamm said: "elderly people who are terminally ill have a 'duty to die and get out of the way"[738]. With Lamm's idea, the dignity of the human person is replaced with the assessment of human life and health on benefits and monetary basis. With this mentality, the vulnerable and those in need of care will be left to suffer and die unnecessarily because their lives are considered to have no cash value.

The Catechism of the Catholic Church defines justice as a virtue that consists in the firm and constant will to give to others their due[739]. Respecting the dignity of the human person by allowing them to exercise their right to health and have equal access to care is the observance of the definition and nature of justice. "The human *person* is and ought to be the principle, the subject and the end of all social institutions"[740]. When an institution loses sight of the human person and anchors the distribution of its health resources on principles that contradict the principle of the dignity of the human person, such society cannot act justly and can hardly have an ethical health care system. Such idea leads to the *depersonalisation* of health care and cannot be morally permissible. "The dignity of a person must be recognized in every human being from conception to natural death"[741].

Peace», in Truth, Justice, Charity, and Liberty, n. 139, (1963), in C. CARLEN (ed.), *The Papal Encyclicals...*

[737] Cfr. R. A. CAPONE, «AMA Reconsiders opposition to physician-assisted suicide», in *Ethics & Medics*, 41(2016), 1-3; R. D. LAMM, «Saint Martin of Tours in a New World of Medical Ethics», *Cambridge Quarterly of Healthcare Ethics* 3.2 (1994), 159-167.

[738] R. A. CAPONE, «AMA Reconsiders opposition...».

[739] Cfr. THE CATECHISM OF..., n. 1836, 445.

[740] Ibid., n. 1881, 453.

[741] CONGREGATION FOR THE DOCTRINE OF THE FAITH, «Instruction Dignitas personae on Certain Bioethical Question» in E. J. FURTON – P. J. CATALDO – A.

4.1.2. The Principles of Common Good and Solidarity

The social doctrine of the Catholic Church promotes the principle of the common good. According to the Church's doctrine, common good is achieved where there are complete social conditions which permit and facilitate the full realization of people either as groups or as individuals[742]. This idea of the common good, which is also present in the Vatican II document, *"Guadium et Spes"*[743] "presupposes respect for the person as such"[744]. This implies that in the distribution of health care resources, which is a vital part of the common good, "the public authorities are bound to respect the fundamental and inalienable rights of the human person"[745]. Doing this is essential for the public authorities because "the attainment of common good is the sole reason for the existence of civil authorities"[746]. In addition, the civil authority cannot claim to promote common good without respecting the dignity of the human person, because following the Catholic doctrine "for the common good, since it is intimately bound up with human nature, can never exist fully and completely unless the human person is taken into account at all times"[747]. Not respecting the rights and dignity of the human person may lead to a *denaturalization* of the common good since it is in its nature "that every single citizen has the right in it"[748]. Pope Francis likewise evidences that the authentic human development has a moral character. Thus, it presumes full respect for the human person[749]. The common good essentially respects and promotes the fundamental rights of the person. This concretely consists in making "accessible to each what is needed to lead a truly human life: food, clothing, health, work,

---

S. MORACZEWSKI (eds.) *Catholic Health Care...*, 411-423[2].

[742] Cfr. THE CATECHISM OF..., n. 1906, 457.

[743] Cfr. CONCILIO VATICANO II, *Gauduim et Spes*, nn. 26, § 1, Libreria Editrice Vaticana, Città del Vaticano 1998, 892.

[744] THE CATECHISM OF..., n. 1907, 457.

[745] Ibid.

[746] JOHN XXIII, «*Pacem in Terris*, Encyclical Letter of on Establishing Universal Peace», in Truth, Justice, Charity, and Liberty, n. 54, (1963), in C. CARLEN (ed.), *The Papal Encyclicals...*

[747] Ibid., n.56.

[748] Ibid., n. 55.

[749] FRANCIS, «*Laudato Sì Lettera* Enciclica Sulla Cura della Casa Comune», n. 5, Paoline Editoriale Libri, Milano 2015, 5.

education and culture, suitable information, the right to establish family and so on"[750].

It is accepted that the government cannot provide every health care need for everyone, but the principle of common good as we have seen indicates that the primary duty of government is to make accessible to each person what he/she needs to lead a truly and dignified human life. Basic health needs are a vital point without which we cannot talk of leading a truly dignified human life. In the same vein, the Catechism of the Catholic Church rightly points out that the common good is always oriented towards the progress of persons and that "the order of things must be subordinate to the order of persons, and not the other way around"[751]. This is one of the major qualities missing in most parts of the world, where in politics, the syndromes of corruption and selfishness thwart the efforts of the states to respect the above mentioned order which "is founded on truth, built up in justice and animated by love"[752].

Corruption is a great enemy of common good and should be condemned and possibly eradicated from politics in many countries and societies if they want a health system where the good of all and of each person is promoted. The following Church's teaching aptly capture such notion:

> As with any ethical obligation, the participation of all in realizing the common good calls for a continually conversion of the social partners. Fraud and other subterfuges, by which some people evade the constraints of the law and the prescription of societal obligation, must be firmly condemned because they are incompatible with the requirements of justice[753].

The political leaders need to understand that it is a moral obligation to realize the common good. Therefore, the political leaders are to lead by example, embracing conversion to justice and abhorring selfishness, corruption and injustice in their activities of stewardship. This implies being diligent in their duty of promoting and sustaining the policies, programmes and practices that improve the conditions of health and human life. Often the government abandons the Federal Ministry of health in Nigeria, the

---

[750] THE CATECHISM OF…, n. 1908, 457.

[751] Ibid., n. 1912, 458.

[752] Ibid.

[753] Ibid., n. 1917, 459.

doctors who work in the public hospitals are not paid and the hospitals and health centres are abandoned in unhygienic and deplorable conditions. This is not a good example of common good. The principle of common good is closely related to the principle of solidarity, which encourages help given to persons in need, thus being altruists and not egoists. John Paul II teaches that solidarity is "a firm and persevering determination to commit oneself to common good. That is to say to the good of all and of each individual, because we are all really responsible for all"[754]. The principle of solidarity invites everyone to be persons unselfishly concerned for the welfare of all. "Men, both as individual and as intermediate groups, are required to make their own specific contributions to the general welfare"[755]. In line with this Pope's teaching, two American prelates, J. F. Naumann and R. W. Finn explain solidarity in the following terms: "Our sense of "connectedness" to each other person, and moves us to want for them what we would want for ourselves and our most dear loved ones"[756].

Solidarity can be practiced not only by giving aid but also by renouncing what is due to us. In fact it is retained morally licit when one stops burdensome and overzealous medical treatments. This attitude demonstrates our commitment to solidarity which reminds us of our stewardship of health resources which should be done in fairness to others[757]. This thought is epitomized in the following teaching of Pope Paul VI: "the more fortunate should renounce some of their rights so as to place their goods more generously at the service of others"[758]. The Pope encourages solidarity, which spurs those who have more to renounce some of their rights for the sake of the vulnerable and those in need. For some

---

[754] JOHN PAUL II, «*Sollicitudo Rei Socialis,*Encyclical Letter Letter n.36, (1987), for the twentieth anniversary of *Populorum Progressio*», in J. M. MILLER (ed.),*The Encyclicals of John Paul II*, Our Sunday Visitor Publishing Division – Our Sunday Visitor Inc., Huntington, Indiana 1996, 425-477.

[755] JOHN XXIII, «*Pacem in Terris*, Encyclical Letter of on Establishing Universal Peace», in Truth, Justice, Charity, and Liberty, n. 53, (1963), in C. CARLEN (ed.), *The Papal Encyclicals...*

[756] J. F. NAUMANN – R. W. FINN, «Principles of Catholic...».

[757] Cfr. R. A. CAPONE, «AMA Reconsiders opposition...».

[758] PAUL VI, «*Octogesima Adveniens*, Apostolic Letter, On the Occasion of the Eightieth Anniversary of the Encyclical "Rerum Novarum"», n. 23, in http://w2.vatican.va/content/paul-vi/en/apost_letters/documents/hf_p-vi_apl_19710514_octogesima-adveniens.html [10-02-2018].

authors of Catholic bioethics, the Popes' statements encourages voluntary renunciation of rights which could help to set limits to some forms of medical research and treatments that consume resources that could be used for the basic health care provision for others[759]. According to these authors, the principle of common good together with solidarity applied to health care implies the universal provision of basic health services. Common good guarantees access to the basic human rights, which include food, education, clothing, work, quality basic health care etc.[760]. Just distribution of health care and other goods according to the Catholic reflection is a way of manifesting solidarity, which spurs from human and Christian brotherhood[761].

Man is a social and not a solitary being. Consequently, it will be difficult for any individual to live or develop his potentials without being in relation with others. "Solidarity highlights in a particular way the intrinsic social nature of the human person, the equality of all in dignity and rights and the common path of individuals and peoples towards an ever more committed unity"[762]. This gives more reasons for the four Catholic principles of justice that invite humanity to live a just and sane social-connectedness, being our brother's keeper. In fact, the common good depends on such healthy social-connectedness. The Universal Church teaches that "the different human societies also must establish among themselves relationship of solidarity, communication and cooperation, in the service of man and the common good"[763].

For a society to be at the service of human beings, it must have as its primary goal the common good which implies the "the good of all people and of the whole person"[764]. The common good is the responsibility of everyone[765]. This means that every member of society should be involved in the commitment to common good and in its attainment. Thus every member of society which intends to attain common good should imbibe the attitude, acquire the capacity and make effort to "seek the good of

---

[759]   Cfr. P. GATELY – A. BECK – D. A. JONES, *Healthcare Allocation &...*, 31.
[760]   Cfr. Ibid., 34.
[761]   Cfr. THE CATECHISM OF..., n. 1939, 462.
[762]   PONTIFICAL COUNCIL FOR JUSTICE AND PEACE, *Compendium of the...*, n. 192, 109.
[763]   Ibid., n. 150, 83.
[764]   Ibid., n. 165, 93.
[765]   Cfr. Ibid., n. 133, 74.

others as though it were one's own good"[766]. The principle of common good understood in accordance with the Catholic doctrine enjoins that each person should see the other's health care as his or her own health care. This rare altruistic habit should inspire the actions of the members of the society in the distribution of health care resources and in seeing that the poor and the needy are not abandoned in their miserable conditions.

Common good requires that people should enjoy the resources distributed in justice and fairness. The Compendium of the Social Doctrine of the Church explains this issue citing the following teaching of Pope Pius XI:

> The distribution of created goods, which, as every discerning person knows, is labouring today under the gravest evils due to the huge disparity between the few exceedingly rich and the unnumbered propertyless, must be effectively called back to and brought into conformity with the norms of the common good, that is, social justice[767].

Common good entails in this sense fairness in health care resource allocation. The inequality between the rich and the poor, the urban and the rural and other forms of inequalities that reflect injustice in health care distribution should be reduced and eliminated entirely where possible[768]. Everyone should be involved in the commitment to the common good, but the state should specifically lead the movement. In fact, since common good is the reason for the existence of the state[769] any state that has no intention of attaining common good has no reason to exist. Health care allocation is the responsibility of the state which should endeavour to do this in fairness. This implies making sure that no one is left without the basic health care needs and health needs. "The goal of life in society is in fact the historically attainable common good"[770].

---

[766] Ibid., n. 167, 95.

[767] Pius XI, «*Quadragesimo Anno*, Encyclical Letter on Reconstruction of the Social Order, n. 49 (1931)», in C. Carlen (ed.), *The Papal Encyclicals...*, 415-443.

[768] Cfr. Pontifical Council for Justice and Peace, *Compendium of the...*, n. 167, 95.

[769] Cfr. Ibid., n. 168, 95.

[770] Ibid.

While pursuing the common good, man should, however, not lose sight of the ultimate end of the person, which is God the creator. So common good should not be deprived of its transcendental dimension that goes beyond the historical dimension[771]. The universal right to use of the goods of the earth, which is based on the principle of universal destination of goods affirms that every human person must have access to such well-being necessary for his or her full development. This underlies the reason why the right to the common use of good is considered the first principle of the social order. Following the above affirmations, no one should be denied access to the use of common good. Therefore, we affirm that health as a common good should be accessible to all.

4.1.3. The Principle of Preferential Option for the Poor and the Vulnerable

Preferential option for the poor and the vulnerable is one of the key concepts of Catholic belief. The Bible and most of the parables told by Jesus present "an assertion that in human history the Christian God is on the side of the poor and oppressed, and poses a challenge and judgement to the rich and powerful"[772]. The Catholic health care ethics invites us to dedicate more attention to the health care needs of the poor, the uninsured, the underinsured and all those who cannot afford their basic health needs by themselves. Such ethics is motivated by the biblical injunctions, especially on the invitation of Jesus: "I was ill and you cared for me" [Mt 25:36]. "The biblical mandate to care for the poor requires us to express this in concrete action at all levels of Catholic health care. This mandate prompts us to work to ensure that our country's health care delivery system provides adequate health care for the poor"[773]. Pope Francis hopes in the establishment of social initiative that can give the poor regular access to basic resources like health care goods and he notes that so far, the world has failed in this[774].

---

[771] Cfr. Ibid., n. 170, 96.

[772] P. GATELY – A. BECK – D. A. JONES, *Healthcare Allocation &...*, 32.

[773] UNITED STATES CONFERENCE OF CATHOLIC BISHOPS, «*Ethical and Religious...*», 389-400².

[774] Cfr. FRANCIS, «*Laudato Sì Lettera...*», n. 109.

The poor and most vulnerable were always at the center of Jesus' preaching for social justice and Jesus always identified with them [Matthew 25, 31-46; Matthew 11, 4-6; Luke 6, 21-22; Luke 8, 47; Luke 16, 1-9]. Pope Leo XIII in his encyclical letter *Rerum Novarum* called for attention for the poor, emphasizing that workers should receive just wages and work in conditions that reflect the principle of dignity of the human person[775]. The Catholic social doctrine in accordance to Jesus' teaching has always invited the governments, Catholic and non-Catholic health workers to give more attention to those whose social conditions forced to the margins of our society, the vulnerable who are victims of discrimination and other forms of injustice. Their rights to health care should be safeguarded and their equal access to and utilization of quality health care resources must be guaranteed. Pope Francis describes the issue of providing health care for the poor as a global "social debt"[776]. Expressing this as the duty of the governments, John XXIII writes: "Considerations of justice and equity can a times demand that those in power pay more attention to the weaker members of society, since these are at a disadvantage when it comes to defending their own rights and asserting their legitimate interests"[777].

Defending the poor and the vulnerable is a duty demanded by justice. Pope Paul VI in his teaching on the principle of the preferential option for the poor and the vulnerable writes: "Legislation is necessary, but it is not sufficient for setting up true relationships of justice and equity. In teaching us charity, the Gospel instructs us in the preferential respect due to the poor and the special situation they have in society"[778].The mainstream Catholic theological vision wants health care resources to be allocated fairly with special attention to the poor and the vulnerable. The Church teaches that authentic human society requires respect for justice and that charity, which requires and facilitates the practice of justice, is the greatest social commandment[779]. The United States Bishops as recalled by Pope Francis invite all to give greater attention to the needs of the poor, the weak and

---

[775] Cfr. LEO XIII, «*Rerum Novarum*, Encyclical Letter on Capital and Labour (1891) », nn. 1-64, in C. CARLEN (ed.), The Papal Encyclicals..., 241-261.

[776] FRANCIS, «*Laudato Sì Lettera...*», n. 30, 25.

[777] JOHN XXIII, «*Pacem in Terris*, Encyclical Letter of on Establishing Universal Peace», in Truth, Justice, Charity, and Liberty, n. 56, (1963), in C. CARLEN (ed.), *The Papal Encyclicals...*

[778] PAUL VI, «*Octagesima Adveniens*, Apostolic...»., n. 23.

[779] THE CATECHISM OF..., nn. 1886-1889, 453-454.

the vulnerable[780]. Similarly, the Italian Episcopal Conference calls for attention to the situation of suffering and pains. Such attention should have no limits following the spirit of the parable of the Good Samaritan. The bishops remind Christians of the injunction by Christ to love ourselves and to be responsible for the life and health of one another[781].

Some already mentioned Catholic authors indicate the duty of the policy makers concerning the poor and the vulnerable: "The concept of the preferential option for the poor challenges policy makers, and this means that the Church should challenge the dogmatic introduction of market forces into a healthcare setting where this militates against the poorest in society"[782]. Preferential option for the poor and the vulnerable is supported by other important principles of Catholic social thoughts contained in the principles of solidarity and common good. These principles encourage care for the most vulnerable members of the society, "whether they are vulnerable because of their stage of human development, a chronic illness, their economic stratum, or another difference"[783]. People in these conditions, "in spite of the limitations and sufferings affecting their bodies and faculties, they point up more clearly the dignity and greatness of man"[784]. Being poor or vulnerable does not reduce the dignity of the person in this condition and does not imply that he or she merits less or inferior quality of health care. Appreciating the immense dignity of the poor and the vulnerable according to Pope Francis, today, is an ethical imperative essential for effectively attaining the common good[785]. Preferential option for the poor and the vulnerable is a logical application of the common good. The above affirmation emphasizes the concern for the vulnerable and the attitude of the society towards them in health care distribution and it recalls the proverb: "A nation's greatness is measured by how it treats its

---

[780] FRANCIS, «*Laudato Sì*, Lettera...», n. 52, 40.

[781] Cfr. CONFERENZA EPISCOPALE ITALIANA, Ufficio Nazionale per la pastorale della salute, Messaggio per XXVI Giornata Mondiale del Malato, 11 febbraio 2018.

[782] P. GATELY – A. BECK – D. A. JONES, *Healthcare Allocation &...*, 33-34.

[783] R. A. CAPONE, «AMA Reconsiders opposition...».

[784] JOHN PAUL II, «*Laborem Exercens*, Encyclical Letter on Human Work», n. 22 (1981), in J. M. MILLER (ed.), *The Encyclicals of John Paul II*, Our Sunday Visitor Publishing Division – Our Sunday Visitor Inc., Huntington, Indiana 1996, 165-214.

[785] Cfr. FRANCIS, «*Laudato Sì*, Lettera...», n. 158, 120-121.

weakest members"[786]. Helping the poor and the vulnerable is not an option but a basic question of justice.

4.1.4. The Principle of Subsidiarity

The principle of subsidiarity "is among the most constant and characteristic directives of the Church's social doctrine"[787]. The principle implies helping them in what they cannot do but not substituting them in what they can do. The *compendium of the social doctrine of the Church*, citing the Papal Encyclical *Quadragesimo Anno*, underlines that the principle of subsidiarity is retained as "the most important principle of "social philosophy"[788]. According to the document of the Church's doctrine, based on the principle of subsidiarity, "all societies of a superior order must adopt attitudes of help (*"subsidium"*) – therefore of support, promotion, development – with respect to lower-order societies"[789]. The Catholic social teaching sustains giving aid to the most vulnerable without suppressing their human dignity. We maintain that the principle of subsidiarity is very important in health justice and renders the distribution of health care resources just and more appreciable when it is founded on the fundamental principle of the dignity of the human person. Pope John Paul II asserts the principle of subsidiarity. His view concerning this principle is expressed in his encyclical letter *Centesimus Annus*, to mark the 100th anniversary of Pope Leo XIII's *Rerum Novarum*. According to his teachings:

> A community of higher order should not interfere in the internal life of a community of a lower order, depriving the latter of its functions, but rather should support it in the case of need and help co-ordinate its activity with the activities of the rest of society, always with a view to the common good[790].

---

[786] J. F. NAUMANN – R. W. FINN, «Principles of Catholic…».

[787] PONTIFICAL COUNCIL FOR JUSTICE AND PEACE, *Compendium of the…*, n. 185, 104.

[788] Cfr. Ibid., n. 186, 105.

[789] Ibid., n. 186, 105.

[790] JOHN PAUL II, «*Centesimus Annus*, Encyclical Letter on The Hundredth Anniversary of *Rerum Novarum*», n. 48, (1991), in J. M. MILLER (ed.), *The Encyclicals of…*, 587-650.

Helping others in what they cannot do and not substituting them in what they can do is an essential quality of this principle. This means that each person should try as much as he or she can to do for himself or herself what is possible. It also means that each person should be responsible for his or her health where he or she can. The vulnerable, that is those who are not capable of helping themselves, should be assisted in accordance with the principles of subsidiarity, respecting their dignity. Pope Benedict XVI points out the most essential quality of the principle of subsidiarity by emphasizing that it respects personal dignity because it recognizes in the person a subject who is capable of offering something of his own to others[791]. Subsidiarity according to his teaching is primarily the help given to the human person through the autonomy of intermediate bodies. This principle is symbolized in the acts of charity and is guided by the criterion of fraternal cooperation that exists between believers and non-believers[792]. The Catholic notion of subsidiarity in health care according to J. F Naumann and R. W. Finn includes determining health care at the lowest level rather that at the higher strata of society. The Catholic Prelates indicate:

> Subsidiarity is that principle by which we respect the inherent dignity and freedom of the individual by never doing for others what they can do for themselves and thus enabling individuals to have the most possible discretion in the affairs of their lives[793].

These authors reecho the warning of recent Popes that sweeping the principle of subsidiarity under the carpet "can lead to an excessive centralization of human services, which in turn leads to excessive costs and loss of personal responsibility and quality of care"[794]. Pope John Paul II calls for attention to the right application of this principle because it's wrong application will worsen the condition of the poor. The Pope's invitation to precaution is expressed in the following words:

---

[791] Cfr. BENEDICT XVI, «*Caritas in Veritate*», Lettera Enciclica, Sullo Sviluppo Umano Integrale nella Carità e nella Verità, n. 57, Libreria Editrice Vaticana, Città del Vaticano 2009, 95-96.

[792] Cfr. Ibid., n. 57, 95-96.

[793] J. F. NAUMANN − R. W. FINN, «Principles of Catholic…».

[794] Ibid.

> By intervening directly and depriving society of its responsibility,
> the Social Assistance State leads to a loss of human energies
> and an inordinate increase of public agencies, which are
> dominated more by bureaucratic ways of thinking than by
> concern for serving their clients, and which are accompanied
> by an enormous increase in spending[795].

The caution by the Pope shows the delicate nature of this principle. There is the need to be prudent especially in the application of this principle to the distribution of health care resources because health is an important element that is intrinsically connected to life. The Catholic teaching retains that subsidiarity cannot be separated from the important principle of the dignity of the human person. If this separation occurs, it means the principle will be lost and it will become a mere bureaucracy, which does not help those in need but may rather worsen their situations. The Universal authority according to John XIII should not interfere in the sphere of action of the public authority of the individual states, thus arrogating their functions and limiting their duties. "On the contrary, its essential purpose is to create world conditions in which the public authorities of each nation, its citizens and intermediate groups, can carry out their task, fulfill their duties and claim their rights with greater security"[796]. The public authorities of individual states should not be substituted but helped to carry out their duties in fairness. This teaching is affirmed by the Catholic social teaching, which in accordance to the principle of subsidiarity urges the community of a higher order not to interfere in the internal affairs of a community of a lower order, depriving the latter of its function, except in the bid to support the society of lower order in case of need and help. This should always be done with a view to the common good[797].

The call for attention against derailment in the application of this principle has always been in the teaching of the Church. Pope Pius XI in his Encyclical Letter recommended that: "every social activity ought

---

[795] JOHN PAUL II, «*Centesimus Annus*, Encyclical Letter on The Hundredth Anniversary of *Rerum Novarum*», n. 48, (1991), in J. M. MILLER (ed.), *The Encyclicals of...*

[796] JOHN XXIII, «*Pacem in Terris*, Encyclical Letter of on Establishing Universal Peace», in Truth, Justice, Charity, and Liberty, n. 140, (1963), in C. CARLEN (ed.), *The Papal Encyclicals...*

[797] Cfr. THE CATECHISM OF..., n. 1883, 453.

of its very nature to furnish help to the members of the body social, and never destroy and absorb them"[798]. The warnings by the Popes draw attention to the function of the principle of subsidiarity to protect people from abuses by higher-level social authority. The principle also reminds the higher authorities of their duty to assist and encourage the individuals and intermediate groups to carry out diligently their duties[799]. The absence of the principle of subsidiarity may lead to the suppression and non-acknowledgement of private initiative. This injures the dignity of the person whose right to express himself through his personal capability is denied. The principle of subsidiarity encourages every individual to contribute to the common good. On the one hand, it is true that every individual has the right to enjoy the common good; on the other hand, it is right and just for every individual according to his or her capacity to contribute to the common good. Rights are rightly accompanied by duties and this is one of the "appropriate methods for making citizens more responsible in actively "being a part" of the political and social reality of their country"[800].

4.2. The Competence of the Magisterium in Proffering Solutions to Problems in the Secular Spheres: Focus on the distribution of Health Care Resources in the Nigerian Health System

Some ask if the Catholic Church has the professional competence in the secular fields like health, politics and economics, to warrant her offering technical solutions to problems in these areas. Such question may be directed to us by asking if our dissertation is claiming the Catholic principles are better and more efficient than the economic and political policies, health plans and programmes and laws on ground in Nigeria? If we are claiming that the Catholic Magisterium is more competent than the Federal Ministry of Health Nigeria and the Nigerian government in handling distribution of health care resources? Why do we think the

---

[798] PIUS XI, «*Quadragesimo Anno*, Encyclical Letter on Reconstruction of the Social Order, n. 49 (1931)», in C. CARLEN (ed.), *The Papal Encyclicals...*

[799] Cfr. PONTIFICAL COUNCIL FOR JUSTICE AND PEACE, *Compendium of the...*, 187, 105-106.

[800] Ibid., n. 187, 106.

Magisterial teaching can work where Nigerian government's attempts have failed?

It is clear that when the Catholic Magisterium treats problems pertinent to the above-mentions spheres of human reality, it does not do this as an expert in these disciplines that proffers technical analysis or solutions. The contribution of the Magisterium can be described as a moral vision of the social reality. In the same way, this doctoral thesis intends to be a moral vision of the social realities of Nigeria considered in chapter one and chapter two of the same doctoral thesis. This as we have preannounced is to be done in the light of the Catholic principles. The ethical perspective according to the Church is indispensable. Pope Francis in agreement with this view advocates: "we see the need for an increased awareness of our ethical responsibility toward humanity"[801]. The Pope reinterates: "While the Church applauds every effort in research and application directed to care of our suffering brothers and sisters, she is also mindful of the basic that "not everything technically possible or adorable is thereby ethically acceptable"[802]. Coming from one with professional knowledge or being technically feasible does not give a solution an all-encompassing quality. The global view of man could be easily acquired through an ethical procedure. We would like to give further responses by taping from the richness of the Catholic doctrine. Pope John Paul II addressed similar questions stating:

> The Church does not have technical revolutions to offer for the problem of under development as such, as Pope Paul VI already affirmed in his Encyclical. For the Church does not propose economic and political systems or programs, nor does she show preference for one or the other, provided that human dignity is properly respected and promoted, and provided she herself is allowed the room she needs to exercise her ministry in the world[803].

---

[801] FRANCIS, Unite to care, «Address to the International Conference on Regenerative Medicine, April 28, 2018», in *The National Catholic Bioethics Quarterly*, 18(2018), The National Catholic Bioethics Center, Philadelphia, 503-505.

[802] Ibid.

[803] JOHN PAUL II, «*Sollicitudo Rei Socialis*, Encyclical Letter, (1987), for the twentieth anniversary of *Populorum Progressio*», n. 41, in J. M. MILLER (ed.), *The Encyclicals of...*

Paul VI maintains that the Church is an "expert in humanity"[804], for this, even when she does not fully give technical solutions to the challenges of the world today, she renders services to all the peoples of the world by teaching them about the truth, justice and love. The social doctrine of the church has always thought that whatever affects the dignity of the human persons cannot be seen as a mere technical issue because such simplification would not give, but rather, hide the real quality and identity of such issues, thereby paving way for reductionism "and this would be an act of betrayal of the individuals and peoples whom development is meant to serve"[805]. Paul VI insists that when treating the issue of development and obviously matters regarding the distribution of health care resources in a country like Nigeria, our decision "cannot be restricted to economic growth alone. To be authentic, it must be well rounded; it must foster the development of each man and of the whole man"[806]. Those who uphold the utilitarian principle in Nigeria would not accept this view because it is not gain oriented. But what Paul VI teaches is the truth about man and the satisfaction of his quest for happiness. Surely, the Church does not force anyone to accept her teaching but addresses her message "to faithful of the Catholic world, and to all men of good al will"[807]. There are many in Nigeria who are non-Catholics, but will find the principles proposed by our dissertation very interesting because they are people of good will. More so, because it appeals to reason and it is credible.

John Paul II tries to prove the legitimacy of the interventions of the Church "about the nature, conditions, requirements and aims of authentic development, and also about the obstacles which stand in its way"[808] declaring that, "in doing so, the Church fulfils her mission to evangelize, for she offers her first contribution to the solution of the urgent problems

---

[804] Paulo VI, «*Populorum Progressio*, Encyclical letter (1967),» n. 13, in http://w2.vatican.va/content/paul-vi/en/encyclicals/documents/hf_p-vi_enc_26031967_populorum.html [11-12-2019].

[805] John Paul II, «*Sollicitudo Rei Socialis*, Encyclical Letter, (1987), for the twentieth anniversary of *Populorum Progressio*», n. 41, in J. M. Miller (ed.), *The Encyclicals of...*

[806] Paulo VI, «*Populorum Progressio*, Encyclical letter (1967)», n. 14.

[807] Ibid., n.1.

[808] John Paul II, «*Sollicitudo Rei Socialis*, Encyclical Letter, (1987), for the twentieth anniversary of *Populorum Progressio*», n. 41, in J. M. Miller (ed.), *The Encyclicals of...*

of development [...] As her instrument for reaching this goal, the Church uses her social doctrine"[809]. There are so many people in Nigeria afflicted by poverty and some are denied their right to health care and access to health needs. The lack of recognition of the dignity of every human person creates a big moral questions in Nigeria. Accordingly, we are offering our contribution to the solution of these problems by proposing the application of the Catholic principles to the distribution of health care resources in Nigeria. John Paul II also prefers the application of the Catholic principles to social realities because he think they help to obtain lasting solutions. According to him:

> In today's difficult situation, a more exact awareness and a wider diffusion of the "set of principles for reflection, criteria for judgment and directives for action" proposed by the Church's teaching would be of great help in promoting both the correct definition of the problems being faced and the best solution to them[810].

The Church's social teaching does not represent in anyway her intention to claim to be better in spheres of competence of the state or other institutions, but as Pope Paul VI aptly remarks, the Church: "Has long experience in human affairs [...] sharing the noblest aspirations of men and suffering when she sees these aspirations not satisfied, she wishes to help them attain their full realization. So she offers man her distinctive contribution: a global perspective on man and human realities"[811]. The Catholic social doctrine is not an ideology, neither is it a set ideas in defence of the Catholic faith.

> But rather the accurate formulation of the results of a careful reflection on the complex realities of human existence, in society and in the international order, in the light of faith and of the Church's tradition [...] And since it is a doctrine aimed at guiding people's behavior, it consequently gives rise to a "commitment to justice," according to each individual's role, vocation and circumstances[812].

---

[809] Ibid., n. 41.

[810] Ibid., n. 41.

[811] PAULO VI, «*Populorum Progressio*, Encyclical letter (1967)», n. 13.

[812] JOHN PAUL II, «*Sollicitudo Rei Socialis*, Encyclical Letter, (1987), for the

The social doctrine of the Catholic Church is prompted by sense of responsibilty as revealed by John Paul II: "Pastoral solicitude also prompts me to propose analysis of some events of recent history"[813]. The Pope also asserts: "Part of the responsibility of Pastors is to give care consideration to current events in order to discern the new requirements of evangelization. However, such an analysis is not meant to pass definitive judgements since this does not fall *per se* within the Magisterium's specific domain"[814].

The Second Vatican Council's document, *Gaudium et Spes* presents a scenario identical to the Nigerian setting where "the order of values is jumbled and bad is mixed with the good, individuals and groups pay heed solely to their own interests, and not to those of others. Thus it happens that the world ceases to be a place of true brotherhood"[815]. Issues like corruptions and poverty related problem such as hospital detention and the denial of basic health care needs to the poorest and the most vulnerable are situations which represent the face of the Nigerian health care system. The involvement of the Catholic principles in the Nigerian health care resource allocation we think is very important because the Church, "trusting in the design of the Creator, acknowledges that human progress can serve man's true happiness"[816]. Hence, she proposes a realistic and ethical vision of the social reality to help people live happily as willed by God. In accordance with this view, Pope Paul VI enumerates conditions that do not favour the human dignity and others that indicate its recognition:

> What are less than human conditions? The material poverty of those who lack the bare necessities of life, and the moral poverty of those who are crushed under the weight of their own self-love; oppressive political structures resulting from the abuse of ownership or the improper exercise of power, from the exploitation of the worker or unjust transactions. What are truly human conditions? The rise from poverty to the acquisition

---

twentieth anniversary of *Populorum Progressio*», n. 41, in J. M. MILLER (ed.), *The Encyclicals of...*

[813] JOHN PAUL II, «*Centesimus Annus*, Encyclical Letter on The Hundredth Anniversary of *Rerum Novarum*», n. 3, (1991), in J. M. MILLER (ed.), *The Encyclicals of...*

[814] Ibid., n.3.

[815] CONCILIO VATICANO II, *Gauduim et Spes* ..., n.37.

[816] Ibid., 37

of life's necessities; the elimination of social ills; broadening
the horizons of knowledge; acquiring refinement and culture.
From there one can go on to acquire a growing awareness of
other people's dignity, a taste for the spirit of poverty, an active
interest in the common good, and a desire for peace. Then man
can acknowledge the highest values and God Himself, their
author and end[817].

Another strong reason why the Church's moral vision is necessary in the
Nigerian health care system is because the human institutions are not neutral.
There are some consequences of their actions or activities which can influence
the life of man and can lead him to ignore the vocation of every human
person to acknowledge the ultimate values and God the maker of all things.
Suffice it to mention that the main intention of the Catholic social teaching
is not to defend religion as some think, instead its reflections are centered on
the human person to better his quality of life. The Church is conscious of the
fact that it is impossible to find in man and from man an exhuastive answer
about the mistery of man. For this she turns to the incarnate verb: the only
one who is capable of revealing man to man[818]. It is only through Revelation
that we can know the greatness of the human person[819].

The main guide of the Catholic social doctrine is the human person
and his dignity. Specifically, when the Catholic social doctrine makes
reference to man, it does not refer to abstract or metaphysical man, it
rather intend every concrete man and woman, including those in Nigeria.
If the Church abandons the concrete man, that means she has ignored her
mission. Affirming this John Paul II writes: "The Church cannot abandon
man for his "destiny" [...] We are speaking precisely of each man on this
planet"[820]. The Pope discloses that at the centre of most of the activities of
the Second Vatican Council "was precisely this man in all the truth of his
life, in his conscience, in his continual inclination to sin and at the same
time in his continual aspiration to truth, the good, the beautiful, justice
and love"[821]. He further remarks:

---

[817]   Paulo VI, «*Populorum Progressio*, Encyclical letter (1967)», n. 21.

[818]   Cfr. Concilio Vaticano II, *Gauduim et Spes* ..., n. 22.

[819]   Ibid., 24

[820]   John Paul II, «*Redemptor Hominis*, Encyclical letter (1967) », n. 14, in J. M.
Miller (ed.), *The Encyclicals of...*, 31-96.

[821]   Ibid., n.14.

> Since this man is the way for the church, the way for her daily
> life and experience, for her mission and toil, the Church of today
> must be aware in an always new manner of man's "situation".
> That means that she must be aware of his possibilities, which
> keep returning to their proper bearings and thus revealing
> themselves. She must likewise be aware of threats to man and
> all that seems to oppose the endeavour "to make human life ever
> more human" and make every element of this life correspond
> to man's true dignity-in a word, she must be aware of all that is
> opposed to that process[822].

Proclaiming the truth of the dignity of the human person is the core
of the social doctrine of the church. The church has the responsibility of
defending and taking care of every man, especially the afflicted, the poorest
and the weakest. Consequently, she has to illuminate the conscience of
every human being so that each person can understand what the dignity
of the human being entails. We believe the application of the Catholic
doctrine, in her special quality of having attention for every human person,
especially the weak and the most vulnerable can help Nigeria to have a
better health care system.

4.3. Dialogue with the Islamic World regarding Justice

A question that should not be overlooked in our reflection on the
Nigerian health care system is the simultaneous presence of two major
monotheistic religions in Nigeria: Christianity and Islam. We sustain that
there are notable convergences regarding the principles of justice, although
in some aspects, like the conception of person, these convergences are not
clearly evident. Regarding the presence of Christians and Muslims in
Nigeria: "A 2012 survey by the Pew Research Center's Forum on Religion
and Public Life estimated the population to be 49.3 percent Christian and
48.8 percent Muslim, while the remaining 2 percent belong to other or no
religions"[823]. The above report mentions also that:

---

[822] Ibid.

[823] International Religious Freedom Report for 2018, United States Department of
State, Bureau of Democracy, Human Rights, and Labor in https://www.state.
gov/wp-content/uploads/2019/05/NIGERIA-2018-INTERNATIONAL-
RELIGIOUS-FREEDOM-REPORT.pdf. [06-12-2019].

> The Hausa-Fulani and Kanuri ethnic groups are most prevalent
> in the predominantly Muslim northern states [...] Christians
> and Muslims reside in approximately equal numbers in the
> central region and southwestern states [...] In the southeastern
> states, where the Igbo ethnic group is dominant, Christian
> groups, including Catholics, Anglicans, and Methodists,
> constitute the majority[824].

The Catholic concept of social Justice is contained mostly in its social teaching. The document *Compendium of the Social Doctrine of the Church*, proposes "principles for reflection, the criteria for judgement and directives for action which are starting point for the promotion of an integral and solidary humanism"[825]. The document is "fruit of careful Magisterial reflection and an expression of the Church's constant commitment in fidelity to the grace of salvation wrought in Christ and in loving concern for humanity's destiny"[826]. The Catholic teaching on Social Justice "is proposed also to the brethren of other Churches and Ecclesial Communities, to the followers of other religions, as well as to all people of good will who are committed to serving the common good"[827].

Shariah is an Arabic word which identifies Islamic law which leads a good Muslim to through this life to paradise[828]. The Nigerian 1999 Constitution recognizes Shariah law, despite the fact that it provides that section 10 of the same Constitution states that: "The government of the Federation or of a State shall not adopt any religion as State Religion"[829]. Islamic canon law or shariah is founded on the doctrines of *Quran* and *Sunnah*. Muslims believe that growth in the spiritual and material spheres can be assured at the personal and societal levels through "reliance by human beings solely on divine guidance"[830].

---

[824] Ibid.

[825] Pontifical Council For Justice And Peace, *Compendium of the...*, n. 7, 3.

[826] Ibid., n. 8, 4.

[827] Ibid., n. 12, 6.

[828] Cfr. A. E. Mayer, «Legge Islamica» in D. M. Cosi – L. Saibene – R. Scagno (eds.), *Enciclopedia delle Religioni*, Città Nuova, Milano 2004, 398-414.

[829] Cfr. O. Awofeso, «Political Islam and Democracy in Nigeria: Compatibility or Incompatibility?» in *International Journal of Interdisciplinary Research Method*, 3(2016), 24-33.

[830] M. M. Khan – M. I. Bhatti, «Islamic Economics: Divine Vision of Distributive Justice», in Developments in Islamic Banking, Palgrave Macmillan, London

Some authors remark that "the concept of distributive justice per se only came about as an independent economic issue with the increased socio-economic problems in the Muslim world"[831]. The primary aim of the Islamic concept of distributive justice is to resolve economic issues like financial inequalities. The Catholic concept of distributive justice has the holistic well-being of the human person as it primary objective. However, the Islamic model is not against the Catholic concept, there is only a distinction based on their respective perspectives. They are similar as regards the intention of creating social balance. Just as in the Catholic social teaching, "Islam demands for socioeconomic inequalities to be minimized through fair distributional system of resources, factor payments and transfer payment"[832]. M. M. Khan and M. I. Bhatti affirm that "Islamic Economics is an ideological discipline that primarily aims at fostering equality, justice, fairness, brotherhood, mercy, compassion, solidarity and freedom of choice in human society"[833]. The features of Islamic model of economics gives an idea of what are its principles of distributive justice. There is certain level of similarity with the Catholic principles of distributive justice. For instance, solidarity is specifically identified as a Catholic principle and equality, justice, fairness, brotherhood, mercy and compassion are all fundamental features of Catholic social teaching. If these features are intended in Islam as it is conceived in Catholic social doctrine, our proposal would be acceptable to Muslims who correctly intend and interpret the *Quran* and *Sunnah*.

In the Catholic world, the issue of justice is fundamental and many Catholic scholars and prelates consider it a duty to defend justice. The Catholic world has a fair number of literature in the area of social justice. Dissimilarly, as revealed by some already cited authors: "To Muslim theologians and philosophers, justice is an abstract and idealist concept. They made no serious attempt to view it from a positive concept and analyse it from existing social conditions"[834]. For this, literature in this area is limited and "the absence of academic works in the formulation of a theory of Distributive justice" spurred contemporary Muslim scholars like

---

2008, 7-37.

[831] S. Begum – A. Rahim, «A Conceptual Framework of Distributive Justice in Islamic Economics», *AL ALBAB – Borneo Journal of Religious Studies (BJRS)*, 1(2015), 19-38.

[832] Ibid.

[833] M. M. Khan – M. I. Bhatti, «Islamic Economics: Divine».

[834] S. Begum – A. Rahim, «A Conceptual Framework...».

Umar Chapra (1981) and Nejatullah Siddiqui (1986) to initiate "creative ways to incorporate the relevance of justice in distributive functions". The current situation gives an impression of Islam with "great emphasis on justice"[835] [836].

The Islamic approach to distributive justice is similar to Catholic belief because Muslims agree that "Absolute ownership rest with the Creator and thus all men have equal rights over His bounties"[837]. The Catholic social teaching affirms the right to the common use of goods is the primary principle of the entire ethical and social order[838]. Catholic social teaching retains that it is a matter of justice to help the poor and the vulnerable. By the same token, the Islamic ethics recommends that the most disadvantaged members of society should be given aid, through individual obligation, personal piety and "state responsibility for social welfare"[839].

The concept of "person" is not explicit in the Islamic notion of distributive justice. However, we think there is enough evidence to claim that a faithful Muslim will see good reasons to accept the Catholic social principles. Again, the concept is person could be said to be implicit in the ideas developed by Muslim scholars because being 'a person' is a universal feature.

4.4. Catholic Principles and some Questions on Distribution of Resources in Nigeria

4.4.1. Health Care and Common Good in Nigeria

The understanding of the Catholic social doctrine prompts us to underline in this part of our work that it is the duty of the Nigerian

---

[835] A. H. ANSARI, «Distributive Justice in Islam: An Expository Study of Zakah for Achieving a Sustainable Society», *Australian Journal of Basic and Applied Sciences*, 5(2011), 383-393.

[836] S. BEGUM – A. RAHIM, «A Conceptual Framework...».

[837] Ibid.

[838] Cfr. JOHN PAUL II, «Address to the Plenary Session and to the Study Week on the Subject 'Cosmology and Fundamental Physics' with Members of Two Working Groups who had Discussed 'Perspectives of Immunisation in Parasitic Diseases' and 'Statements on the Consequences of the Use of Nuclear Weapons' 3 October 1981», n. 4, in *Papal Addresses to...*

[839] S. BEGUM – A. RAHIM, «A Conceptual Framework...».

government to make accessible to the Nigerian citizens basic health care and all other elements necessary for leading a truly human life. The Universal Church teaches particularly that the provisions of the health care and other common goods should be done in accordance to respect for the person as such. Hence, public authorities in Nigeria are invited to respect the fundamental and inalienable rights of the human person[840]. In addition, Pope John Paul II reminds us that "the leaders of civil society fulfil their mission when they seek above all the common good with absolute respect for the dignity of the human person"[841]. Are the Nigerian civil leaders adhering to this?

Some scholars have asked questions about the ethical rationale for publicly financed health[842] The various arguments and answers relevant to this and other debates refer to the following points:

> (1) the ultimate purpose of a human life or human society; (2) the role of health and its distribution is society in advancing this ultimate purpose; (3) the role of access to or utilisation of health care in maintaining or improving the desired level and distribution of health among members of society, and (4) the role of public financing in ensuring the ethically justified access to and utilisation of health care by member of society[843].

The points listed in the above citation are vital issues of distributive justice. Because of the divergent distributive preferences of public goods, especially health care goods, there is a need to define social value judgements to govern health care resource allocation decision-making process. In the third chapter of this work, while treating the concept of justice, we mentioned that distributive justice, is mainly refers to the fair allocation of benefits and burdened. Thus, the principle of distributive justice according to many is very important to health care organizations

---

[840]   Cfr. PONTIFICAL COUNCIL FOR JUSTICE AND PEACE, *Compendium of the...*, n. 1907, 457.

[841]   JOHN PAUL II, «Address to the plenary Session on the Subject 'Intergenerational Solidarity', 11 April 2002», n. 4, in *Papal Addresses to the Pontifical Academy of Sciences 1917 – 2002 and to the Pontifical Academy of Social Sciences 1994 – 2002*, The Pontifical Academy of Sciences, Vatican City 2003, 435-437.

[842]   J. HURLEY, «Ethics, economics, and ...».

[843]   Ibid.

and can help to improve their acceptability, by increasing transparency in decision-making processes. One of the theories of distributive justice which we treated in chapter three that fits in here is procedural justice, essentially defined as due process. This theory is described as means of reaching fair outcomes because it does not approve arbitrary decisions, since it represents the belief in fair procedures.

The Nigeria case as the first chapter of this dissertation disclosed is such that over $16 billion of oil revenues were stolen between 1979 and 1983 during the reign of President Shehu Shagari by some civil authorities. Also in the same chapter, it was observed that Transport Minister during the period indicated above, Alhaji Umaru Dikko, was alleged to have mismanaged about N4 billion of public fund budget to buy an important good like food for the nation[844]. These are not qualities of commendable stewardship of the common good and respect for the dignity of the human person. Fair procedure is totally missing in a situation such as this. The stolen and squandered fund could have given many Nigerians the opportunity of satisfying their health needs and the rice, if purchased by Umaru Dikko, would have fed many Nigerian Children who died of hunger during that period. It is sad to note that children die in Nigeria from preventable diseases more than in any other country in Africa[845]. The moral obligation of quality stewardship is very crucial because as the health capability approach affirms, in line with our thesis, what is done by the government, whatever decision made in terms of health and other social goods has inevitable consequences on the real person in his real health situations. Regarding this, some already mentioned Catholic author asserts: "Rendering health care is not just a matter of commutative justice, a simple exchange of goods and services between the provider and the patient. Rather, it must be governed by the principles proper to distributive justice, and implied here is access to health care by all members of society"[846].

The Catholic person-centered principles represent the best approach of the distributive justice to assure that every member of the society especially the weakest and the most vulnerable, has access to health care and utilizes

---

[844] M. M. Ogbeidi, «Political Leadership and…».

[845] Cfr. L. O. Olusegun – T. R. Ibe – M. M. Ikorok, «Curbing maternal and…».

[846] D. M. Gallagher, «The Common Good», in E. J. Furton – P. J. Cataldo – A. S. Moraczewski (eds.), *Catholic Health Care…*

the available health care resources. These principles guarantee the right to health and access to care of all especially of those who are ignored where the principles do not exist or are not applied, as it is the case in Nigeria. In this sense, we think that if procedures justice is applied respecting the principles of the dignity of the human person, the results of the procedures are acceptable without any resistance[847]. The Catholic Magisterium teaches that the "human rights correspond to the demands of human dignity and entail, in the first place, the fulfilment of the essential needs of the person in the material and spiritual spheres"[848].

Does the Nigerian government do this? How does the Nigerian government respond to the health needs of her citizens? We will give more answers to these questions subsequently when we will treat issues of implementation of policies and other matters concerning health and social justice in the Nigerian health care system especially the problem of distribution of health care resources. It is however obvious that considering health as a common good implies that it is not the responsibility of only one person or a group of persons (the political leaders) to provide it. In fact the social teaching of the Church indicates that health, as a common good is the responsibility of every member of the society (each person according to his or her capacity). This is also sustained by the health capability approach in its view that individuals should be aided to be personally responsible for their health[849]. This may sound new to some Nigerians who are used to the idea that the government should provide everything for everyone. The paradox of the such mentality is that the government provides much less than it should, when the citizens expect more than it has as its responsibility to provide. The people should not expect everything from the government and the government should not abandon the individuals to provide all their health needs. The health capability approach captures this our idea aptly as it explains that health capability is not limited to the individual capability, but includes also other related situations or conditions that enable optimal health[850]. Striking a right balance is just what is needed.

---

[847] M. DEUTSCH, «Justice and Conflict», in M. DEUTSCH – P. T. COLEMAN (eds.), *The Handbook of...*, 45.
[848] PONTIFICAL COUNCIL FOR JUSTICE AND PEACE, *Compendium of the...*, n. 154, 85.
[849] J. P. RUGER, «Health Capability: Conceptualization...».
[850] Ibid.

4.4.2. Lack of Political Will to implement the formulated Health Care Policies, Programs and Plans and the Consequences on the performance of the Nigerian Health System

This part of our dissertation undertakes to unearth the factors that constitute obstacle to the implementation of health policies and plans in Nigeria and to suggest the application of the Catholic principles of distributive justice as possible solution to the problem(s). Many believe that the indifferent attitudes of some political leaders is prominent among the enigmas of health policies' implementation in Nigeria. The second chapter of the present dissertation shows that numerous brilliant health policies have been formulated in Nigeria, but according to various opinions, the paradox is that there is no interest of those responsible to implement them. In certain cases where the policies are implemented, only negligible parts of them are implemented. This is evident in the fact that the health sector in Nigeria has no significant results and development to show for the implementation of health policies and plans. Instances abound; the evolution of health care in Nigeria treated in the second chapter this doctoral thesis points out that the Nigerian government employed the Basic Health Service Scheme (BHSS) founded on Primary Health Care (PHC) approach in 1979[851]; health for all, starting from the primary level was motivation for the National Health Policy of 1988, with which the Federal Government launched the Primary Health Care. Also, the National Development Plan (1975 - 1979) was put in place to make health care accessible and available at the grassroot levels. Other policies, plans and programs of this nature adopted by the Nigerian government are: The National Primary Healthcare Development Agency (NPHCDA) launched in 1992, the Ward Health System established in 2001, to help in the bid to achieve the millennium development goal (MDG) targets of Nigeria[852], National Health Policy, National Health Insurance Scheme, National Health Bill, National Health Act 2014 and National Strategic Health Development Plan.

With these, the government had the intention of bringing health service to all. But this goal has not been realized[853]. In fact, most Nigerians,

---

[851]   Cfr. D. M. N. McDɪᴋᴋᴏʜ, *The Nigerian Health…*, 91.

[852]   Cfr. A. O Aɪɢʙɪʀᴇᴍᴏʟᴇᴍ – I. Aʟᴇɴᴏɢʜᴇɴᴀ – E. Eʙᴏʀᴇɪᴍᴇ – C. Aʙᴇᴊᴇɢᴀʜ, «Primary Health Care…».

[853]   Cfr., Ibid.

especially at the grassroot level, remain without access to decent minimum health care[854]. This situation suggests that mere formulation of policies and plans is not the most important thing to do, because the effective implementation is also very important too and has to be considered. The paradoxes of policy implementation in Nigeria include: corruption, lack of continuity in government policies, lack of human and material health resources, poor leadership programme, tribalism and ethnic 'wars', indifferent attitude to need and interest of poor and the problems of the governed and lack of will on the part of the political leaders to implement the formulated policies. The application of the Catholic principles of justice, especially in policies relevant to the distribution of health care resources, according to our work can help the country to address the above cited problems and to achieve the noble goals of the Nigerian health care system.

The social teaching of the Catholic Church indicates that the attainment of the common good is the reason for the existence of the civil authority[855]. This implies the primary duty of government to make available and accessible to each person or groups what they need to lead a truly and dignified human life. Basic health needs are important qualities for reaching fulfilments both as individuals and as groups. How are the Nigerian civil authorities responding to their duty toward their citizens with regard to health as a common good? Some Nigerian authors reveal that the performance of the government's health care agencies in this regard is unsatisfactory. One of the problems of the Nigerian government as we have seen is the lack of will to implement the health policies and plans already in existence. Some authors expressing the failures of the Nigerian health sector due to the nonchalant attitude of the political leaders argue that:

> Despite sound policies and interventions to develop the Nigerian Health sector, it has witnessed several challenges that continue to reduce the progress and achievement of universal access to health care. Some of the factors that affect the overall performance of the health system include; inadequate health facilities/structure, poor human resources and management,

---

[854] Cfr. B. S. AREGBESHOLA – S. M. KHAN, «Primary Health Care...».

[855] Cfr. JOHN XXIII, «*Pacem in Terris*, Encyclical Letter of on Establishing Universal Peace», in Truth, Justice, Charity, and Liberty, (1963)», n. 45, in C. CARLEN (ed.), *The Papal Encyclicals...*

poor remuneration and motivation, lack of fair and sustainable health care financing, unequal economic and economic and political relations, the neo-liberal economic policies of the Nigerian state, corruption, illiteracy, very low government spending on health, high out-of-pocket expenditure in health and absence of integrated system for diseases prevention, surveillance and treatment, inadequate mechanism for families to access health care, shortage of essential drugs and supplies and supervision of health care providers are among some of the persistent problems of the health system in Nigeria[856].

The Catholic social doctrine asserts that the "authority is exercised legitimately when it seeks the common good of the group concerned and if it employs morally licit means to attain it"[857]. Nevertheless, the list of challenges of the Nigerian health sector shows that citizens are not enjoying the common good, as they should. Thus, the Nigerian government is reminded that "the public authorities are bound to respect the fundamental and inalienable rights of the human person"[858]. The right to health is a fundamental right of the human person, of every individual to get the just share of the common good. Health is a part of the common good. Not recognizing this truth implies injustice that gives rise to serious moral questions.

The problem with the Nigerian health care system considered above, centers more on the political leadership. This is a salient point because the political will is considered the principal factor to government policy formulation strategies. A group of political leaders capable of and willing to implement policies hitherto formulated is very crucial to improve the Nigerian health care system and the health situations of many Nigerians. This represents one of the major reasons why most African countries of weaker economic and other powers perform better than Nigeria in the health sectors. In chapter two of this work, we cited many examples regarding the supremacy of the smaller and economically weaker African countries over Nigeria in this regard. Despite its large human, economic

---

[856] G. Timothy – O. Irinoye – U. Yunusa – A. Dalhatu – S. Ahmed – A. Suberu, «Balancing Demand and Efficiency in Nigerian Health Care Delivery System», *European Journal of Business and Management*, 6(2014), 50-56.

[857] The Catechism of…, n. 1903, 456.

[858] Ibid., n. 1907, 457.

and natural resources, Nigeria has continued to be ranked among the poorest and least developed countries of the world especially in health performance. This reveals how those holding political powers are lagging behind in respecting the rules of common good.

The social teaching of the Catholic Church observes that the most complete realization of the common good is found in those political communities where the state defends and promotes the interest of their citizens. Defending and promoting the wellbeing of the citizens according to the Church is the role of the state[859]. The poor performance of Nigeria in the health sector is not due to the lack of policies. We make this affirmation because, we believe that if the formulated health policies in Nigeria were appropriately implemented, the key health indicators and major causes of death and main pathologies in Nigeria we saw in chapter one would have been better than what they are today. For instance, as revealed by some Nigerian authors we made reference to in the first chapter of this thesis, one of the determinant factors of life expectancy is government's expenditure on health[860]. We also learnt from the same chapter that the life expectancy in Nigeria is very low, due to the poor performance of the government in its duty[861]. There are many policies capable of ameliorating the health conditions of the Nigerian populace, but the paradox is that they are only on paper and not translated into practice. Most often, when some of the policies are implemented, this is done to suit the interest of that in power and not for the interest of the governed or for the common good. This attitude is glaringly evident in all the three levels of government in Nigeria.

4.4.3. Available and Unavailable Resources and the Modalities of Distribution of Health Care in Nigeria

Our thesis is of the view that distributive justice is necessary to achieve a just health care system in Nigeria both at the social policy and the practical levels. There are some who think it may not be necessary for health professionals to apply distributive justice in their various operations. But the third chapter of this work has proved it is a crucial element for health workers despite the fact that they are not directly occupied with determining

---

[859]   Cfr. THE CATECHISM OF..., n. 1910, 458.

[860]   Cfr. P. I. SEDE - W. OHEMENG, «Socio-economic determinants...».

[861]   Cfr. Ibid.

the base package to be available for distribution. The health workers are directly in contact with the patients. Often, in a country like Nigeria, there are cases where requests supersede the available resources. In some other cases, there is the dilemma of whether to charge the rich more in order to balance the deficit amounting from the inability of the poor to settle their bills. Most hospitals and governments agencies in Nigeria handle many cases where distributive justice becomes the central issue, thus unavoidable. Some documents highlight the health care facilities present in Nigeria. As revealed by recent documents like the *Malaria Operational Plan FY 2017*:

> Nigeria has a total of 34,173 health facilities: 30,098 primary, 3,992 secondary, and 83 tertiary. The private sector constitutes 33% of all health facilities in Nigeria. Private health facilities include private not-for-profit, private for-profit, pharmacies, proprietary patent medicine vendors (PPMVs), and mobile clinics[862].

The just mentioned document indicates that the private health care system provides health care services for a substantial proportion of the Nigerian population. It discloses that "approximately 76% of all secondary facilities and about 20 % of primary health care facilities are private. Forty-two percent of all fever cases seek treatment first in the private sector"[863]. The private owned clinics and hospitals are commonly found in the urban areas. The document on the President's Malaria Initiative affirms that "The estimated 34,173 health facilities nationwide are fairly evenly distributed between the urban and rural areas"[864]. Dissimilarly, the *Nigerian Health Sector Market Study Report* admits that:

> On the supply side, Nigeria has a significant deficit in well-equipped and staffed healthcare facilities. With an estimated 5 beds per 10,000 population, Nigeria will need additional 117, 000 beds costing approximately USD12 billion to reach the Sub-Saharan African average of 12 beds per 10,000 and an additional 350, 000 beds costing approximately USD37 billion to reach the global average 26 beds per 10,000[865].

---

[862] *President's Malaria Initiative, Nigeria: Malaria Operational Plan FY 2017*, 15.

[863] Cfr. Ibid, 15.

[864] Ibid., 15.

[865] NIGERIAN HEALTH SECTOR, *Market Study Report*, March 2015, 20.

The insufficient quantity of health facilities in Nigeria and the problems it creates, show that some principles, theories and approaches of justice treated in chapter three, guided by the Catholic principles are inevitable in making and implementing distributive policies in the Nigerian health care system. Writing about the theories of distributive justice, T. L. Beauchamp and J. F. Childress acknowledge that "policies for health care access and distribution in many countries provide an example of the problems that confront these theories"[866]. The condition of health care distribution in Nigeria has the characteristics expressed by these authors. Nigeria is acclaimed "the giant of Africa", but her budgets in comparison to those of other African countries like South Africa, Kenya, Senegal, Ghana and Angola, do not show this greatness of Nigeria. While other smaller and less affluent countries respect the Abuja declaration by allocating about 15% of their annual budget to the health sector, Nigeria's annual budgetary allocation to the health sector has not surpassed 6%. As our work has earlier revealed, most Nigerians, especially the most vulnerable, including women and children are deprived of the basic health care and some die unnecessarily due to curable and preventable diseases. The Catholic principle of solidarity spurs us to provide quality health care services for the poor that reflect their innate human dignity "thus enabling an increasingly adequate, incisive, and even personalized response to needs of the sick"[867]. The government has the duty to protect human life, ensure that the common good is achieved and the moral obligation to promote and nurture the culture of solidarity that motivates people to act unselfishly and charitably for the good of those in need. In this pursuit, the primordial principle of the life and dignity of the human person continues to be a fundamental point.

Inequality in the distribution of health care resources in Nigeria is an ethical issue. According to John Rawls, there is injustice where there is inequity that does not benefit every citizen. The initial chapter of this dissertation presented a *"World Bank Report"* to highlight the disparity in the distribution of resources in Nigeria particularly in a very high geographical concentration of economic and health opportunities of the nation in the big cities[868]. There is failure in the realization of just distribution of health care

---

[866]   T. L. BEAUCHAMP – J. F. CHILDRESS, *Principles of Biomedical...*, 230.
[867]   FRANCIS, Unite to care ..., 503-505.
[868]   Cfr. THE WORLD BANK, *Nigeria Economic Report...*, 2.

resources in Nigeria because of variations highlighted in chapter one. This dereliction of duty gives rise to medical deprivation in rural areas where most persons of the poorest class live[869]. For this, the *"World Bank Report"* admits that poverty rates tend to be high in Nigeria, notably in rural areas[870]. The Catholic social vision believes that if the principle of solidarity is properly understood and applied, it can help to reduce various forms of inequalities that bring about inequities that hurt the dignity of the poor and the vulnerable person. Thus, the social vision of the Catholic Church affirms that "solidarity with our neighbor is also about the promotion of equality of rights and equality of opportunities; hence we must oppose all forms of discrimination"[871].

Regarding the problem of inequalities in the distribution of resources, a Catholic scholar A. Fisher thinks that sometimes the problem is not with the quantity of resources available, but with how the resources are distributed. The 'how', according to him is often the crux of the problem[872]. This is remarkably true and it is a big question to be addressed in Nigeria, where our study in chapter one revealed that there was no correlation between the increased rates of **GDP** that exceeded the population growth and the rate of poverty reduction[873]. Concerning this, a United Nation report affirms:

> No matter what level of resources they have at their disposal, progressive realization requires that governments take immediate steps within their means towards the fulfillment of these rights. Regardless of resource capacity, the elimination of discrimination and improvement in the legal and judicial systems must be acted upon with immediate effect[874].

---

[869] Cfr. S. I. OKAFOR, «Spatial Aspects of ...», 263-274.

[870] Cfr. The World Bank, *Nigeria Economic Report...*, 9.

[871] CATHOLIC BISHOPS OF ENGLAND AND WALES, «*The Common Good and the Catholic Church's Teaching*», n. 10, 1996, in http://www.catholicsocialteaching.org.uk/wp-content/uploads/2010/10/THE-COMMON-GOOD-AND-THE-CATHOLIC-CHURCH_1996.pdf [20-04-2018].

[872] Cfr. A. FISHER., «The ethics of health care (Lecture delivered to the annual sympotium of the Guild of Catholic Doctors on April 24, 1993)», *Catholic Medical Quarterly*, 44(1993), 13-20.

[873] Cfr. THE WORLD BANK, *Nigeria Economic Report...*, 9.

[874] UNITED NATIONS HUMAN RIGHTS, OFFICE OF THE HIGH COMMISSIONER, *Special Rapporteur on the right to health*, in http://www.who.int/mediacentre/

Lack of application of the right principles of justice as the criterion for distribution of resources can lead to misdistribution of the resources. Common good requires that distribution of resources be done in fairness. Thus, equity is an essential quality of a just distribution of health care resources. Equity implies the elimination of all forms of inequalities and unhealthy discriminations from the practice of health care resource allocation[875].

Furthermore, studies considered in the second chapter of this dissertation reveal that most public hospitals in Nigeria are under-equipped in terms of material and human resources and they are poorly managed. Whereas some private hospitals have good architectural presentation and are fundamentally equipped. The private health facilities attend to patients quickly and their services are often efficient. With these qualities, they attract more people than the public hospitals. Most countries that have little resources manage them well to achieve encouraging results. On the other hand, some countries, are richly endowed with resources, but there is lack of will to distribute them fairly among the people. At times, the responsibility to decide and distribute are in the hands of people who lack the required acumen. As aptly remarked by some, one of the major problems of the developing countries like Nigeria, is not only lack of health resources but also the misdistribution of available resources[876]. This does not help in the improvement of the health status of the people. In Nigeria, the decision-making on the health care resource allocation should be made based on ethical principles for the allocation of resources found in the Catholic social teaching. Additionally, Universality is a quality that is inevitable for the Nigerian health system. Universality is crucial to the right to health because it is all embracing and strives to provide primary health care for all. As a feature of an ethical health system, we recommend it for distribution of resources in the Nigerian health system.

Determinations on distribution of health care resources in Nigeria which has been centralized in the hands of bureaucratic political leaders has never given proper attention to the respect for the right to basic health

---

factssheets/fs323/en/ [02-01-2018].

[875] Cfr. PONTIFICAL COUNCIL FOR JUSTICE AND PEACE, *Compendium of the...*, n. 167, 95.

[876] Cfr. R. AKHTAR (ed.) *Health Care Patterns and Planning in Developing Countries*, Greenwood Press, New York 1991, 73.

needs of the vulnerable. In contrast to the attitude of the Nigerian political leaders, the social teaching of Church states: "each person must have access to the level of well-being necessary for his full development"[877]. The content of the Catholic doctrine is expressed in universality and availability which represent features of a just health system. Universality implies availability; this means that at least the basic health care services must be available and affordable for all. In line with this, Pope John Paul II affirms: "Human beings normally need a basic minimum of health and material goods in order to be able to live in a manner worthy of their human and divine vocation"[878]. The universal Church considers the right to the common use of goods as the "first principle of the whole ethical and social order"[879]. The right to public good is one of the major characteristics of the Christian social doctrine. The four pillars of procedural theory of distributive justice are perfectly in line with the Catholic doctrine in the pursuit for an ethical health system. According to procedural justice, to ascertain that the right to common good was respected, one should ask if, in the process of distribution, there are the following: consistency (fairness), impartiality, giving voice and transparency. This implies assuring that fair procedures were in place and that they were rightly observed[880].

An economic policy that pays attention to giving the required allocation to health care as we considered in chapter one makes positive impact on the life expectancy because it helps to tackle the problems of morbidity and mortality[881]. Following the major health indicators and the budgetary allocations of Nigeria to the health sector, it appears that the right to health and the dignity of the human person has never been a priority for the country's leaders[882]. It appears so because most plans and

---

[877] Pontifical Council for Justice and Peace, *Compendium of the...*, n. 172, 97.

[878] John Paul II, «Address to the Plenary Session and to the Study Week on the Subject 'Cosmology and Fundamental Physics' with Members of Two Working Groups who had Discussed 'Perspectives of Immunisation in Parasitic Diseases' and 'Statements on the Consequences of the Use of Nuclear Weapons' 3 October 1981», n. 4, in *Papal Addresses to the Pontifical Academy of Sciences 1917 – 2002 and to the Pontifical Academy of Social Sciences 1994 – 2002*, The Pontifical Academy of Sciences, Vatican City 2003. 249-252.

[879] Ibid.

[880] Cfr. J. Summer, «Principles of Healthcare...».

[881] Cfr. P. I. Sede, W. Ohemeng, «Socio-economic determinants...».

[882] Cfr. M. M. Ogbeidi, «Political Leadership and...».

policies are not based on person-centered ethical principles. Nigeria needs a political ideology founded on social justice, equitable distribution of income, health resources and access to basic medical care for all especially, the vulnerable as taught by the Catholic social teaching. There are very wide disparities between the rich and the poor, and the rural and urban areas in terms of access to medical services. The proper introduction of the Catholic principles can help to confront the unjust inequalities and make the Nigerian health care system appreciable.

In terms of performance in the health sector, especially in the distribution of resources and the general management of the health system, Nigeria does better than only 3 countries globally: Democratic Republic of Congo, Central Africa Republic and Myanmar[883]. Comparably, these countries are far behind Nigeria in terms of economic, human and other potentials. Nigeria is expected to take the lead seeing its important position in Africa, but unfortunately, it is classified among the last group. Pointing out some of the causes of the unimpressive output of the Nigerian healthcare system, many authors agree on the issue of bad leadership. Consequently, they think there is need for structural change in order to state clearly the nature of leadership responsibility for healthcare strategy and implementation. According D. Eboh, "there is no credible leadership and management accountability in the present Nigeria's health care system. Doctor's dual roles as experts clinicians as well as the key strategic managers have not encouraged greater innovation and proper accountability in service development and delivery process"[884]. For this, the author suggests, there should be proper checks and balances, the trained strategic managers should hold the positions for management leadership and not doctors who are already occupied with delivery of health services. A doctor is commonly identified and evaluated by his clinical competencies and not managerial skills[885]. "One of the fundamental duties of civil authorities [...] is so to co-ordinate and regulate social relations that the exercise of one person's right does not threaten others in the exercise of their own rights"[886].

---

[883] Cfr. D. Eboh, *Strategic Concept for...*, 35.

[884] Ibid.

[885] Cfr. Ibid. 35-36.

[886] John XXIII, «*Pacem in Terris*, Encyclical Letter of on Establishing Universal Peace», in Truth, Justice, Charity, and Liberty, (1963)», n. 62, in C. Carlen (ed.), *The Papal Encyclicals...*

Accordingly, the Nigerian government has the responsibility of helping the health care system to ameliorate its performance, thus improving the life of the people. The governmental health agencies should assure that the medical personnel are placed in positions where they are qualified to be for the good of the population.

> The common good requires that civil authorities maintain a careful balance between coordinating and protecting the rights of the citizens on the one hand, and promoting them, on the other. It should not happen that certain individuals or social groups derive special advantage from the fact that their rights have received preferential protection[887].

Another important moral issue that cannot be ignored is that of allocating more funds to arms and ammunitions in the name of security, while allocating less to the health sector. Health is wealth. A nation with healthy citizens is a wealthy nation. The Nigerian government seem not to understand these sayings that are part of the culture and traditions of many in Nigeria. Most of the crisis we have in Nigeria that warrant the need for security could be traced to the youths who are jobless, illiterates, abandoned with no hope and left with crime as the only option. Nigerians usually say that "a hungry man is an angry man". Most of the youths commit various crimes because their health and other needs are unmet, so they are hungry and consequently angry.

The western world who encourage the buying of the weapons they produce should discourage the African leaders from buying them and encourage them to invest in health to provide health care needs to their people. The Catholic principles of solidarity and subsidiarity invite world powers to do such. This could also be a way of resolving the problem of "mass exodus" of many young Africans and especially Nigerians who cross the sea, not like the Israelites, but with very unsafe means risking their lives. Unfortunately, many who would have been future leaders of Africa have died in this perilous adventure and others have suffered all sorts of injustice at the hands of the human traffickers. The western world gives money as philanthropists to help the African nations and take it back through the selling of arms and other businesses with some corrupt African leaders. This is against the principles of dignity of the human person, common

---

[887]   Ibid., n. 65.

good, solidarity and subsidiarity. The Church's Magisterium on the principle of solidarity affirms that we all are responsible for all. The Church also teaches that being our brother's keeper is a divine injunction to all, Christians and non-Christians alike. There is no perfect health system in the world. That being so, the valid suggestions that are being mentioned are to aid Nigeria's healthcare system to achieve a more impressive performance and not to attack the government or the health system. We are optimistic in our proposal of the Catholic principles because "the Catholic Church knows from its social teaching that all this is possible, and that no social trend, however negative, is beyond reversal"[888]. The health indicators in Nigeria are obviously too bad, among the worst in the world, but that does not mean that there could be no remedy. The rebirth of the Nigerian health care system will be possible through a diligent application of the Catholic moral principles. We are convinced about this belief particularly because the Catholic doctrine is not strange to health care in Nigeria. Christianity, as chapter two of this thesis acknowledges, is at the origin of the health care service in Nigeria[889].

4.4.4. The Catholic Principle of Subsidiarity and the Distribution of Health Care Resources in Relation to Community Health in Nigeria

The principle of subsidiarity as sustained by the Catholic social doctrine affirms that "it is impossible to promote the dignity of the person without showing concern for the family, groups, associations, local territorial realities"[890]. Doing without them or 'helping them without them' is a reductionist approach to giving aid because; it does not recognize the people's dignity as human persons. Procedural justice treated in chapter three is in synergy with the Catholic principles of subsidiarity because, the crucial aspects of this secular theory retain as very important the involvement of all parties in the decision-making and execution of the agreements. It also affirms that the decision-making process must be trustworthy, and the outcomes must address the personal situation of those for whose interest agreements are reached. Likewise, acceptability as a feature of a just health care system requires that

---

[888] CATHOLIC BISHOPS OF ENGLAND AND WALES, *The Common Good...*, n. 28.

[889] Cfr. D. M. N. McDIKKOH, *The Nigerian health...*,73.

[890] PONTIFICAL COUNCIL FOR JUSTICE AND PEACE, *Compendium of the...*, n. 185, 104-105.

laws, policies and programmes be people-centered. With this, it intends that the need of the people must always be considered and the population should be engaged in planning and executions since the health care services are for them. This can help also to guarantee a standard quality of services because when people are guided by experts to choose for themselves, they can hardly decide to choose inferior qualities. Including the people in deliberations and in sorting their problems, and not doing for them what they are capable of doing themselves, are the major characteristics of the Catholic principle of subsidiarity. On the one hand, it is good to help people in their needs, and on the other hand it is not good to absorb them. Subsidiarity is the most effective antidote against any form of paternalistic assistance[891].

Subsidiarity implies that people should be encouraged by the society and the authorities to develop what they have to offer to the community. They should neither be suppressed nor substituted. The administration of the public goods such as health care according to the Catholic social doctrine should be a "shared responsibility of each individual with regard to the common good"[892]. Depriving people of the opportunity to contribute to the achievement of the common good means undermining the principle of subsidiarity. Worse still, when this is done with the intention of monopolizing the distribution of a common good, such as health care. The Catholic moral tradition believes that in order to put into practice the principle of subsidiarity, there must be a sincere resolution by the political leaders to respect and promote the dignity of the human person and the family and to set an appropriate method that can enable citizens, as individuals or groups, to participate more actively and responsibly in the political and social reality of their country[893]. Affirming this idea the US Catholic Bishops' Conference indicates that:

> The responsible stewardship of health care resources can be accomplished best in dialogue with people from all levels of society, in accordance with the principle of subsidiarity and with respect for the moral principle that guide institutions and persons[894].

---

[891]   Cfr. BENEDICT XVI, «*Caritas in Veritate…*», n. 57, 96.

[892]   Ibid., n. 189, 107-108.

[893]   Cfr. PONTIFICAL COUNCIL FOR JUSTICE AND PEACE, *Compendium of the…*, n. 187, 105-106.

[894]   UNITED STATES CONFERENCE OF CATHOLIC BISHOPS, *Ethical and Religious…*,

There are however cases of exceptional nature where only the public authorities can intervene to guarantee a return to normalcy. In such cases, the government should wedge in, for the purpose of restoring justice and peace. However, the principle of subsidiarity retains that the presence of the public authorities should not be permanent. They should give way to the people once they have done their job, that is, once there are no longer cases of emergency or cases of a exceptional nature. Furthermore, the Universal Church teaches that "in any case, the common good correctly understood, the demands of which will never in any way be contrary to the defence and promotion of the primacy of the person and the way this is expressed in society, must remain the criteria for making decisions concerning the application of the principle of subsidiarity"[895]. The principle of subsidiarity is concretely expressed, and put into action, in the principle of participation, which according to the social teaching of the Catholic Church is the characteristic implication of subsidiarity. Participation, the Church affirms, "is a duty to be fulfilled consciously by all, with responsibility and with a view to the common good"[896]. The *Catechism of the Catholic Church* affirms that the obligation to participate is inherent in the dignity of the human person"[897].

Providing primary health care is the duty of the government because the principle of solidarity includes the provision of health care by the state to the poorest members and zones of the country. This becomes imperative with those health care goods that only the state can provide, and that will remain unprovided if the state does not procure them. The government is the authority within the state that is responsible for the common good. This however does not imply that it should arbitrarily take over the distribution of all the elements of the common good. Rather, the state should in accordance with the principle of subsidiarity promote and encourage the achievement of the common good by the lower communities, especially the family[898].

---

part 1, Introduction.

[895] Ibid., n. 188, 106-107.

[896] Ibid., n. 189, 107-108; Cfr. THE CATECHISM OF…, nn. 1913-1917, 458-459.

[897] THE CATECHISM OF…, nn. 1913-1917, 458-459.

[898] Cfr. D. M. GALLAGHER, «The Common Good», in E. J. FURTON – P. J. CATALDO – A. S. MORACZEWSKI (eds.), *Catholic Health Care…*

The principle of subsidiarity demands that the state leaves space to the intermediate communities in the distribution of health care resources because "subsidiarity means decisions being taken as close to the grass roots as good government allows"[899]. The state can oversee and harmonize their activities for the achievement of the set goals. The consideration of the powers and contribution of those at the grass root levels are very necessary for the realization of the common good. Thus, the community health care system in Nigeria should be promoted in this spirit. The communities should be encouraged by funding the community health system, training the health workers, providing infrastructure and other instruments that will allow the people to participate in the realization of the common good. The people should be helped in what they cannot do, but never substituted in what they can do themselves. Giving the people, that is, the communities a chance in the distribution of the common good according to the principles of subsidiarity is a matter of justice.

By allowing the communities to perform in the activity of distribution of resources necessarily implies recognizing their dignity. Regarding this, Rawls affirms that justice as fairness means assisting the less privileged without suppressing their liberty. In this sense, Rawls' theory of "justice as fairness" proves to be a good instrument to achieve, together with the Catholic principles, an ethical community health system in Nigeria. The administrative structure of the Nigerian health care system would need a reformation in this regard. The Federal and State governments should not continue to grab the 'lion's share' of the budgetary allocation to the health care sector leaving the local governments, which are closer to the people, with a handful portion of the allocation. The higher level of the state think it has the duty to do for the lower level, represented by the people, what they need to do for themselves. They think, after all, we provide everything for them, so why do they need the money. But the people should be allowed through the community health system to be part of the solutions to their health problems. It is however quite appalling that most often, the presumed help does not get to these individuals at the grassroots or community levels. This and similar situations create possibilities of injustice borne by the people.

---

[899] Catholic Bishops of England and Wales, *The Common Good...*, n. 5.

4.5. Health Care and Social Justice in Nigeria: Some Concrete Issues about Health Care Distribution in Nigeria in the Light of the Catholic Principles

4.5.1. Health Care Services in Nigeria and the Dignity/Integrity of the human person – Health Inequalities between Persons

Most of the questions we have seen in the previous parts of this work, especially in chapters one and two, are conditions concerning social justice in Nigeria. The effects of health indicators and the major causes of death and the prevalent pathologies in Nigeria hit more the poor and the most vulnerable in the country. The first among the vulnerable in Nigeria according to our dissertation are women and children. They suffer more than any other class, the problem of inequity in the Nigerian health care system. Equity in health ensures the reduction of the avoidable differences in health and its determinants[900]. Inequality in health refers to health status differences which are unnecessary, avoidable, unfair and unjust[901]. In line with equity, other features of an ethical health system such as universality, availability and accessibility indicate that the basic health needs of everyone should be met without any form of distinction. These qualities of an ethical health system stand for the reduction of inequalities in the distribution, availability, accessibility and affordability of health care resources.

There are authors who conceive equitable access as giving equitable provision to people of equal health care needs regardless of their income or socio-economic status. In Nigeria, "little is known regarding income-related vertical inequality in financing healthcare services"[902]. That being the case, a notable difference persists between individuals and zones in terms of health care. To correct the inequality in healthcare financing in Nigeria, the just cited authors think, "It is imperative to assess in a systematic manner the prevailing healthcare financing inequality"[903]. The

---

[900]   Cfr. A. O. LAWANSON – OLAIDE SEKINAT OPELOYERU, «Equity in healthcare financing», *Journal of Hospital Administration*, 5(2016), 53-59.

[901]   Cfr. P. A. BRAVEMAN – S. KUMAYIKA – J. FIELDING – T. LaVEIST – L. N. BORRELL – R. MANDERSCHEID – A. TROUTMAN, «Health Disparities and Health Equity: The Issue Is Justice», *American Journal of Public Health*, 101 (2011), 149-155.

[902]   A. O. LAWANSON – OLAIDE SEKINAT OPELOYERU, «Equity in healthcare...».

[903]   Ibid.

egalitarian theory of justice is often associated with vertical equity in healthcare financing. The egalitarian approach affirms that in a public financed system, it is just to offer equal opportunity of access to persons in equal need irrespective of their economic capacity and ability to pay[904]. The vertical equality approach requests a clear connection between the healthcare payments and ability to pay. In this connection, it is assumed that persons with unequal ability to pay make appropriately dissimilar payments. The vertical principle is in favour of giving treatment in accordance with ability to pay. This means that the poor and the vulnerable can receive equal treatment as the rich with the same medical needs, but paying an amount, which corresponds to their economic status, in other words, paying less than the rich do. This approach appears to be in favour of the vulnerable and the poorest.

Understood as such, we can say that it is closer to the ideas of the Church's social teaching which sustains the "obligation of every individual to contribute to the good of society, in the interests of justice and in pursuit of the "option for the poor". Pope John Paul II in line with the Catholic doctrine calls the attention of "those who have the responsibility of government and those who make the decisions that affect society to be particularly careful by reflecting on future long-term decisions and by thinking how to create economic and social balances"[905]. This is the context most likely to foster human fulfilment for everyone, where each individual can enjoy the benefit of living in an orderly, prosperous and healthy society. "A society with insufficient regard for the common good would be unpleasant and dangerous to live in, as well as unjust to those it excluded"[906]. This is what the Church means when it interprets the principle of solidarity in terms of us all being responsible for one another.

In Nigeria, applying the Catholic principles is imperative because according to the aforementioned authors, Nigeria is lagging behind. The authors sustain clearly that: "There is inequality in financing health care in Nigeria"[907]. To correct this problem of inequality and to install the right concept of health care financing in Nigeria, the above-cited authors

---

[904] Ibid.

[905] JOHN PAUL II, «Address to the plenary Session on the Subject 'Intergenerational Solidarity', 11 April 2002», n. 3, in *Papal Addresses to...*

[906] CATHOLIC BISHOPS OF ENGLAND AND WALES, *The Common Good...*, n. 19.

[907] A. O. LAWANSON – O. S. OPELOYERU, «Equity in healthcare...».

propose a thesis similar to that of the social teaching of the Catholic Church. According to them: "The pro-poor strategies need to be stepped up to really cater for the plight of the vulnerable in the society and drastically reduce the healthcare financing burden they currently share"[908]. Thus, the Catholic principle of preferential option for the poor and the vulnerable is an important key to the reduction of health care inequalities in Nigeria. Rawls' idea of justice as fairness is in line with the Catholic thought because it looks out for everyone and sustains the thesis that no one should be left behind in the distribution of resources, especially the needy. Correspondingly, the second Vatican document, *Gaudium et Spes* condemns all forms of discriminations and excess social and economic differences between individuals which often cause scandal as well as "militate against social justice, equity, and the dignity of the human person"[909].

The Egalitarian conviction is similar to the teaching of the Church because it sustains the non-discriminatory ideals of a just health system. The theory, just like Catholic health care ethics, supports the idea of giving services that permit every individual to have access to a decent minimum range of health care. The Egalitarian theory recommends a fair opportunity to access health care service. It also accepts that not every health care service is possible. For this, it asks that the minimum decent health care be provided. This Egalitarian position is identical to what we are advocating for the Nigerian health system through the Catholic principles.

The criteria of 'social worthiness' is often applied in Nigeria where the socially privileged receive more medical attention and before the less privileged. There are notable differences in the treatments given to the two classes of persons. On this, the Catholic health care ethics agrees that the ruling principle should be that of equal right of every human person to life, which is not relative to personal or social worth. This Catholic position is affirmed by the Egalitarian principle when it sustains that health care must be distributed in such a way that inequality between persons in terms of lifetime health is reduced[910]. The religious belief that all men are equal before God leads intelligibly to the non-acceptance of criteria of social worthiness. The *Compendium of the Social Doctrine of the Catholic Church*

---

[908]   Ibid.

[909]   Concilio Vaticano II, *Gaudium et Spes*…, n. 29, 899-900.

[910]   Cfr. R. Cookson – P. Dolan, «Principles of justice …».

confirms this when it states: "The Church sees in men and women, in every person, the living image of God himself"[911]. Some unjust treatments women and children receive in Nigeria as we have seen in the first and second chapters of our work indicts the Nigeria society regarding injustice. The Catholic moral tradition believes that life is a value incommensurate with others. This implies that life is a value not negotiable by battering a person's worth against another's.

Equality as sustained by Egalitarian theory of distributive justice sustains it is not correct for an individual's right to healthcare resources to be influenced by his or her social status, in terms of age, sex, quality of life and racial origin. Social worthiness or social productiveness, creates a big ethical problem if applied as the criterion for healthcare allocation. The author G. Outka, adherent to the Catholic doctrine, rightly points out that:

> If one agrees, for whatever reasons, with the agapeic judgment that each person should be regarded as irreducibly valuable, then one cannot succumb to a social productiveness criterion of social of human worth. Interests are to be equally considered even when people have ceased to be, or are not yet, or perhaps never will be, public assets[912].

The Universal Church teaches that: "Human rights are to be defended not only individually but also as a whole: protecting them only partially would imply a kind of failure to recognize them"[913]. This means that every person, including women and children, has the right to health care in an equal manner. Therefore, it will be unjust to respect and protect the right to health of some while neglecting that of others. The libertarian approach is of the view that demand from self-paying or insured persons is the condition for making available any form of health care service. So, they agree that even the need for health care is not enough to guarantee the provision of services where there is insufficient number of payers. This approach obviously discriminates against those who do not have ability to

---

[911] PONTIFICAL COUNCIL FOR JUSTICE AND PEACE, *Compendium of the …*, n. 105, 61.

[912] G. OUTKA, «Social Justice and Equal Access to Health Care», in S. E. LAMMERS, A. VERHEY, (eds.), *On Moral medicine*, William B. Eerdmans Publishing Company, Grand Rapids, Michigan 1988, 632-642.

[913] Cfr. PONTIFICAL COUNCIL FOR JUSTICE AND PEACE, *Compendium of the…*, n. 154, 85.

pay. Making accessible health care resources based on the socio-economic class is unjust and it does not represent the idea of a fair distribution of health care resources. Equity is the key word and should be based on the respect for the dignity of every human person, rich and poor alike.

The poor and the vulnerable must be protected because they are always the victims. In accordance with this idea, the Catholic principle of solidarity highlights particularly the equality of all in dignity and rights[914]. The Church's teaching emphasizes more on this because it is affirmed that there are gross inequalities between persons in various societies. Concerning this, the social teaching of the Catholic Church advises that there is the need for the ethical principles to bring under control this phenomenon, to avoid the dangerous impact of perpetrating injustice. Such advice is what our dissertation is proposing for the Nigerian health care system, because health inequalities in the country is a phenomenon that is getting out of hand. There is the need to act in accordance with what the Catholic social teaching enjoins: health care is part of the common good and, as such, demands equality in its distribution. To do this, the Nigerian government and the health agencies should be guided by the idea that "the equality of men rests essentially on their dignity as persons"[915]. Thus, the good of every individual must be considered in the distribution of the common good.

Life experiences show that no one is born with all he or she needs in life. Ergo, we need others for some of our needs. The distinctions that are the fruits of our natural endowments which are not distributed equally are in accordance with God's plan for each person and the society. The differences encourage human beings to be kind and generous towards one another in the sharing and distribution of goods. Nevertheless, some differences or inequalities are in accordance with man's will and plan. For this, the Catholic moral tradition retains that some inequalities are sinful and they have grave impacts on millions of men and women and are contrary to the Gospel. Consequently, the Catholic social teaching condemns the excessive economic and social disparity between individuals because they do not foster social justice, equity and the dignity of the human person. Where there is equal dignity of individuals as persons, it is possible and easier to strive for fairer and more humane conditions[916].

---

[914] Cfr. Ibid., n. 192, 109-110.

[915] THE CATECHISM OF…, n. 1935, 461.

[916] Cfr. Ibid., nn. 1936-1938, 461-462.

4.5.2. Injustice in Health Care: Inequality between Urban and Rural Areas in Nigeria

There are permissible differences and inequalities; those due to natural endowment, and in accordance with God's plan. On the other hand, there are inequalities that are unjust and that give rise to moral debates, such as health inequalities between individuals, urban and rural, the young and old, the healthy and the sickest. For the Catholic social teaching, the former is morally permissible, while the latter is not. The social concern of the Catholic Church has always been fashioned in the way that it gears towards an authentic development of man and the society[917]. The concept of right to health care as understood by the Catholic principles retain that the right to health care is rooted in the dignity of the human person. Such right is respected only when the dignity of the human person is the main reason for making decisions, policies and programmes for the distribution of health care resources and this crucial point cannot be forgotten. Thus, the concept of the human person has consistently been the guiding principle of the Church's social vision. An authentic development of man and the society will be difficult to achieve if the inequalities between persons, zones and populations continue to be excessive. The inequalities created unjustly by man, do not respect the dignity of the human person, which represent the core of the Catholic social doctrine.

Here, we are treating the issue of unjust differences or inequalities between the urban and the rural areas. "In Nigeria, 66% of the poor live in the rural areas where incomes are up to 30% lower than in urban areas"[918]. In addition, it has been ascertained that there is a lopsided distribution of health facilities between urban and rural areas in Nigeria. The urban areas, where the educated and the rich live, always receive the lion share of the common good. An article by some Nigerian authors reveal that: "Serious inequalities in health outcomes (including mortality and fertility) exist between rural and urban areas; northern and southern states; and across income groups"[919]. Maldistribution of health resources

---

[917] Cfr. JOHN PAUL II, «*Sollicitudo Rei Socialis*, Encyclical Letter, (1987), for the twentieth anniversary of *Populorum Progressio*», n. 1, in J. M. MILLER (ed.), *The Encyclicals of...*

[918] D. EBOH, *Strategic Concept for...*, 22-23.

[919] G. TIMOTHY – O. IRINOYE – U. YUNUSA – A. DALHATU – S. AHMED – A. SUBERU, «Balancing Demand and...».

is one of the major causes of health inequalities in Nigeria. Often there is a concentration of health facilities and health professionals in the urban areas. "Even when some doctors, laboratory technologist and nurses are posted to the health centres in the rural areas, they either influence/ refuse posting or resume and put up nonchalant attitude to work because of poor health infrastructural development in these areas"[920]. The US Bishops affirm that "a just health care system will be concerned both with promoting equity of care – to assure that the right of each person to basic health care is respected – and with promoting the good health of all in the community"[921].

Affirming the inequality in the distribution of health care resources in Nigeria, S. I. Okafor asserts that there are spatial imbalances in the country's health care delivery system. According to him, one of the factors contributing to this is the degree of the centralized control of provision and the policies on health care provision. With this pattern, health care resources are allocated intensively to the central areas ignoring the local needs[922]. Explaining further on the factors, he writes:

> Many factors influence health care delivery systems and resultant spatial patterns in nation-states [...] the first factor affects the responsiveness of health care delivery systems to local needs. At the same time, it could cause disparities in the quantity and quality of provision between different areas[923].

The imbalance which manifests in the low level of available healthcare facilities/infrastructures in the rural areas, compel the rural dwellers to engage in long travels; spending a lot of time and money to have access to the better facilities situated only in the urban area[924]. Pope John Paul II commenting on such differences in allocation of resources states:

---

[920] S. I. EFE, «Health care problem and management in Nigeria», *Journal of Geography and Regional Planning*, 6(2013), 244-254.

[921] UNITED STATES CONFERENCE OF CATHOLIC BISHOPS, «*Ethical and Religious…*», part 1, introduction.

[922] Cfr. S. I. OKAFOR, «Spatial Aspects of Health Care Provision in Nigeria», in R. AKHTAR (ed.) *Health Care Patterns…*

[923] Ibid.

[924] S. I. EFE, «Health care problem…».

> We are therefore faced with a serious problem of unequal distribution of the means of subsistence originally meant for everybody, and thus also an unequal distribution of the benefits deriving from them. And this happens not through the fault of the needy people, and even less through a sort of inevitability dependent on natural conditions or circumstances as a whole[925].

The Pope's comment reveals that, unfortunately, the common good, which is for everyone, is enjoyed by few persons and that many others who are in need are denied the right to use what belongs to them as citizens. The unequal distribution of health care resources violates the rights to life and health of many Nigerians. Therefore, it is an issue that must be addressed by the society. A return to governing by concern for the common good of all is very important to solve this problem. Some people think the Nigerian government should embrace the location-allocation models, which help in improving geographical accessibility of health care facilities. Efforts should be made to choose the most suitable location for the rural and urban primary health care centers. The issue of geographical location according to G. Rushton is very essential for developing countries "because a large proportion of their population is rural and their transport and communication systems are often poorly developed and costly to use"[926].

At the root of inequality in the distribution of health care resources in Nigeria is the lack of application of the moral principles especially those proposed in this dissertation. For instance, some authors already cited in this work assert that cough and dehydration from diarrhoea are big threats to the children's life as they are among the major causes of childhood morbidity and mortality, but if the medical attention is timely, there could be an important reduction in the rates of child deaths[927]. This is the truth about the various diseases that claim the lives of many

---

[925] Cfr. JOHN PAUL II, «*Sollicitudo Rei Socialis*, Encyclical Letter, (1987), for the twentieth anniversary of *Populorum Progressio*», n. 9, in J. M. MILLER (ed.), *The Encyclicals of…*

[926] G. RUSHTON, «Use of Location-Allocation Models for Improving the Geographical Accessibility of Rural Services in Developing Countries», in R. Akhtar (ed.) *Health Care Patterns and Planning in Developing Countries*, Greenwood Press, New York 1991, 147-170.

[927] Cfr. H. V. DOCTOR – R. BAIRAGI – S. E. FINDLEY – S. HELLERINGER – T. DAHIRU, «Northern Nigeria Maternal …».

poor Nigerian children, especially those who live in the rural areas where medical attention arrives late, if it arrives at all. This happens due to some evitable factors, but unfortunately, they are not controlled because the medical interventions are not timely. In some cases, some children in the rural areas die in the hands of their poor mothers who do what they can to save their children on their own, having lost hope on the government's health care provision.

The applications of the Catholic principles of distributive justice can help to checkmate such situation. The health care facilities are retained as part of common good by the Catholic social teaching, thus they should be accessible to all especially those in most need of them. In a similar vein, the egalitarian approach to health has the basic assumption that each individual is eligible to an equal claim in health care. For this model, as a matter of justice, everyone has a just claim to receive the resources necessary for him or her to be healthy[928]. Rawls' theory is literally in line with the egalitarian theory and the Catholic principles in the ongoing arguments. According to Rawls, laws guiding distribution of resources should be founded on the principles of equality and social and economic inequalities. This implies assigning equal rights and duties to individuals and permitting inequalities only in cases where they are for the good of all, especially if they are compatible with the ethical principle of preferential option for the poor and the vulnerable[929]. The need principle belongs to the same stream of thought because it accepts "need" as a justifiable reason for discrimination in the distribution of health care resources. Our thesis agrees the need principle and some above-mentioned models can be combined with the Catholic principles to reduce the gross unjustifiable inequalities between the urban and rural areas in Nigeria and to address the health problems of those ignored because of their status.

If the dignity of the human person and the respect for the inalienable right to life were understood in Nigeria as taught by the Catholic social teaching, the situations of unjust inequalities described above would never have been as bad as they are. The inalienable right to life and the right to health are not to be respected depending on whether one is poor or rich, rural or urban dweller. They should simply be respected unconditionally. The dignity of every human person as the Church teaches stems from his

---

[928]   Cfr. R. L. SHELTON, «Human rights and…».

[929]   Cfr. M. GRONEBAUM, *John Rawls' Theory…*, III.

relation with God. Therefore, it does not depend on the person's social or economic conditions. Morality demands that we act rationally to pursue what is good and reject what is evil. Unjust inequalities in this sense should be avoided to embrace equity in health care allocation. This has to be done uninterruptedly because "our obligation to be moral is *unconditional* and therefore not something that we may choose to suspend at our convenience. Morality is about living well in all areas of our lives and at every moment of our lives, without exception. It is not a game that we can switch off at our whim"[930].

In line with the foregoing, Jacques Maritain retains that a human right legitimately belongs to a human being by virtue of having a human nature[931]. Furthermore, the philosopher Jacques Maritain, in line with the Catholic doctrine, affirms that the absolute dignity of the human person derives from his relationship with the Absolute[932]. The present dissertation proposes the principles of the Catholic social teaching with the intention of generating for Nigeria national initiatives in health care reform aimed at distributing health care resources in a fair, equitable, accessible, affordable manner and realizing an ethical health care system. A health care system in which the human person is seen as the summit of all the activities. Good health obviously contributes to our ability to seek our own fulfillment and that of others. This is why it will be difficult to ignore the fair provision of health care when we want our nation to progress. A wealthy nation is a nation with healthy citizens. Respect for the human person demands that everyone should look upon his neighbour as another self. This should be done always (thinking about the 'neighbour's' life and the means necessary for living it with dignity). The duty of being a good neighbour and one's brother's keeper according to the Catholic doctrine becomes more urgent when it involves the disadvantaged, that is, the poor and the vulnerable[933].

---

[930] T. HSIAO, «Why Recreational Drug Use Is Immoral», in E. J. FURTON (ed.), *The National Catholic Bioethics Quarterly*, Philadelphia, 17(2017), 605-614.

[931] Cfr. D. A. SCRANDIS, «Jacques Maritain on the Rights of Man and the Common Good», in E. J. FURTON (ed.), *The National Catholic Bioethics Quarterly*, Philadelphia, 17(2017), 615-621.

[932] Cfr. Ibid.

[933] Cfr. THE CATECHISM OF…, nn. 1931-1932, 460-461.

4.5.3. Medical Detention and other Unethical Practices
in Nigerian Hospitals and Clinics: A Moral Vision
from the Perspective of the Catholic Principles

Medical detention is the practice of detaining people in hospitals and clinics for non-payment of hospital bills. This practice is widespread in Nigeria and its negative impacts on the poor and most vulnerable arouses serious moral questions. Some affirm that hospital detention deters health care use and increases the violation of human rights, especially the right to health of the poor. Such practice represents a health system that lacks the 'virtue of solidarity' which according to the Catholic teaching:

> Finds its deepest roots in Christian faith, which teaches that God is our Father and that all men and women are brothers and sisters. From this belief flows Christian ethics, an ethics which excludes every form of selfishness and arrogance and seeks to unite persons freely in pursuit of the common good[934].

The practice of hospital detention also indicates lack of the virtue of 'charity' which is a fundamental value of the Church's social doctrine; it occupies a special place among the human values, because it represents the first category of life in society[935].

Studies on this issue make known that many Nigerians experienced financial hardship in settling their medical bills[936]. Consequently, most

---

[934] JOHN PAUL II, «Address to the Study Week on the Subject 'Science for Development in a Solidarity Framework, 27 October 1989», n.4, in *Papal Addresses to the Pontifical Academy of Sciences 1917 – 2002 and to the Pontifical Academy of Social Sciences 1994 – 2002*, The Pontifical Academy of Sciences, Vatican City 2003, 306-310.

[935] JOHN PAUL II, «Address to Plenary Session on the Subject 'The Study of the Tension Between Human Equality and Social Inequalities from the Perspective of the Various Social Sciences', 25 November 1994», n.9, in *Papal Addresses to the Pontifical Academy of Sciences 1917 – 2002 and to the Pontifical Academy of Social Sciences 1994 – 2002*, The Pontifical Academy of Sciences, Vatican City 2003, 405-410.

[936] Cfr. O. S. ILESANMI – A. A. FATIREGUN, «The direct cost of care among surgical inpatients at a tertiary hospital in south west Nigeria», *The Pan African Medical Journal*, 18(2014), 3, in https://doi.org/10.11604/pamj.2014.18.3.3177 [24-8-2018]; Cfr. O. P. EZEOKE – O. E. ONWUJEKWE – B. S. UZOCHUKWU,

poor people are held in the hospitals and clinics for long periods where their freedom and movements are restricted. While in detention, they are denied care and other vital services. Expressing concern over atrocities against the human life and dignity in Nigeria, the Catholic Bishops' Conference of Nigeria note: "We have found the outright disdain for the sanctity of human life totally at variance with both our cultural traditional norms and our religious sensibilities"[937]. The Catholic Bishops' Conference of Nigeria describes the situations of inequalities and indignities as intolerable and emphasized that the majority of Nigerians cannot continue to live under so much poverty and inequality[938].

The unjust practice of hospital detention in Nigeria prevails because some apply libertarian theory to the distribution of health care resources, forgetting that many Nigerians are very poor and cannot provide for their necessities health-wise. The libertarian approach believes that only the ability to pay is a measure to determine one's willingness to receive treatment. Often services should be rendered only if there are persons capable of paying. This is applied in Nigeria and it is one of the root causes of inequalities/injustice being meted out to the poor and the most vulnerable in Nigeria. Such situation, as we have seen in the previous chapter of this thesis, is created where there is a confusion about the issue of right to health; between what the government should control and provide under the distribution of common good and what should be left to the market place[939].

Hospital detention according to some, does not only cause deep psychological distress for the poor, it also opens doors that lead to abject

---

«Towards Universal Coverage: Examining Cost of Illness, Payment, and Coping Strategies to Different Population Groups in Southeast Nigeria», *The American Journal of Tropical Medicine and Hygiene*, 86(2012), 52-57; Cfr. U. B. ANYAEHIE – E. D. NWAOBODO, «Administrative responsibilities of Community-funded health insurance scheme in Nigeria», *Nigerian Medical Practitioner*, 45(2004), 26-28; Cfr. A. LEIVE – K. XU, «Coping with out-of-pocket health payments: empirical evidences from 15 African countries», *Bull World Health Organ*, 86(2008), 817-908.

[937] CATHOLIC BISHOPS CONFERENCE OF NIGERIA, «Our Dignity, Our Nation and Our Citizenship», Statement by the Catholic Bishops Conference of Nigeria (CBCN), in https://www.cbcn-ng.org/docs/g26.pdf [20-6-2018].

[938] Ibid.

[939] Cfr. This doctoral thesis 3.4.1. Right to Health and Access to Care.

poverty. Medical detention is a phenomenon present both in the public and private health facilities in Nigeria. Often mothers in need of life-saving emergency caesarean sections and their babies are particularly vulnerable to this practice in Nigeria. They are hospitalized under emergency condition and after birth and post-natal period of stay in the hospital, if the husband or family is unable to pay, the woman and her child are held while awaiting payment. Often, they stay in this condition of physical and psychological torture without knowing when they would be set free. "Detention is an abuse of women's and children's rights and contravenes national and international laws"[940]. In general, the poorest members of the society that were admitted to the health facilities for emergency medical treatment are the victims of this practice. The victims being the poorest and the most vulnerable makes the practice gravely immoral and an act of injustice. Hospital detention is a practice which thwarts the dignity of the poor. For the Nigerian bishops, "the dignity of the human person is inalienable. It can neither be detached from the personality of the individual nor taken away by anyone, not even by the state. It is inherent. From this inherent dignity derive some basic rights"[941].

One of the basic rights is the right every individual has to a minimum decent health care irrespective of his or her economic status. The position of the Nigerian Bishops, in line with Rawls' theory, is in contrast with utilitarianism which maximizes advantages for the most but not for all[942]. For instance, Rawls' theory affirms that every person possesses an inviolability based on justice and such inviolability should be held above the societal welfare. This means that this personal inviolability cannot accept to be

---

[940] D. DEVAKUMAR – R. YATES, «Medical Hostages: Detention of Women and Babies in Hospitals», *Health and Human Rights Journal*, 18(2016), 1; Cfr. R. YATES, Women and children first: an appropriate first step towards universal coverage, *Bull World Health Org*, 88(2010), 474-475; Cfr. B. A. O.-ADENIRAN – I. F. ADEWOLE – N. IWERE – P. MAHMOUD, «Promoting Sexual and Reproductive Health and Rights in Nigeria through Change in Medical School Curriculum», *African Journal of Reproductive Health*, 8(2004), 85-91.

[941] CATHOLIC BISHOPS CONFERENCE OF NIGERIA, «*Nigeria: Citizenship Rights and Duties*», A Communiqué at the End of the First Plenary Meeting of the Catholic Bishops' Conference of Nigeria (CBCN) at Daughters of Divine Love Retreat and Conference Centre (DRACC), Abuja, 4-10 March, 2107, in https://www.cbcn-ng.org/docs/g26.pdf [20-6-2018].

[942] Cfr. M. GRONEBAUM, *John Rawls' Theory…*, V.

compromised by advantages in favour of the majority[943]. More so, in contrast with the QALY and other utilitarian oriented approaches, we affirm in line with the principle of equity that when economic gain outweighs the value of human life and health, the dignity of the human person risks being compromised. Such criterion can hardly guarantee a just health system.

Hospital detention is a practice that must be denounced because the detention of the poor means discriminating against them. Such discrimination is contrary to what the common good stands for. "Common" means that it is "all-inclusive". This implies that by common good it is meant that no one should be excluded. Hence, "if any section of the population is in fact excluded from participation in the life of the community, even at a minimal level, then that is a contradiction to the concept of the common good and calls for rectification"[944]. In line with the ongoing arguments, the US Bishops explain: "The common good is realized when economic, political and social conditions ensure protection for the rights of all individuals and enable all to fulfil their common purpose and reach their common goals"[945]. The situation of many in some societies today is similar to that of the poor Lazarus. "Like Lazarus at the door of the rich man, millions of people are in dire need while a great part of the world's resources are employed in areas which have little or nothing to contribute to the improvement of life"[946]. This exactly is what happens between the rich and the poor, between the urban and poor rural areas. It is also glaring in the world today where more funds are dedicated to war and nuclear weapons than to life saving projects. Responding to this miserable condition, John Paul II recalls that "The Church has forcefully affirmed that solidarity is a grave moral obligation, for nations as well as for individuals"[947].

Some have traced the problem of medical detention to the high rate of poverty in Nigeria. Many citizens are unemployed. Those working in the public offices in some states are not always paid on time and most are underpaid. Pensioners pass through various kinds of humiliation before

---

[943] Cfr. J. RAWLS, *A Theory of Justice…*, 3.

[944] CATHOLIC BISHOPS OF ENGLAND AND WALES, «*The Common Good…*», n. 19.

[945] UNITED STATES CONFERENCE OF CATHOLIC BISHOPS, «*Ethical and Religious…*», n.80.

[946] JOHN PAUL II, «*Address to the…*», n.4, 306-310.

[947] Ibid.

receiving what is their due. Many Nigerians are at present experiencing financial hardship and the governments both at the federal and state levels seem not to have solutions to this perennial problem. Others associate the illicit and immoral practice of hospital detention with high out-of-pocket payments required for health care in both public and private health facilities in Nigeria. A study in South Eastern Nigeria showed that there was no evidence of differences across socio-economic groups in terms of illness occurrence, inequality in expenditures, payment mechanisms used and income sources to confront the burden of payments. There was no clear evidence to show that policy makers cared to protect the poor and the vulnerable groups against the financial risk of ill-health. Rather the policy makers and facility managers assumed that households have the capacity to cope with health care payments. Consequently, no provision was made for fee exemptions[948]. The situation described by this study is one of the major causes of medical detention in Nigeria and it shows that little is done to curb it. Thus, B. A. Lanre-Abass thinks that "care ethics has implications for medical practice in Nigeria"[949].

Medical detention is an issue of the health-poverty link in Nigeria. The Federal government of Nigeria retains that the hospitals do not have any right to detain patients. Therefore, the government retains that medical detention is illicit. We think that this is not enough because the problem has to be solved by addressing the root-cause. Poverty is the root-cause of the inability of citizens to pay their hospital bills. Hence, a lasting solution should be made possible through poverty alleviation and the government must be involved. Furthermore, the practice of medical detention should be explicitly proscribed in domestic law. There are no legal or moral justifications for hospital detention of the poor and the vulnerable who

---

[948] Cfr. O. E. ONWUJEKWE – C. A. ONOKA – B. S. C. UZOCHUKWU – E. N. OBIKEZE – N. EZUMAH, «Issues in equitable health financing in South Eastern Nigeria: Socio-economic and geographic differences in households' illness expenditure and policymakers' views on the financial protection of the poor», *Journal of International Development*, 21(2009), 185-199; Cfr. O. E. ONWUJEKWE – B. UZOCHUKWU, «Socio-economic and geographic differentials in costs and payment strategies for primary healthcare services in Southeast Nigeria», *Health Policy*, 71(2005), 383-397.

[949] B. A. L.-ABASS, «Poverty and maternal mortality in Nigeria: towards a more viable ethics of modern medical practice», *International Journal for Equity in Health*, 7(2008) https://doi.org/10.1186/1475-9276-7-11 [14-8-2018].

are unable to pay their bills. There should be an explicit ban on hospital detentions in the private and public hospitals in order to respect the right and dignity of the poor and the vulnerable.

The legal ban as we have said is very important but not enough and cannot perfectly solve the problem. The poverty alleviation could be an effective solution from the point of view of eliminating the root-cause. In addition, the programme of health care for all can help in tackling the grave moral problem of medical detention. The government's will to apply correctly the policies regarding health financial system could be a proper means of solving this issue. It is widely accepted that the attainment of Universal Health Coverage (UHC) is achieved when every member of the society has access to and utilizes the health care they need without going through financial hardship. A proper understanding and application of the Catholic principles with the corresponding characteristics of the secular principles, theories and approaches of distributive justice can go a long way to address the above mentioned problems. For instance, considering the human person always as an end and not means to an end will always help the governments and health officials to make the right choices.

R. A. Capone in line with our dissertation sustains the necessity to apply the Catholic principles in confronting the issue at stake. According to him:

> Catholic social teaching has a rich tradition of intellectual responses to societal and economic problems [...] The Church teaches, for example, that the common good consists of those conditions "which allow people, either as group or individuals, to reach their fulfilment more fully and more easily" in other words, to flourish both materially and spiritually[950].

It follows that the solution to medical detention proffered earlier will hardly be effective if they are not deeply rooted in the moral principles of the Catholic doctrine. If the human person is not at the centre of the legal fight against medical detention or the focus of poverty alleviation, it will be difficult to identify the way forward. The Catholic principle of preferential option for the poor has the dignity of the person as the fulcrum of its application. The Catholic moral tradition sustains that the poor, the marginalized and in all cases, those whose living conditions do not permit

---

[950] R. A. CAPONE, «AMA Reconsiders opposition…»; PONTIFICAL COUNCIL FOR JUSTICE AND PEACE, *Compendium of the…*, n. 160, 91.

their proper development, should be treated with particular attention. Thus, it invites all institutions and authorities to adopt the doctrine of preferential option for the poor and not medical detention.

For the Catholic social teaching, it is imperative that the principle of the preferential option for the poor be reaffirmed in all its forces[951]. Preferential option for the poor is our social responsibility. Pope John Paul II in line with the Catholic moral tradition remarks: "this love of preference for the poor, and the decisions which it inspires in us, cannot but embrace the immense multitudes of the hungry, the needy, the homeless, those without health care and, above all, those without hope of a better future"[952]. The love for the poor opens our mind to the truth that humanity is one family despite our various differences. It also helps societies to understand that "the poor are not a burden; they are our brothers and sisters"[953].

In the Catholic social teaching, the care for the poor; charity is juxtaposed with justice, that is, giving each his or her due. In this juxtaposition, the aid given to the poor is not considered as charity but justice, that is, paying a debt of justice. This means that the care for the poor, especially in the areas of distribution of health care resources is what is already due in justice. Going by this Catholic teaching, the detentions of patients who cannot afford to pay their bills, which is practiced in Nigeria, is particularly immoral and it connotes violence and injustice. The poor is unable to pay because someone, somewhere, has refused to make a fair distribution of the common good. Therefore, the Universal Church recommends that the duty of giving health care for the poor and the vulnerable be fulfilled diligently[954]. The American Catholic Bishops following the mainstream social teaching of the Catholic Church affirm: "The common good is realized when economic, political and social conditions ensure protection for the fundamental rights of all individuals and enable all to fulfil their common purpose and reach their common goals"[955].

---

[951] Cfr. PONTIFICAL COUNCIL FOR JUSTICE AND PEACE, *Compendium of the...*, n. 182, 102.

[952] JOHN PAUL II, «*Sollicitudo Rei Socialis*, Encyclical Letter, (1987), for the twentieth anniversary of *Populorum Progressio*», n. 42, in J. M. MILLER (ed.), *The Encyclicals of...*

[953] CATHOLIC BISHOPS OF ENGLAND AND WALES, *The Common Good...*, n. 10.

[954] Cfr. PONTIFICAL COUNCIL FOR JUSTICE AND PEACE, *Compendium of the...*, n. 184, 103-104.

[955] UNITED STATES CONFERENCE OF CATHOLIC BISHOPS, Ethical and Religious

The position of the aforementioned Catholic Bishops Conference corresponds to the teaching of Pope John XIII that sustains that the common good is best protected when personal rights are respected. The Roman Pontiff indicates that: "The chief concern of the civil authorities must therefore be to ensure that these rights are recognized, respected, coordinated, defended, and promoted, and that each individual is enabled to perform his duties more easily"[956]. Hence, the principle of common good is said to attain its fullest meaning only when "it stems from the dignity, unity and equality of all people"[957]. The teaching of the Catholic Church is in line with the aim of bioethics and medical ethics, that is, the "good, the health of the individual person and the health of society"[958]. The underlying force of this position is the principle of the common good; the good of the individual person and the good of society, where the good of the individual is included in the good of the society and the individual person is considered as an end and not as a means in the pursuit of the common good. Using the individual as a means is not consistent with the Catholic principles. The person in the Catholic social teaching is always considered as an end in himself. To ensure the common and individual good in health care in Nigeria, we need the Catholic principles, especially those inherent to dignity and the value of the human person.

This Catholic principle of solidarity is needed when the poor cannot afford to pay for their hospital bills. Solidarity according to the Catholic social doctrine is demonstrated primarily in the distribution of goods. Socio-economic problems can be resolved with help of all forms of solidarity, like solidarity between the rich and the poor. More so, the principle of solidarity presupposes the effort to reduce conflicts and settle conflicts by negotiation[959]. There is a firm connection between solidarity and other

---

Directives for Catholic Health Services (2009)[5] in E. J. FURTON — P. J. CATALDO — A. S. MORACZEWSKI (eds.), *Catholic Health Care Ethics. A Manual for Practitioners*, The National Catholic Bioethics Center, Philadelphia 2009, 389-400[2].

[956] JOHN XXIII, «*Pacem in Terris*, Encyclical Letter of on Establishing Universal Peace, in Truth, Justice, Charity, and Liberty, (1963)», n. 60, 107-129, in C. CARLEN (ed.), *The Papal Encyclicals*...

[957] PONTIFICAL COUNCIL FOR JUSTICE AND PEACE, *Compendium of the*..., n. 164, 93.

[958] D. BEAUREGARD, «Virtue in Bioethics», in E. J. FURTON — P. J. CATALDO — A. S. MORACZEWSKI (eds.), *Catholic Health Care*..., 27-29[2].

[959] Cfr. THE CATECHISM OF..., nn. 1940-1941, 462.

Catholic principles and values proposed by our work for a just health care system in Nigeria. Affirming this relationship, the compendium of the social teaching of the Church states:

> The message of the Church's social doctrine regarding solidarity clearly shows that there exists an intimate bond between solidarity and the common good, between solidarity and the universal destination of goods, between solidarity and equality among men and peoples, between solidarity and peace in the world[960].

More so, according to the Catholic social teaching, "the principle of solidarity requires that men and women of our day cultivate a greater awareness that they are debtors of the society of which they have become part"[961]. This message reminds those that practice medical detention in the Nigerian health facilities of the truth that we are all debtors of the society in which we live. Therefore, we are all invited to be responsible for all in accordance with the principles of common good and solidarity. The common good, the universal Church teaches, concerns the life of all[962], including the life of those detained because they are poor and so unable to pay for the treatments they received. Related to this line of thought is the following affirmation of John Paul II: "At stake is the dignity of the human person, whose defence and promotion have been entrusted to us by the Creator, and to whom the men and women at every moment of history are strictly and responsibly in debt"[963].

The common good as the Church teaches is always oriented towards the progress of persons. This, according to the Catholic doctrine, implies that "the order of things must be subordinate to the order of persons, and not the other way around"[964]. The human person, irrespective of his social or economic condition cannot be valued less than money and other material goods. This order that is founded on truth, built up in justice,

---

[960] PONTIFICAL COUNCIL FOR JUSTICE AND PEACE, *Compendium of the…*, n. 194, 111.

[961] Ibid., n. 195, 112.

[962] Cfr. THE CATECHISM OF…, n.1906, 457.

[963] JOHN PAUL II, «*Sollicitudo Rei Socialis*, Encyclical Letter, (1987), for the twentieth anniversary of *Populorum Progressio*», n. 38, in J. M. MILLER (ed.), *The Encyclicals of…*

[964] Cfr. THE CATECHISM OF…, n.1912, 458.

and animated by love, indicates how the hospital detention of the poor is not in accordance with justice and charity. The dignity of the human person is not respected wherever the poor are detained because they cannot afford to pay for the health care services received. The issue of detention of the poor patients thus, is a very delicate issue. It is an ethical issue that should be confronted with seriousness. Respecting the human person means respecting his rights. It is a moral obligation for all authorities and societies to respect the rights of the human person since these simply flow from his dignity as a human person. The authorities and the societies are not the authors of these rights because the rights are prior to the authorities and societies. Thus, everyone has just the duty to recognize the rights. Rights to life and health care of the poor and the vulnerable in this case are there to be recognized by respecting and protecting them. Failure to do this, makes questionable the legitimacy of any authority because, these are among the rights considered as the basis of the moral legitimacy of every authority[965]. The Social teaching of the Church constantly invites us "to be especially at the service of our brothers and sisters who are most in need of aid in order to lead a life that corresponds to their nature and their incomparable dignity"[966]. The Church is firm in its struggle to reaffirm the transcendent dignity of the human person and constantly to defend human rights and freedom"[967].

The past experiences of unethical conduct of clinical trials in Nigeria makes it imperative for all those involved in health care in Nigeria to be aware of the requirements for ethical conduct of clinical research in Nigeria[968]. The above situation makes clear the presence of ethical

---

[965] Cfr. Ibid., n.1930, 460.

[966] JOHN PAUL II, «Address to the Plenary Session on the Subject 'Human Genome; Alternative Energy Sources for Developing Countries; the Fundamental Principles of Mathematics; and Artificial Intelligence', 28 October 1994», n.8, in *Papal Addresses to the Pontifical Academy of Sciences 1917 – 2002 and to the Pontifical Academy of Social Sciences 1994 – 2002, The Pontifical Academy of Sciences*, Vatican City 2003, 358-363.

[967] JOHN PAUL II, «Address to the Plenary Session on the Subject 'Democracy – Reality and Responsibility', 23 February 2000», n.3, in *Papal Addresses to the Pontifical Academy of Sciences 1917 – 2002 and to the Pontifical Academy of Social Sciences 1994 – 2002, The Pontifical Academy of Sciences*, Vatican City 2003, 427-430.

[968] Cfr. P. I. OKONTA, «Ethics of clinical trials in Nigeria», *Nigerian Medical*

challenges in the Nigerian Health care system. **P. I.** Okonta emphasizes this affirming that "the conduct for the development and licensing of drugs is a very important aspect of healthcare"[969]. There was a case of unethical conduct of clinical trials in Nigeria against Pfizer in 1996, when "there was an outbreak of cerebro-spinal meningitis in Tudun Wada in Kano State. Children were predominantly affected by the outbreak. The state government mobilised resources to combat the meningitis epidemic. Also, international organisations like the Medecins Sans Frontieres (MSF) were there to assist in treating patients. Pfizer brought in a team to conduct a research on its test drug TROVAFLOXACIN (TROVAN) – a quinolone antibiotic. Pfizer recruited a total of 200 children into the study in two arms- one arm had the test drug Trovan orally and the control arm was given Ceftriaxone or Chloramphenicol. Within 3 weeks of commencing the study, the required numbers of participants were recruited and the study concluded. The study was however criticised severely for falling short of ethical standards. The allegations were that:

1. Pfizer never obtained ethical clearance before conducting the study;
2. Pfizer did not obtain informed consent before recruiting participant and did not inform the study participants that the drug was an experimental drug;
3. Pfizer capitalised on the poor, illiterate and desperate situation of the people; and,
4. Pfizer left the town after conducting the study despite the fact that the epidemic was still ongoing"[970].

The total number of 88 Nigerian families continued their lawsuit in the United States of America against Pfizer, the world's largest drug maker,

---

Journal, 55(2014), 188-194.

[969] Cfr. Ibid.

[970] Cfr. Ibid; K. AHMAD, «Drug company sued over research trial in Nigeria», *Lancet*, 358(2001), 815, in https://doi.org/10/1016/S0140-6736(01)06011-1 [14-0-2018]; D. MALAKOFF, «Nigerian Families Sue Pfizer, Testing the Reach of U.S. Law», *Science*, 293(2001), 1742, in https://doi.org/10.1126/science.293.5536.1742 [14-82018]; J. LENZER, «Appeals court rules that Nigerian families can sue Pfizer in US», *BMJ*, 338(2009), 458, in https://doi.org/10.1136/bmj.b458 [14-8-2018].

who allegedly conducted an illegal drug trial in Kano State, Nigeria, in 1996, during an outbreak of bacterial meningitis in the state[971]. Addressing questions on : What make individuals or groups vulnerable? And why vulnerability is a major question in bioethics? R. Macklin writes: "A simple answer to both questions is that vulnerable individuals and groups are subject to exploitation, and exploitation is morally wrong"[972]. The author affirms that even if the vulnerable groups are not harmed during an intervention or a non-intervention, once they are exploited, it a grave moral issue. Some of the ethical challenges in the conduct above include:

1. Justifying the medical and social relevance of the clinical trials to the host community
2. The quality of informed consent
3. The standard of care
4. Post-trial availability of interventions[973].

Because of some unethical conducts that unveil the level of injustice in the Nigerian health care system, the Federal Ministry of Health Abuja Nigeria, sustains that Health Research Ethics Committee (HREC), must be given the possibility to exercise its authority in the review of prescribed application materials and in the approval or disapproval of all health research activities covered by the National Code of Health Research Ethics[974]. Accordingly, we think that ethical theories in line with the Catholic principles can be a good guide for the Ethics committee in

---

[971]   Cfr. D. MALAKOFF, «Nigerian Families Sue ...» ; J. LENZER, «Appeals court rules that Nigerian families can sue Pfizer in US», *BMJ*, 338(2009), 458, in https://doi.org/10.1136/bmj.b458 [14-8-2018]; ID., «Secret report surfaces showing that Pfizer was at fault in Nigerian drug tests», *BMJ*, 332(2006), 1233, in https://doi.org/10.1136/bmj.332.7552.1233-a [14-8-2018]; ID., «Nigerian judge orders arrests of Pfizer officials», *BMJ*, 336(2008), 11, in https://doi.org/10.1136/bmj.39444.446725.DB [14-8-2018].

[972]   R. MACKLIN, «Bioethics, Vulnerability and Protection», *Bioethics*, 17(2003), 5-6.

[973]   Cfr. P. I. OKONTA, «Ethics of clinical ... »; K. AHMAD, «Drug company sued ... »; C. LORENZO – V. GARRAFA – J. H. SOLBAKK – S. VIDAL, «Hidden risks associated with clinical trial in developing countries», *Journal of Medical Ethics*, 36(2010), 111-115.

[974]   Cfr. FEDERAL MINISTRY OF HEALTH ABUJA, NIGERIA, The national code for health research ethics, Federal Ministry of Health Abuja 2007.

Nigeria. "Ethical theories and principles are the foundations of ethical analysis because they are the viewpoints from which guidance can be obtained along the pathways to decision making"[975].

The Federal Ministry of Health, Abuja, Nigeria, recognizes respect for persons and their rights to make a choice as an important ethical consideration to be respected in participation in research and their access to health services in Nigeria. It also states that "another ethical consideration is justice". Justice according to the Federal Ministry of Health, Abuja, Nigeria, implies weighing the costs and benefits for the participants to ensure "that they receive the expected benefits of the research outcomes proportionate to the burden they bear during the research process. It upholds the need to distribute equally the risks and benefits of participating in research"[976]. Similarly a Nigeria ethicist, B.C. Nwachukwu-Udaku points out that "Justice as solidarity with the weak requires that we accept people even if vulnerability seems to constitute a major definition and hallmark of their existence. We should accept people for who they are, and not for what is happening to them"[977]. The words of B. Haring explain well the concept expressed above: "To another, not his goods, but his dignity and personal rights are due before all else"[978]. B. Haring's view is in harmony with the Catholic principles which are represented in the following statement of B. C. Nwachukwu-Udaku: "Justice as solidarity with the weak is also against all forms of exclusion which seems to be the order of the day in the world's economic system"[979].

---

[975] A. S. JEGEDE – A. S. FAYEMINO, «Cultural and Ethical Challenges of Assisted Reproductive Technologies in the Management of Infertility among the Yoruba of Southwestern Nigeria», *African Journal of Reproductive Health*, 14(2010), 114-127.

[976] FEDERAL MINISTRY OF HEALTH (FMoH) ABUJA, NIGERIA, Guidelines for Young Persons' Participation in Research and Access to Sexual and Reproductive Health Services in Nigeria 2014.

[977] B. C. N.-UDAKU, *From What We Should Do To Who We Should Be – Negotiating Theological Reflections and Praxis in the Context of HIV/AIDS Among the Igbos of Nigeria*, AuthorHouse United States of America 2001, 244.

[978] B. HARING, *The Law of Christ*, The Newman Press, Westminster 1996, 65.

[979] B. C. N.-UDAKU, *From What We* ...

4.5.4. The Negative Influence of Corruption (An Enemy of the Common Good) on the performance of Nigerian Health Sector and the Life of the People

Corruption is inherent to the political inefficiency in the administration of common good in Nigeria. Corruption and ineptitude make political leaders govern with selfish and egoistic interests. The governed are the least to be considered in decision-making in a polity where corruption reigns. In such a political organization, the vulnerable are not represented by anyone and their interests mean nothing, so they are deprived of their fundamental rights, including the right to life and the right to health. The Nigerian political leadership has been accused of perpetrating corruption which has wrecked various sectors of the country's vital activities and its national values. The pitiable state of Nigeria's socio-economic development has been a direct consequence of the logic the Nigerian political leadership class has always applied in carrying out their duties, the mentality of self-services. The Nigerian Catholic Bishops are clear in their view on corruption among the political leaders and those who are supposed to fight corruption in the country. Their state on such issues that threatens common good reads:

> Several recent incidents have contributed to undermine the faith of Nigerians in the credibility of the fight against corruption. To restore the faith of the people in this war, we call on the Federal Government to allow independent investigation into recent allegations of corrupt mis-conduct against senior members of the administration[980].

The Nigerian Prelates insist that "there is enough in our Constitution to guarantee citizens' rights and dignity"[981], but the lack of will to correctly interpret and implement the constitution and corruption among the political leaders has made it difficult for many Nigerian to have their rights defended or guaranteed.

Most of the Nigerian past and present leaders are mired in the pursuit of selfish and personal goals at the expense of broader national interest. Against this background, John Paul II in his social teaching warns that

---

[980] Catholic Bishops Conference of Nigeria, «Our Dignity, Our...».

[981] Ibid.

"if there is no ultimate truth to guide and direct political activity, then ideas and convictions can easily be manipulated for reasons of power"[982]. This attitude is common in Nigeria and has grave impact on the Nigerian health care system and the health conditions of many individuals in the country. Such attitude according to the Church disrupts the cooperation between the authorities and the people. The *compendium of the social doctrine of the Church* instructs that corruption among the political leaders and in the entire political arena creates serious problems. Citing instances the document asserts that corruption disrupts the smooth running of the State by creating negative influence on the rapport between those who govern and the governed. Furthermore, "it causes a growing distrust with respect to public institutions, bringing about a progressive disaffection in the citizens with regard to politics and its representatives, with a resulting weakening of institutions"[983].

The above statement explains the kind of relationship that exist between the political leaders and the citizens in Nigeria. The people feel oppressed by those who should protect them. Hence, they do not believe the words and promises of the "politicians" because they see them as being fishy and deceitful. The people feel robbed and this makes them lose all respect for the political representatives. Such a situation according to the social doctrine constitutes "an obstacle to bringing about the common good of all citizens"[984]. Considering the harm political corruption can cause, John Paul II describes it as a grave enemy and obstruction in a democratic state like Nigeria[985]. Instances of corruption in Nigeria, especially among the political leaders abound as we have demonstrated in chapter one. The effect of corrupt practices on the health conditions of the poor masses in Nigeria is devastating. The *compendium of the social doctrine of the Church* aptly describes the concrete problems associated to a society subjected to corruption and moral degradation stating that "mention must be made of illiteracy, lack of food security, the absence of structures and services,

---

[982] Cfr. JOHN PAUL II, «*Centesimus Annus*, Encyclical Letter on The Hundredth Anniverssary of *Rerum Novarum*, (1991) », n. 46, in J. M. MILLER (ed.), *The Encyclicals of...*

[983] PONTIFICAL COUNCIL FOR JUSTICE AND PEACE, *Compendium of the...*, n. 411, 231.

[984] Ibid.

[985] Cfr. JOHN PAUL II, «*Sollicitudo Rei Socialis*, Encyclical Letter, (1987), for the twentieth anniversary of *Populorum Progressio*», n. 44, in J. M. MILLER (ed.), *The Encyclicals of...*

inadequate measures for guaranteeing basic health, the lack of safe drinking water and sanitation, corruption, instability of institutions and political life itself"[986]. In the same vein, John Paul II declares: "Christian ethics gives rise to the conviction that it is unjust to squander resources which might be necessary for the lives of others. Today a new awareness of this moral imperative is needed, given the present conditions of such large portions of the human race"[987]. These are typical problems faced by Nigerians every day. The Nigerian leaders are therefore invited to sit down and do some soul-searching on the pains corruption is inflicting on the citizens.

In Nigeria, most often some projects are agreed on and funded, but never completed. In some other cases, they are funded but never commenced. The funds allocated for the projects go into private pockets, while the poor and the vulnerable continue to wait endlessly and most die while waiting. Similarly, some projects are created purposefully as a means of siphoning the public fund and resources into private accounts and ends. Personal aggrandizement sadly has replaced selfless service, which is the hallmark of a just society. The Pontifical Council for Justice and Peace indicates what happens eventually, stating: "The costs are borne by the citizens: the price of corruption is paid by using monies intended for the legitimate use of society"[988]. The governed, the poor and the vulnerable bear the consequences of the corrupt practices of the leaders. For this, we say that corruption militates against the common good and violates human rights especially the right to life and the right to health.

The above-mentioned lifestyles of the Nigerian political elites are immoral and are acts of injustice. Hence, the Catholic doctrine enjoins that "Fraud and other subterfuges, by which some people evade the constraints of the law and the prescriptions of societal obligation, must be firmly condemned because they are incompatible with the requirements of justice"[989]. Many are convinced that, most Nigeria political leaders do not show interest for the wellbeing of their citizens. Most often, the national programmes aimed at addressing some critical health issues in

---

[986] PONTIFICAL COUNCIL FOR JUSTICE AND PEACE, *Compendium of the...*, n. 447, 252.

[987] JOHN PAUL II, «Address to the..., n.4, 306-310.

[988] PONTIFICAL COUNCIL FOR JUSTICE AND PEACE, «*The Fight against Corruption*», n. 3, in http://www.vatican.va/roman_curia/pontifical_councils/justpeace/documents/rc_pc_justpeace_doc_20060921_lotta-corruzione_en.html [22-04-2018].

[989] THE CATECHISM OF..., n. 1916, 459.

Nigeria succeed only because they receive economic support from, and are piloted by, external agencies. Any government that does not care about the common good should be questionable because it has no moral basis to exist. According to the Catholic doctrine, by the very fact of being corrupt, the civil authority loses every moral basis for its legitimacy because the common good is the reason for the existence of any public authority and corruption as the Church affirms militates against the common good. Corruption is also contrary to social solidarity. It exalts selfishness whereas "social solidarity implies putting aside the simple pursuit of particular interests, which must be evaluated and harmonised in keeping with a hierarchy of balanced values; ultimately, it demands a correct understanding of the dignity and right of the person"[990]. The common interest sought in line with the respect for dignity of the human person is the way to justice and fairness.

To enjoy a just and fair health system therefore, Nigeria has to be purged of corruption which has caused her health system to be characterized by inadequate health facilities/structure, poor human resources and management, poor remuneration and motivation, lack of fair and sustainable health care financing, unequal economic relations, low government spending on health, high out-of-pocket expenditure in health, inadequate mechanism for families to access health care, shortage of essential drugs and supplies and inadequate supervision of health care providers[991]. Some authors sadly remark that:

> In spite of huge government spending coupled with bilateral assistance in the health sector, the patterns of health status in Nigeria mirror many other Sub-Sahara African nations but are worse than would be expected given Nigeria's GDP per capita. The health sector is in shambles[992].

Corruption has been defined by the social teaching of the Catholic Church as a great enemy of common good. This means that common

---

[990] JOHN PAUL II, «Address to the…», n. 4, 435-437; Cfr. ID., «*Centesimus Annus*, Encyclical Letter on The Hundredth Anniverssary of *Rerum Novarum*, (1991) », n. 13, in J. M. MILLER (ed.), *The Encyclicals of…*

[991] G. TIMOTHY – O. IRINONYE – U. YUNUSA – A. DALHATU – S. AHMED – A. SUBERU, «Balancing Demand, Quality…».

[992] Ibid.

good is threatened every day in Nigeria because; corruption has become a euphemism for explaining political leadership in Nigeria in relation to the management of public good. This is far from the way the Catholic social teaching intends the stewardship of the public good. According to the Catholic doctrine, the management or administration of common good "requires the constant ability and effort to seek the good of others as though it were one's own good"[993]. This is the attitude the Nigerian leaders are called to imbibe in order to ensure a transparent and responsible stewardship of the people and goods entrusted to them. The 'national cake' is not reserved only for the ruling class because "everyone also has the right to enjoy the conditions of social life that are brought about by the quest for the common good"[994].

The Nigerian political leaders as well as all other Nigerians guilty of working against the common good are invited to eschew theft and corruption and to imbibe the culture of justice, fairness, altruism, transparency and all the qualities of the common good sustained by the Universal Church. The Pontifical Council for Justice and Peace in line with the entire Church's Magisterium affirms that "without transparency, corruption is made that much easier"[995]. Accordingly John Paul II states: "it is a well-known fact that the availability of resources is obstructed by various social, economic and political factors, to the extent that some people fear that the point will even be reached when it will be impossible to feed all the world's population"[996]. What the Pope underlines here is typical of Nigeria in terms of distribution of health care and other resources. The situation has changed from bad to worse in Nigeria and many fear it will continue to become wore because they do not see any sign of improvement. Nevertheless, fear should not prevail as the Roman Pontiff has affirmed. This doctoral thesis hopes to reawaken the hope of Nigerians. There is the need to evaluate the problems of the distribution of health care resources and the entire activities of the health care system in Nigeria to know the

---

[993] PONTIFICAL COUNCIL FOR JUSTICE AND PEACE, *Compendium of the...*, n. 167, 95.

[994] Ibid.

[995] PONTIFICAL COUNCIL FOR JUSTICE AND PEACE, The Fight Against..., n. 3.

[996] JOHN PAUL II, «Address to the Study Week on the Subject 'Resources and Population' 22 November 1991», n.2, in *Papal Addresses to the Pontifical Academy of Sciences 1917 – 2002 and to the Pontifical Academy of Social Sciences 1994 – 2002, The Pontifical Academy of Sciences*, Vatican City 2003 331-335.

correct way of applying the Catholic principles to ameliorate the health conditions of Nigerians.

The Nigerian government and its health agencies are invited to adopt the method of transparent stewardship of the people's resources. In accordance with the Catholic social doctrine, the Nigerian political leaders are invited to always consider the divine origin of every 'authority' and the inseparability of their political activities and the will of God for them and the people they govern. This is clearly stated in the statement by the Catholic Bishops of England and Wales:

> The Church's social teaching places the political within the larger context of humanity's relationship with God. Social and political action is important, but realising our full human dignity as children of God, made in his image and likeness, also requires each of us to undertake an inner spiritual journey. The future of humanity does not depend on political reform, social revolution or scientific advance. Something else is needed. It starts with a true conversion of mind and heart[997].

4.6. Some Barriers to accessing Healthcare in Nigeria and their Implications for the Poor and Vulnerable

4.6.1. Financial Barriers: Poverty as a Barrier to accessing Health Care in Nigeria

Accessibility, Availability and Universality are some of the features of an ethical health system which ensures minimum decent health care for all. These characteristics of equity in health make accurate analysis of the various barriers: physical, economic, social and others, that cause individual and other differences/inequalities, in order to reduce them. Explaining some salient points inherent to the problems of poverty and other economic barriers to receiving adequate health care in Nigeria, M. I. Olatubi, O. O. Oyediran, I. O. Adubi and O. C. Ogidan remark:

> Nearly two-thirds of Nigerian's live below the poverty line; eighty percent work in the informal sector. Even not all those that work in the formal setting are able to access the scheme.

---

[997] CATHOLIC BISHOPS OF ENGLAND AND WALES, *The Common Good...*, n. 3.

Most states of the country up till now have not enrolled their workers on the scheme. As the national health system mostly covers the formally employed only 3 percent of the population is covered by the NHIS. Private prepaid schemes are unreachable for the poor as premiums are unaffordable. With the overburdened public system unable to deliver, people have no option but pay for health care out-of-pocket. By default, the private health sector has grown rapidly over the past decades and now provides over 65 percent of health care services[998].

Poverty in Nigeria and in most parts of the world represents one of the major motives of the denial of the right to health care to those who cannot afford to pay for services. In Nigeria, failure to pay in most cases means absence of treatment even when the person is in dire need of it. This libertarian mentality is clear in the practices of paying for a card, presenting a guarantor (for payments), depositing money before receiving any attention and other economic requirements that are part of the preliminary procedures before seeing the doctor and the commencement of treatment in most Nigerian hospitals. In these practices, if a person does not pay, the nurses or the hospital attendants will not allow him or her to see the doctor. Apart from the cases of emergency, it is either "payment before service" or the compulsory provision of a guarantor. In some private and public hospitals, the nurse or the medical personnel according to the unwritten codes may face some disciplinary measures if he or she allows a patient or the patient's family member to reach the doctor without the above mentioned compulsory preliminary passages. Therefore, what counts more is money and not the health or life of the sick person. Addressing issues of this nature, some authors affirms that "without doubt, there are questions of resource allocation here that involve the more general ethical question of

---

[998] M. I. OLATUBI – O. O. OYEDIRAN – I. O. ADUBI – O. C. OGIDAN, «Health Care Expenditure...»; Cfr. A. S. BAKARE – S. OLUBOKUN, «Health care expenditure and economic growth in Nigeria: An empirical study», *Journal of Emerging Trends in Economic Management Science*, 2(2011), 83-87; Cfr. A. TEMITOPE, «Effect of Health Investment on Economic Growth in Nigeria», *IOSR Journal of Economics and Finance*, 1(2013), 39-47; Cfr. Y. JAMEELAH – O. TAIWO – R. O. YUSSUFF, «Public Health Expenditure and health outcome in Nigeria: the impact of governance», *European Scientific Journal*, 8(2012), e – ISSN 1857 – 7431.

achieving distributive justice within the public health and private medical care sectors"[999] in Nigeria.

Similarly, Pope Paul VI, reminded the participant the Plenary Session and to the Study on the Subject 'The Econometric Approach to Development Planning' 13 October 1963 that the main reason for their activity was to:

> Gather together the latest result of a new branch of science, econometry, and to present them to political economists in order to aid them in formulating those plans for a more stable security and for greater development which can contribute so much to the well-being and peace of nations[1000].

The Pope's injunction is equivalent to the affirmation that any economic development programme or plan that derails from the well-being of the individual and society cannot be for the good of the human person and as such can hardly be morally permissible. Here it is obvious how Catholic understanding of health care distribution is in clear contrast with the Utilitarian principle. This opposition is one of the reasons why we affirm that utilitarianism cannot guarantee a just health system in Nigeria. For instance, according to the utilitarian theory, those who have little or nothing to offer to the society are not to be considered in the distribution of resources. Contrarily, the Catholic principles stands for an approach that carries everyone along and that does not cut off individuals because of their social worth. While the utilitarian theory is for the allocation of funds to where the majority have access to care, the Catholic principles support the motion of giving everyone the equal opportunity of having access to the minimum decent health care and assuring heath care services for the most deserving. Thus, we maintain that the health condition of the sick,

---

[999]   O. AKINLOYE – E. J. TRUTER, «A review of management of infertility in Nigeria: framing the ethics of a national health policy», *International Journal of Women's Health*, 3(2011), 265-275, in http://dx.doi.org/10.2147/IJWH.S20501 [22-8-2018].

[1000]   PAUL VI, «Address to the Plenary Session and to the Study on the Subject 'The Econometric Approach to Development Planning' 13 October 1963», in *Papal Addresses to the Pontifical Academy of Sciences 1917 – 2002 and to the Pontifical Academy of Social Sciences 1994 – 2002, The Pontifical Academy of Sciences*, Vatican City 2003, 180-182.

the dignity of the human person should guide the distribution of resources in Nigeria and not the utilitarian gain oriented mentality that places the human person as means to an end.

Identifying some problems of resource allocation in Nigeria, O. Alubo argues that "for-profit motive and high fees" are among the limitations of private medicine in tackling the prevailing burden of disease and death in Nigeria. This according to him prevents most people from affording health services in Nigeria, where there is high and rising poverty and unemployment[1001]. It is always necessary to make a distinction between "price and dignity" because such Kantian distinction logically shows that price applies to things while dignity applies to persons. Just as the Catholic teaching sustains, the order of things should be subordinate to the order of person. The person should be at the center of every health care distribution decision and not other material things. The person should make use of things and not be used for or be a slave of things. "The Catholic social vision has as its focal point the human person", because she believes that "each person possesses a basic dignity that comes from God, not from any human quality or accomplishment, not from race or gender, age or economic status". Hence, she teaches:

> The test therefore of every institution or policy is whether it enhances or threatens human dignity and indeed human life itself. Policies which treat people as only economic units, or policies which reduce people to a passive state of dependency on welfare, do not do justice to the dignity of the human person[1002].

Respect for the human person is fundamental for all societies and for all human activities because the human person is "the origin and the purpose of all social institutions"[1003].

[1001] Cfr. O. ALUBO, «The Promise and limits of private medicine: health policy dilemmas in Nigeria», *Health Policy Plan*, 16(2001), 667-676; Cfr. A. E. ORIMADEGUN – K. S. ILESANMI, «Mothers' understanding of childhood malaria and practices in rural communities of Ise-Orun, Nigeria: implications for malaria control», *Journal of Family Medicine and Primary Care*, 4(2015), 226-231. https://doi/10.4103/2249-4863.154655 [30-7-2018].

[1002] CATHOLIC BISHOPS OF ENGLAND AND WALES, *The Common Good...*, n. 3. n. 9.

[1003] JOHN PAUL II, «Address to the Study Week on the Subject 'Resources and Population' 22 November 1991», n. 6, in *Papal Addresses to...*; CONCILIO

In line with the Catholic moral principles of the dignity of the human person, preferential option for the poor and the vulnerable and the principle of solidarity, we retain that the economic condition should not be a reason for denying anyone the access to and utilization of the decent basic health care. In accordance with the Catholic principle of common good, for instance, every individual by the virtue of his or her citizenship in a particular community ought to have some basic rights, such as the right to minimum healthcare. A country that sustains a policy that makes it impossible for her citizens to access the basic health care because they cannot afford to pay it, cannot be said to be a just and fair society.

With the foregoing arguments, it is difficult to mention or describe Nigeria as a just and fair society as far as the provision for the minimum decent heath care is concerned. This is because the system is predominantly out-of-pocket spending. The slogan: "pay before service" is very common in Nigeria for issues of hospital bills. You must deposit some money before you start receiving attention. In the case of emergency after treatment, the person is detained if the hospital authorities discover he or she and the family members cannot afford to pay the hospital bills. This situation makes it difficult and often impossible for those who cannot pay because of poverty to have access to even the basic health care.

The above arguments show that even where facilities are available to make accessible health care services for women and children in Nigeria, because of the poor distribution of health care resources and due to poor governance, it has been revealed that most mothers and their children are denied the opportunity to utilize the services because they are poorly accessed. Consequently, this vulnerable group, helplessly resort to "traditional healers, over-the-counter drug peddlers or self-medication"[1004].

VATICANO II, *Gaudium et Spes*, n. 25.

[1004] S. T. ADEDOKUN – V. T. ADEKANMBI – O. A. UTHAM – R. J. LILFORD, «Contextual factors associated with health care service utilization for children with acute childhood illness in Nigeria», *PLoS ONE*, 12(2017), e0173578, in https://doi.org/10.1371/journal.pone.0173578 [3-8-2018]; Cfr. V. O. ADIKA – S. BALARABE – J. J. AGADA – N. NNEOMA, «Mothers Perceived Cause and Health Seeking Behaviour of Childhood Measles in Bayelsa, Nigeria», *Journal of Research in Nursing and Midwifery*, 2(2013), 6-12; Cfr. T. A. OKEKE – J. C. OKEIBUNOR, «Rural-urban Differences in Health-seeking for the Treatment of Childhood Malaria in South-east Nigeria», *Health policy*, 95(2009), 62-68, in https://doi.org/10.1016/j.healthpol.2009.11.005 [3-8-2018]; Cfr. O.

Usually the under-current motive for the projects like Universal Health Coverage or other programmes made to guarantee primary health care services is to protect the right to health and access to minimum decent health care of the poor, the weak and the most vulnerable. When we say the most vulnerable, we mean those who are not capable of promoting and or protecting their rights and interest.

Since the citizens are not enjoying the fruits of Universal Health Coverage and similar, we think the Nigerian health care system needs to be galvanized by the Catholic principles in order to be liberated from their actual situation. The government and the health care agencies in Nigeria need to imbibe the person-centered/common good approach of the Catholic social teaching.

> The foundation of this teaching is the dignity of the human person. In virtue simply of our shared humanity, we must surely respect and honour one another. Each individual has a value that can never be lost and must never be ignored. Moreover, each of us is made in the image and likeness of God. Society must therefore first of all respect and protect human life itself - at all its stages from conception to its natural end. This is the bedrock of our civilisation[1005].

Assimilating and applying concretely the Catholic principles is an objective the Nigerian government and Health sector should pursue to be able to adequately harness and justly distribute the available health and other resources in accordance with the principle of common good. The government has the duty to establish health insurance scheme, sustained by the state, which should be designed in such a way that the vulnerable could benefit from it. This will really go a long way to promote and provide healthcare for the economically deprived citizens.

B. Akogun – K. K. John, «Illness-related Practices for the Management of Childhood Malaria among Bwatiye People of North-eastern Nigeria», *Malaria Journal*, 4(2015); Cfr. L. J. Mangham – B. Cundill – O. Ezeoke – E. Nwala – B. S. C. Uzochukwu, «Treatment of uncomplicated malaria at public health facilities and medicine retailers in south-eastern Nigeria», *Malaria Journal*, 10(2011), 155.

[1005] John Paul II, Address to the…, n.6, 331-335; Concilio Vaticano II, *Gaudium et Spes*, n. 2.

The issue of poverty alleviation is very important because many Nigerians are convinced of the fact that one of the fallouts of poverty is poor nutrition. This in turn translates into poor health that places pressure on health care resources. Similarly, there are some who aptly highlight the strongly and persuasive link between poverty and health, saying that, a commitment to health necessarily implies a commitment to reducing poverty[1006]. The fight against poverty in Nigeria cannot be done by avoiding the poor or considering them a problem but by seeing them as potential principal builders of a more human future for everyone. This can find "a strong motivation in the option or preferential love of the Church for the poor"[1007]. Hence, in line with the Church's motion, we think it is necessary to tackle the problem of poverty through investments and empowerment of the citizens so that there would not be an excessive pressure on the resources. With an improvement in the economic and general conditions of the citizens, it will be easier to achieve a fair distribution of resources. The Catholic social teaching in this regard stands for principles that can bring about a good and fair society. Principles that can help in organizing the society in such a way as to improve the lot of its members.

If caring for the sick is a prime moral and cultural principle, helping Nigerians to have access to minimum health care is the moral obligation of the government. The care given to the sick must be guided by the ethical principle of the dignity of the human person. Usually, the financial barrier is a limiting barrier to access to health care by individuals in the low socio-economic bracket. The just mentioned class often make those giving care to lose sight of their dignity as human person. Therefore, they are treated with lack of respect. The Catholic principle of the preferential option for the poor and the most vulnerable encourages that the help to be given be focused on the poor and the vulnerable who make up a high rate of the percentage of the Nigerian population. The poor and the vulnerable in Nigeria will continue to risk financial catastrophe if they receive the health care they need without the help of society through universal coverage. Many as we have seen pass through the humiliation of medical detention. A good financing system is very important in this regard.

[1006] Cfr. P. BRAVEMAN – S. GRUSKIN, «Poverty, equity, human rights and health», *Bulletin of the World Health Organization*, 81(2003), 539-545.

[1007] PONTIFICAL COUNCIL FOR JUSTICE AND PEACE, *Compendium of the…*, n. 449, 253.

One of the major characteristics of a good financing system is the capacity to realize a fair distribution of the burden of the health care services, thus protecting the people from heavy spending on health services, which may result in catastrophe for the families. A sound financing system is also expected to reduce the barriers to health care services by ensuring a fair distribution of public expenditures. Nigeria is really lagging behind in this. A. O. Lawanson remarks that while government expenditures on health in some developing countries are increasing to match with the increment of the health care needs, others Nigeria inclusive appear to be on the decline[1008]. This failure by the government translates into increasing burden on the population, especially on the poor and the vulnerable. The government cannot pursue the objective of human welfare concentrating on the material wellbeing; allocating more money to arms in the name of security, while it is giving less attention to other important values like health. Following this line of thought, the Catholic Bishops of England and Wales vehemently affirm:

> The Church also rejects the view that human happiness consists only in material wellbeing, and that achieving this alone is the goal of any government. If a government pays too much attention to material welfare at the expense of other values, it may advocate policies which reduce people to a passive state of dependency on welfare. Equally, if a government gives too little priority to tackling poverty, ill-health, poor housing and other social ills, the human dignity of those who suffer these afflictions is denied. In every society respect for human dignity requires that, so far as possible, basic human needs are met. The systematic denial of compassion by individuals or public authorities can never be a morally justified political option[1009].

It is therefore necessary to have appropriate principles that can help the Nigerian government and the health agencies to garner their efforts, funds and energies and direct them to the projects and values that promote and protect the dignity of the human person.

[1008] A. O. LAWANSON – O. S. OPELOYERU, «Equity in healthcare...».

[1009] CATHOLIC BISHOPS OF ENGLAND AND WALES, *The Common Good...*, nn. 2-3.

4.6.2. Infrastructural and Institutional Barriers

Infrastructural and Institutional barriers are among the major problems of the Nigerian health care system. The conditions concerning some roads, electricity system, hospital facilities and some other factors related to infrastructures and health institutions in Nigeria are very bad and unbearable. In the report of a study in Nigeria, S. I. Efe sadly remarked that "most of the hospitals visited lack basic modern health facilities. The implication of this, is that it has led to the abysmal poor quality of health care services in the various hospitals and health centers in the state and consequently in Nigeria"[1010]. The report of WHO (2000) "makes *goodness-* the best attainable average level of health in the population-and *fairness-* the smallest feasible differences in health across individuals and groups- standards by which we should judge health systems"[1011]. Both qualities: goodness and fairness are lacking in the Nigerian health care system, if we have to judge by the conditions of the infrastructures and health facilities. This means that the principles of the dignity of human person, solidarity and common good are not properly applied or taking into consideration by those at the helm of economic and socio-political affairs in Nigeria during policy-making. The Catholic social teaching according to Cardinal Basil Hume, warns that the public authority cannot ignore the principles of the dignity of the human person and common good because "every public policy should be judged by the effect it has on human dignity and the common good"[1012].

In Nigeria, it is usual to find hospitals and health care centers in the cities, whereas the rural areas inhabited predominantly by the poor and the vulnerable are without health facilities, roads and other infrastructures. A study on maternal mortality in Anambra State of Nigeria, states clearly that "all major causes of death are avoidable-either by obtaining prenatal and intrapartum care or by anticipating fetopelvic disproportion or abnormal lie"[1013]. This affirmation together with many other similar views

---

[1010] S. I. Efe, «Health care problem …».

[1011] A. Robbins, «The World Health Report 2000: Health Systems: Improving Performance», in *Public Health Reports*, 116 (2001), 268-269.

[1012] Catholic Bishops of England and Wales, *The Common Good…*, n. 3.

[1013] W. O. Chukudebelu – B. C. Ozumba, «Maternal mortality in Anambra State of Nigeria», *International Journal of Gynaecology and Obstetrics*, 27(1988), 365-370.

confirm that "lack of access to health facilities, especially in the rural areas, poor transportation, great distances to nearest health facility, are all implicated in obstructed labour deaths"[1014]. Infrastructures such as roads, good public water, power supplies and practically the basic systems and services are insufficiently provided in Nigeria. Little wonder that Nigeria is listed among countries with the worst health indicators in the world[1015]. This poor performance according to many is due to factors that include "poorly equipped health facilities, insufficient staff, lack of clearly defined roles and responsibilities, inadequate political commitment, and poor accountability"[1016].

Majority of health facilities in Nigeria are not properly equipped and the important infrastructures are in horrible conditions. These situations halt the access to health care of those living in these areas. "This can lead to the risk of "placing the heaviest burden on the poorest and the weakest sectors of society, thus adding injustice to injustice"[1017]. Currently, a high proportion of women have barriers to accessing health care in Nigeria. It is apparent that barriers to accessing health care in Nigeria contribute to the increase in child and maternal mortalities and worsens other health situations of the population. Despite extensive investments, Nigeria still has insufficient health-care delivery infrastructures, poor quality health-care services, and unevenly distribute her human resource capacity[1018]. This shows how the problems of infrastructural and institutional barriers are fruits of bad leadership and bad management.

[1014] Ibid; Cfr. O. O. ADETORO – A. AGAH, «The implications of childbearing in post pubertal girls in Sokoto, Nigeria», *International Journal of Gynaecology and Obstetrics*, 27(1988), 73-77; Cfr. C. C. Ekwempu, «The influence of antenatal care on pregnancy outcome», *Tropical Journal Obstetrics Gynaecology*, 1(1988), 67-71.

[1015] Cfr. F. E. OKONOFUA – A. ABEJIDE – R. A. MAKANJUOLA, «Maternal mortality in Ile-Ife Nigeria: a study of risk factors», *Studies in Family Planning*, 23(1992), 319–324.

[1016] C. C. NNEBUE – U. E. EBENEBE – P. O. U. ADOGU, «Adequacy of resources for provision of maternal health services at the primary healthcare level in Nnewi, Nigeria», *Nigerian Medical Journal*, 55(2014), 235–241.

[1017] JOHN PAUL II, Address to the…, n. 6, 331-335.

[1018] Cfr. B. O. OLAKUNDE, «Public healthcare financing in Nigeria: which way forward?», *Annals of Nigerian Medicine*, 6(2012), 4–10.

The health capability approach of J. P. Ruger which we proposed in the third chapter of this doctoral dissertation underlines the fundamental duty of the society to guarantee conditions for all to be healthy. Health capability approach identifies two crucial elements: desires of good health and ability to pursue it. People must be put in the condition to pursue and to achieve these desires where possible[1019]. It is obvious that the way the distribution of the common good is done in Nigeria penalizes the poor, especially those in the rural areas. For this reason, some insist that there is the need to redistribute the infrastructure in such a way that all Nigerians have a chance of benefiting maximally. This call for change is clear in the teaching of Pope John Paul II:

> In short, a renewed way of life is needed, one which will spread by way of an authentic humanism and will therefore be capable of dissuading public authorities from proposing and legalising solutions which are contrary to the true and lasting common good. It is a manner of living which, by reflecting the real interests of the individual, will help to bring about a world in which love for others is accepted as the general and normative rule[1020].

The Catholic Bishops' Conference of Nigeria in line with the above Church's teaching appeals to the civil authorities in Nigeria to work diligently for "the equitable distribution of our resources for the common good [...] to restore our dignity as human beings"[1021]. The bishops maintain that some Nigerians are denied opportunities to enjoy the social life. Whereas according to the Nigerian Prelates: "Every human person by its very nature stands completely in need of social life in the world and this social life is not something added or accidental to the human person but belongs intrinsically to his dignity as a person"[1022]. Our dissertation in line with this Catholic doctrine pronounced by the Nigerian Bishops, insist that minimum decent health care should be available to every individual and no individual should be denied of this because of his social or economic

---

[1019] J. P. RUGER, «Health Capability: Conceptualization…».
[1020] JOHN PAUL II, Address to the…, n. 9, 331-335.
[1021] CATHOLIC BISHOPS CONFERENCE OF NIGERIA, «Our Dignity, Our…».
[1022] ID., «Nigeria: Citizenship Rights…».

conditions. So, as the Nigerian Bishops emphasize, "the dignity of every Nigerian should be recognised, respected and protected by all"[1023].

4.7. Ethical Consideration of Sexual and Reproductive Health Rights and Practices in Nigeria using the Moral Principles of Catholic Tradition

We have mentioned in the previous parts of this dissertation that one of the general principles of justice is the Dignity/Integrity of the human person. In this section, we will apply this principle to the health situations of those we consider the most vulnerable in Nigeria, namely women, born and particularly unborn children. The consequences of the debacles and failures of the Nigerian health care system, noted in the previous parts of this work (chapters one and two), are often borne by the weakest class, that is women and children. This justifies the particular attention given to them in our work. One of the main issues of concern for children's and women's health in Nigeria is that of sexual and reproductive health rights. Therefore, it is important to consider here the major ethical problems of sexual and reproductive health in Nigeria.

4.7.1. The Issues of Sexual and Reproductive Health Rights in Nigeria

Defining reproductive health, the United Nations International Conference on Population and Development (ICPD) 1994 held in Cairo underlined the importance of being in a condition of complete physical, mental and social well-being, in all that has to do with the functions and processes of the reproductive system[1024]. In the course of the Cairo Conference, sexual and reproductive rights emerged and was adopted as inalienable, integral and indivisible part of universal human rights. L. Omo-Aghoja interpreting the proceedings of the aforementioned ICPD 1994 states: "sexual right means that everyone should have a right to engage

---

[1023] Ibid.

[1024] Cfr. FEDERAL MINISTRY OF HEALTH, ABUJA, NIGERIA, National Reproductive Health Strategic Framework and Plan, 2002-2006, Federal Ministry of Health Abuja 2002, 19, in http://www.policyproject.com/pubs/countryreports/nig_rhstrat.pdf [10-04-2018].

in sex that is enjoyable and safe, and to decide for themselves whether to do so, when, how and with whom"[1025]. This interpretation is such that could lead to arbitrariness, more especially when the adolescents are allowed to engage in sexual activities for enjoyment; using contraceptives; performing abortion and engaging in sex with whom they decide and how they want.

Right to reproductive health does not mean lawlessness in engaging in sex, neither does it mean devaluation of sex. Considering sexual rights in the way L. Omo-Aghoja describes it can also lead to interpreting the human body as an object and limiting the conjugal act to pleasure, losing its profound meanings and values. This according to what the Catholic doctrine intends is a complete misconception of human sexuality. It is not all about sexual intercourse and sex understood as bodily union of a man and a woman is reserved for those who are married. This Catholic notion will be explained better subsequently. Some aptly define sexual and reproductive rights as human rights, but they wrongly include access to affordable contraceptives and safe abortion as human rights of the young people[1026]. The Catholic moral tradition excludes contraception and abortion from the human sexual and reproductive rights.

According to the Federal Ministry of Health Nigeria, reproductive health implies sexual and reproductive rights which include the primary rights of couples and all individuals to decide the number, spacing and timing of the children and to have the possibility to do so[1027]. In the bid to respect the reproductive health rights of its citizens, the Nigerian government has set a goal to improve their quality of health through enhanced reproductive health. Thus, the government gives reproductive health services focusing attention on safe motherhood, family planning, adolescent reproductive health care, STIs, infertility and sexual dysfunction and menopause and andropause[1028]. J. Adinma and E. Adinma agree with us that Nigeria has policies and programmes intended for the improvement of its socio-economic standing and overall development, but with little positive result. The authors believe reproductive health is an important

---

[1025] L. O.-Aghoja, «Sexual and reproductive health: Concepts and current status among Nigerians», *African Journal of Medical and Health Science*, 12(2013), 103-113.

[1026] Cfr. Ibid.

[1027] Cfr. Federal Ministry of Health, Abuja, Nigeria, «National Reproductive Health ...», 19.

[1028] Cfr. Ibid., 6-7.

strategy for the improvement of the slow socio-economic growth of Nigeria. Their affirmation is based on the linkage between reproductive health and socio-economic development established in Millennium Development Goals 3, 4, 5 and 6. Accordingly, they assert that fast tracking Nigeria's development will depend more on the implementation of reproductive health policies and programmes in favour of women and children[1029].

For J. Adinma and E. Adinma, the medical professional in the area of sexual and reproductive health care should stick to ethical principles in their practice because they are in direct contact with the woman's body. For this reason, the authors endorse the intervention of the International Federation of Gynaecology and Obstetrics (FIGO) in collaboration with the Society of Gynaecology and Obstetrics of Nigeria (SOGON), which was aimed at developing a human right based code of ethics inherent to sexual and reproductive health to guide health care professionals that attend to women in doctor-patient relationship[1030]. They emphasize that "an understanding and proper application of the ethical principles is expected to enable these medical practitioners to actualize the ultimate and desired goal of uplifting the sexual and reproductive healthcare and right of women"[1031].

Contrarily, the manner in which the sexual reproductive issues are handled in Nigeria and the types of services that are offered to women especially, raise many ethical problems. These problems we think, could be properly addressed with the application of the moral principles of Catholic tradition. For instance, contraception is prominent among the methods the Nigerian Federal Health Agency offers for family planning. There are also some cultural and non-cultural practices in Nigeria under the reproductive health that infringe on the rights of children and women in particular. Some of these practices are legally banned in Nigeria, but as we will see later in this work, the laws prohibiting them are not strong and clear. We

---

[1029] Cfr. J. ADINMA – E. ADINMA, «Impact of reproductive health on socio-economic development: a case study of Nigeria», *African Journal of Reproductive Health*, 15(2011), 7-12.

[1030] Cfr. ID., «Ethical considerations in women's sexual and reproductive health care», *Nigerian Journal of Clinical Practice*, 12(2009), 92-98; Cfr. T. O. OYEWALE – T. R. MAVUNDLA, «Socioeconomic factors contributing to exclusion of women from maternal health benefit in Abuja, Nigeria», *Curations*, 38(2015), 1-11, in https://doi.org/10.4102/curationis.v38i1.1272 [16-8-2018].

[1031] Ibid.

will treat in this section, some practices in Nigeria regarding maternal and child health and we will consider precisely issues like Female Genital Mutilation (FGM), contraception and abortion in the light of the Catholic moral principles.

4.7.2. The Practice of Female Genital Mutilation and the Dignity/ Integrity of the Nigerian Woman and Girl-Child

As we demonstrated in chapter one of this doctoral thesis, a number of traditional practices in Nigeria infringe on the reproductive rights of the Nigerian woman and girl-child. The commonest of these include Female Genital Cutting (FGC) or Female Genital Mutilation (FGM), forced early marriage, traumatic puberty initiation rites, gender-based violence, and wife inheritance with widowhood rites. A national survey in 1988 showed that 32% of household in Nigeria practice FGM[1032]. As already intimated, we will concentrate of the Female Genital Mutilation.

Female Genital Mutilation is one of those problems bioethics faces in the long-standing African socio-cultural practices. It is a bioethical problem because it violates the human rights to health, physical integrity and individual autonomy so, it is incompatible with the universal human rights. FGM is widely spread and strongly supported and practiced in some countries of Africa such as Nigeria, Ethiopia, Sudan, Egypt and Somalia. In these countries, it is a highly valued ritual[1033]. In Nigeria, the practice of FGM is diffused in the South-East, South-West and South-South regions[1034].

[1032] Cfr. FEDERAL MINISTRY OF HEALTH, Abuja, Nigeria, «National Reproductive Health ...», 15.

[1033] Cfr. I. JEREMIAH – D. G. B. KALIO – C. AKANI, «The Pattern of Female Genitale Mutilation in Port Harcourt, Southern Nigeria», *International Journal of Tropical Disease & Health*, 4(2014), 469-476; Cfr. L. A. ADEKUN – M. ODUWOLE – F. ORONSANYA – A. O. GBOGBAODE – N. ALIYU – W. ADEKUNLE – G. SADIQ – I. SUTTON – M. TAIWO, «Trends in female circumcision between 1933 and 2003 in Osun and Ogun State, Nigeria: a cohort analysis», *African Journal of Reproductive Health*, 10(2006), 48-56.

[1034] Cfr. Ibid; Cfr. I. ABUBAKAR – Z. ILIYASU – M. KABIR – C. C. UZOHO – M. B. ABDULKADIR, «Knowledge, attitude and practice of female genital cutting among antenatal patients in Amino Kano Teaching Hospital, Kano», *Nigerian Journal of Medicine*, 13(2004), 250-253.

It is conducted from days after birth to puberty and beyond. FGM is a strong cultural practice which notably interferes with the health of the woman. Female Genital Mutilation includes procedures that intentionally alter partially or totally or cause injury to the female genital organs for non-therapeutic reasons[1035]. The words used here like physical *cutting* of the body of the woman and *mutilation* imply *disfigurement*, in other words, infliction of serious damage on the girl's or woman's body. J. R. Cook does not agree with the use of the term *mutilation*, which is also applied by WHO to this practice. According to the J. R. Cook, *cutting* is preferred to *mutilation* because the latter may imply a hostile judgment and condemnation of those who seek such practice as mutilators of human beings. Furthermore, the author retains that the name mutilation is culturally disrespectful:

> Because it fails to respect the motivation with which those who request the procedure for their daughters are acting [...] the name is again disrespectful, because it tells women who were subjected to procedures that they have been mutilated, by their parents or other family members[1036].

Some claim it is 'circumcision' and not 'mutilation'[1037], hence they consider it a cultural and religious ritual that should be promoted and not abolished as many authors propose. Such defence and distinction of terms for the purpose of affirming the practice of FGM, has been vehemently rejected by those who campaign for the abolition of the ritual. They argue that the ritual harms the woman both physically and psychologically[1038]. In line with the defence for this practice of FGM, there is a claim that

---

[1035] Cfr. WORLD HEALTH ORGANIZATION, Female Genital Mutilation: An overview. Geneva: World Health Organization, 1998, in http://apps.who.int/iris/bitstream/handle/10665/42042/9241561912_eng.pdf;jsessionid=EC3FD2FFF95F272DAE7FC30D2DE4B07E?sequence=1 [11-04-2018]; Cfr. LARSEN, U. – OKONOFUA, F. E., «Female Circumcision and Obstetric Complication», *International Journal of Gynaecology & Obstetrics*, 77(2002), 255-265. http://dx.doi/10.1016/s0020-7292(02)00028-0 [12-7-2018].

[1036] J. R., COOK, «Ethical Concerns in Female Genital Cutting», *African Journal of Reproductive Health*, 12(2008), 7-11.

[1037] Cfr. O. NNAMUCHI, «'Circumcision' or 'Mutilation'? Voluntary or Forced Excision? Extricating the Ethical and Legal Issues in Female Genital Ritual», *Journal of Law and Health*, 25(2012), 83-119.

[1038] Cfr. Ibid.

circumcision is an ancient practice which has been practiced by Babylonians, Egyptians, and West African Negroes for over 5000 years[1039]. Some afore-mentioned authors therefore think that, to arrive at a complete ethical judgement on the practice of FGM, a distinction has to be made between adult women of sound mind who voluntary submit to the ritual and those forced to undergo the intervention[1040]. The health capability approach suggests ensuring there is a balance between the object of the individual's desire and that which the society or institution offers. This helps to defend the individual's right. In most cases, FGM is practiced in Nigeria under the umbrella of paternalism and societal culture, because decisions are made with the conviction that it is in the best interest of the minor or adult. The health capability approach thinks it is very important to access the impact of the irreducibly social goods on the individual from the individual's point of view and from the societal perspective. It should be made clear as some Nigerian and non-Nigerian authors have observed that:

> Female genital mutilation is associated with profound reproductive health morbidities and mortality. Immediate complications include severe pain, haemorrhage, shock, urinary retention, and ulceration of the genital region, injury to adjacent tissues, tetanus and death. Long term complications include cysts and abscesses, keloid formation, urinary incontinence, gynaetresia, sexual dysfunction, infertility, prolonged obstructed labour and higher rate of episiotomy and caesarean sections[1041].

We retain that the idea of intentionally causing injury to the girl or woman for non-therapeutic reasons renders this procedure an act of

---

[1039] Cfr. L. O. A.-RAHMAN – O. I. MUSA – G. K. OSHAGBEMI, «Community-based study of circumcision practices in Nigeria», *Annals of Tropical Medicine and Public Health*, 5(2012), 231-235; M. A. A.-FALLOUJI – M. P. MCBRIEN, *Circumcision, Postgraduate surgery*, Butterworth-Heinemann, Oxford 2000⁴, 338.

[1040] Cfr. O. NNAMUCHI, «'Circumcision' or 'Mutilation'? ...».

[1041] I. JEREMIAH – D. G. B. KALIO – C. AKANI, «The Pattern of ...»; Cfr. B. C. OZUMBA, «Acquired Gynaetresia in Eastern Nigeria», *International Journal of Gynaecology & Obstetrics*, 37(1992), 105-109; Cfr. E. KRAUSE – S. BRANDNER – M. D. MUELLER – A. KUHN, «Out of Eastern African: Defibulation and sexual function in woman with female genital mutilation», *The Journal of Sexual Medicine*, 8(2011), 1420-1425.

injustice. To this effect, the Catholic moral tradition considers as negative and unjust the procedures that "involve the destruction of human beings or when they employ means which contradict the dignity of the person or when they are used for purposes contrary to the integral good of man"[1042]. For this reason, the Catholic moralists affirm that Female Genital Mutilation (FGM) is illicit[1043].

Before 2015, there was no clear legal prohibition for this procedure in Nigeria. Nevertheless, the Nigerian Constitution (34(1), provides for the respect for the dignity of every human person and accordingly indicates that no person shall be subjected to torture or to inhuman or degrading treatment. In 2015, the Nigerian President, Goodluck Jonathan enacted a law called the 'Violence Against Persons Prohibition (VAPP) Act', meant to stop FGM and other related practices. The pains, bleeding and the fact that FGM is often performed without anaesthetic classifies it as an experience that implies torture. For this, it is condemned by the Nigerian Constitution. It is clear that it will be difficult to reinforce the laws made to curb FGM because it is a practice that has become part and parcel of the peoples' culture. However, being deeply rooted in the people's culture cannot eliminate the truth that FGM is fundamentally a practice that violates the rights and dignity of the Nigerian girl and woman. The girl's and woman's rights and dignity should be respected and protected because as the *Instruction Dignitas Personae* affirms, "dignity is owed to every human being because each one carries in an indelible way his own dignity and value"[1044]. FGM creates some complications that interrupt and disrupt the health and well-being of girls and women[1045], so it goes contrary to the prescription of *Dignitas Personae*.

[1042] Congregation for the Doctrine of the Faith, *Instruction Dignitas Personae*, On certain Bioethical questions, n. 4, Veritas Publications, Dublin, Ireland 2009, 4.

[1043] Cfr. M. P. Faggioni, «Le Mutilazioni Genitali Feminili», in M. C. Basile (ed.), *Vita, Ragione, Dialogo, Scritti in Onore Elio Sgreccia*, Edizioni Cantagalli, Siena 2012, 181-191.

[1044] Congregation for the Doctrine of the Faith, *Instruction Dignitas Personae…*, n. 6, 5.

[1045] Cfr. Ndugbu, K. U., «The Pervading Public Health Implications of Female Genital Mutilation Among Women (20-40 Years) in a Rural Community in South eastern Nigeria», *Journal of Women's Health Care*, 7(2018), 414. http://dx.doi.org/10.4172/2167-0420.1000414. [13-7-2018].

One of the ideas behind the FGM mentality in Nigeria is that of attenuating the sexual desire of the woman[1046]. This could be seen as an act of humiliation, manipulation of the woman's body and lack of respect for her dignity as a human person. Moreover, some Nigerian authors affirm that FGM has no significant impact of women's sexual behaviour[1047]. The woman at the end is left to be like a fool. The idea of submission of the female to the male, which is strong in the Africa culture, has been traced as one of the motives behind the practice of FGM in Nigeria. This attitude of violation of the rights of the woman is obviously "in contrast with the fundamental truth of the equality of all human beings which is expressed in the principle of justice, the violation of which, in the long run, would harm peaceful coexistence among individuals"[1048]. The Church's doctrine warns against indulging in interventions on the persons that may connote "favouring the will of some over the freedom of others"[1049]. In line with the Catholic doctrine, the egalitarian and Rawls' theories affirm that impartial standard is necessary whenever we are making laws. Hence, all human beings should be treated impartially.

As the World Health Organisation indicates, FGM has no health benefits for the girls and women but rather, it inflicts injuries, both physically and psychologically. It leads to complications in childbirth and often leads to child mortalities[1050]. The Church's doctrine approves the prohibition of harmful practices like the various forms of FGM, which violate the dignity of the human person. Thus, prohibiting all forms of unjust discrimination and marginalization of women and children. Such prohibition according to *Dignitas Personae* "bear witness to the inalienable value and intrinsic dignity of every human being and are a sign of genuine progress in human history"[1051]. The legitimacy of such interdiction is based

---

[1046] H. A. A. UGBOMA – C. I. AKANI – S. BABATUNDE, «Prevalence and medicalization of female genital mutilation», *Nigerian Journal of Medicine*, 13(2004), 250-253.

[1047] Cfr. J. I. B. ADINMA – A. O. AGBAI, «Practice and perceptions of female genital mutilation among Nigerian Igbo women», *Journal of Gynaecology & Obstetrics*, 19(1999), 44-48.

[1048] CONGREGATION FOR THE DOCTRINE OF THE FAITH, *Instruction Dignitas Personae...*, n. 27, 21.

[1049] Ibid., n. 27, 21.

[1050] Cfr. WORLD HEALTH ORGANIZATION, «Female Genital Mutilation...».

[1051] CONGREGATION FOR THE DOCTRINE OF THE FAITH, *Instruction Dignitas Personae...*, n. 36, 5.

on the intention to protect an authentic moral good. The FGM often leads to child mortality, thus violating the inalienable right to life. The procedure in most cases causes infections and other complications that threaten the life of the child. In some cases, FGM is carried out in unhygienic places with inadequate and unsanitary instruments. Incompetent persons who have no medical training often do the intervention (cutting or mutilation). People are not prepared for the risks and complications and many die because of these reasons. The *catechism of the Catholic Church condemns* such careless loss of lives, emphasizing that "life and physical health are precious gifts entrusted to us by God. We must take reasonable care of them, taking into account the needs of others and the common good"[1052].

Apart from the purposes of virginity, purity, modesty and beauty, FGM is conducted in some parts of Nigeria as an initiation ceremony of young girls into womanhood. Most women succumb to FGM because of the fear that their daughters or granddaughter may suffer social exclusion without undergoing FGM. Most hold tenaciously to the practice as if it really confers womanhood to the woman or it adds something to her dignity as a woman and as a person. The dignity of the human person as the Church teaches does not depend on the person's social worthiness. The womanhood of the woman or her dignity does not come from or increase through her initiation through FGM, neither does it reduce if the girl is socially excluded by her peers or the community because she did not undergo the FGM initiation procedure. J. Tham, explaining the position of Dignitas personae on the dignity of every individual asserts: "only persons have humanity and therefore intrinsic dignity". The dignity he further remarks "is intrinsic and present in all human persons from conception to natural death"[1053]. The social doctrine of the Catholic Church sustains that "the fundamental message of sacred scripture proclaims that the human person is a creature of God"[1054]. The Catechism of the Catholic Church continues in the same line affirming that "being in the image of God the human individual possesses the dignity of a person, who is not just something, but someone"[1055]. The dignity of the human person and

---

[1052] THE CATECHISM OF…, n. 2288, 532.

[1053] J. THAM, «Human Dignity in Dignitas Personae: Philosophical and Theological Reflections», in G. MIRANDA (ed.), *Studia Bioethica*, 2(2009), 12-18.

[1054] PONTIFICAL COUNCIL FOR JUSTICE AND PEACE, *Compendium of the…*, n. 108, 62.

[1055] THE CATECHISM OF…, n. 357, 111.

the sacredness of his life surge from man's relationship with the Absolute; being created in God's image and likeness.

Often FGM is carried out on minors with parents, grandparents or other adults assenting to it. In most cases they think their decisions are made in the best interest of the minors. For example, the woman who accepts that the daughter or the granddaughter goes through FGM, to save her from social exclusion thinks her decision is in the best interest of the minor. She prefers to see her daughter pass through the pains of the FGM procedures for the moment to seeing her suffer social exclusion for the rest of her life. Such decision could be said to be one made in good faith. However, one thing is clear; the decision is made from the point of view of the adult[1056]. The question remains whether the decision is right or wrong. With what ethical criteria did the adult make the decision? The Church's Magisterium has always sustained that clear laws be made for the protection of the vulnerable especially children. The Magisterium "constantly points out the need to respect the dignity of children", and accordingly that "the rights of children must be legally protected within juridical system"[1057]. The children are vulnerable persons. A vulnerable person is an individual who due to life circumstances is exposed to dangers and abuse and cannot help him/herself to obtain solutions to his or her problems. Hence, he or she needs others. The principle of preferential option for the poor in this case request that the interests, rights and dignity of the vulnerable be defended. The vulnerable should be protected and not exposed to injustice and risks. The principles of common good, subsidiarity and solidarity in the light of the Catholic social doctrine remind us that we all are responsible for all. Being one's brother's keeper implies making assiduous efforts to know what is the best interest of the other through a moral quandary, especially in the case of a minor or a handicapped person and helping him or her to achieve it where possible. The risks and injustice of the FGM are so glaring that no one can claim to be ignorant of them. FGM is a procedure that is ethically questionable and non-permissible if subjected to strict moral scrutiny.

[1056] Cfr. M. P. FAGGIONI, «Le Mutilazioni Genitali…».

[1057] PONTIFICAL COUNCIL FOR JUSTICE AND PEACE, *Compendium of the…*, n. 244, 143-144.

4.7.3. The use of Contraceptives in Nigeria and its Ethical Implication on the Dignity and Integrity of Adolescents and Women in Nigeria

The reproductive health indicators of Nigeria is one that gives no hope to anyone. For example, Federal Ministry of health indicates that the maternal mortality in Nigeria is estimated to be 1,000 maternal deaths per 100, 000 live births. The just mentioned Ministry of Health admits that "these factors have resulted in low contraceptive prevalence rate of 8.6% and a large pool of people whose needs are unmet"[1058]. Similarly, some who justify contraceptive use in Nigeria claim that "contraceptive use is important to promoting women's health and protecting their rights. It has been shown to reduce maternal morbidity and mortality"[1059]. The Federal Ministry of Health, Abuja, Nigeria, laments that "among adolescents and young persons, contraceptive use is very low, resulting in high prevalence of undesired pregnancies, unsafe abortions and hence high abortion-related morbidity and mortality"[1060]. Some authors who carried out a study in 3 communities in Kaduna state, Nigeria, on the contraceptive knowledge among women of reproductive age reported a relatively high contraceptive knowledge. According the same reports, 64.6% of women know at least one method. The most widely known is pill (54.1%), followed by female sterilization (47.5%) and injectables (47.4%). The study documented that knowledge did not reflect use.

Other methods known to Nigerian women are condom, diaphragm, Norplant, IUD, tubal litigation and vasectomy. According to some Nigerian authors, while the awareness of contraceptive is relatively high in Nigeria, studies reveal that the use by women is not appreciable[1061].

[1058] FEDERAL MINISTRY OF HEALTH, ABUJA, NIGERIA, National Reproductive Health..., 14.

[1059] E. A. ENVULADU – H. A. AGBO – A. MOHAMMED – L. CHIA – J. H. KIGBU – A. I. ZOAKAH, «Utilization of modern contraceptives among female traders in Jos South LGA of Plateau state, Nigeria», *International Journal of Medicine and Biomedical Research*, 1(2012), 224-231. https://doi.org/10.14194/ijmbr.1310 [17-8-2018].

[1060] FEDERAL MINISTRY OF HEALTH, ABUJA, Nigeria, National Reproductive Health..., 14.

[1061] Cfr. S. AVIDIME – L. A.-AKAI – A. Z. MOHAMMED – C. EJEMBI – S. ADAJI – O. SHITTU, «Fertility Intentions, Contraceptive Awareness and Contraceptive

For this, they ask that people be encouraged to use contraceptives and that efforts should be made to increase modern contraceptives uptake in medically underserved settings and to focus on increasing access to health care facilities, because according to them there are many benefits from the use of contraceptives. Some for instance claim that postpartum contraception helps nursing woman recover from the effects of pregnancy and childbirth before embarking on another pregnancy. They also affirm that it promotes child welfare[1062]. The above view is sustained by many Nigerian authors[1063].

Use among Women in Three Communities in Northern Nigeria», *African Journal of Reproductive Health*, 14(2010), 65-70; Cfr. A. EMMANUEL – G. ACHEMA – O. OMALE, «Contraceptive choices of married market women in a north central state of Nigeria», *International Journal of Nursing and Health Science*, 1(2014), 41-45; Cfr. A. S. ADEYEMI – D. A. ADEKUNLE – J. O. KOMOLAFE, «Pattern of contraceptive choice among the married women attending the family planning clinic of a tertiary health institution», *Nigerian Journal of Medicine*, 17(2008), 67-68.

[1062] Cfr. C. EZENYEAKU – I. U. EZEBIALU – J. C. UMEOBIKA – C. A. EZENYEAKU, «Desire to practice postpartum contraception among antenatal women at Awka, Southeast Nigeria», *International Journal of Reproduction, Contraception, Obstetrics and Gynaecology*, 7(2018), 1682, in https://doi.org/10.18203/2320-1770.ijrcog20181895 [16-8-2018]; Cfr. A. I. AJAYI – O. V. ADENIYI – W. AKPAN, «Maternal health care visits as predictors of contraceptive use among childbearing women in a medically underserved state in Nigeria», *Journal of Health, Population and Nutrition*, 37(2018), 19, in https://doi.org/10.1186/s41043-018-0150-4 [17-8-2018].

[1063] Cfr. M. RAJI, «Awareness and utilization of family planning commodities in a rural community of North West Nigeria», *Caliphate Medical Journal*, 1(2013), 103-108; Cfr. C. B. DURU – O. F. EMELUMADU – A. C. IWU – I. OHALE – C. C. AGUNWA – E. NWAIGBO – E. N. NDUKWU, «Prevalence, Pattern and Determinants of Contraceptive Use among Women of Reproductive Age (15-49) In Rural Communities in Imo State, Nigeria», *International Journal of Science and Healthcare Research*, 3(2018), ISSN: 2455-7587; Cfr. I. O. ALENOGHENA – E. C. ISAH – A. R. ISARA – S. S. AMEH – V. Y. ADAM, «Uptake of Family Planning Services Among Women of Reproductive Age in Edo North Senatorial District, Edo State, Nigeria», *Sub-Sahara African Journal of Medicine*, 2(2015),154, in https://doi.org/10.4103/2384-5147.172433 [17-8-2018]; Cfr. E. A. ENVULADU – H. A. AGBO – A. MOHAMMED – L. CHIA – J. H. KIGBU – A. I. ZOAKAH, «Utilization of modern contraceptives among female traders in Jos South LGA of Plateau state, Nigeria», *International*

The above-cited instances show how the use of contraceptive is the most prominent solution the governmental and most non-governmental health agencies offer to the issue of family planning and other sexual rights matters in Nigeria. The Federal Ministry of Health Nigeria for instance reveals how the government has put in place contraceptive logistics and management section with trained staff[1064]. This according to John Paul II shows how the "contemporary culture often regards sexuality in a reductive way, not in harmony with an integral vision of the human person"[1065]. The governmental agencies, especially the Federal Ministry of health Nigeria sustain initiatives for the distribution of condom and other contraceptive devices that are associated with implants and long term or permanent contraception. Thus the federal government's health agency sustains that permanent contraceptives should be made available also to adolescents and young adults[1066].

The afore-stated gives a picture of the use of contraceptive in Nigeria. The previous chapter of this thesis made clear the point that the distribution of health care resources should be carried out in a manner that the resources have positive impacts on real people in real situations. Going by this, one can ask what are the benefits of condoms and contraceptive devices to the lives of Nigerians and what change can it bring in the real situations of women in particular? Since many people are sick and hungry, can the

---

Journal of Medicine and Biomedical Research, 1(2012), 224-231, in https://doi.org/10.14194/ijmbr.1310 [17-8-2018]; O. A. ABIODUN – J. SOTUNSA – O. JAGUN – B. FATUROTI – F. ANI – I. JOHN – A. TAIWO – O. TAIWO, «Prevention of unintended pregnancies in Nigeria ; the effect of socio-demographic characteristics on the knowledge and use of emergency contraceptives among female university students», *International Journal of Reproduction, Contraception, Obstetrics and Gynaecology*, 4(2015), 755-764, in https://doi.org/10.18203/2320-1770.ijrcog20150087 [17-8-2018]; Cfr. E. ASUQUO – N. ORAZULIKE – E. ONYEKWERE – A. EKENOBI – J. ORAGE, «Unintended Pregnancy among Married Antenatal Clinic Attendees in a Tertiary Institution in Nigeria», *British Journal of Medical Research*, 19(2017), 1-11.

[1064] Cfr. FEDERAL MINISTRY OF HEALTH, ABUJA, NIGERIA, National Reproductive Health…, 15.

[1065] JOHN PAUL II, «Address to the Working Group on the Subject 'Scientific Bases of the Natural Regulation of Fertility and Associated Problems' 18 November 1994», n. 3, in *Papal Addresses to…*

[1066] Cfr. FEDERAL MINISTRY OF HEALTH, ABUJA, NIGERIA, National Reproductive Health …, 14.

distribution of condoms place food on their tables? Can such distributions bring healing or ameliorate the health situations of people? Is it right to insist on the provision of contraceptives and encouraging people to use them, when their substance rights such as health care, food, clean environment and other basic need to maintain life are not met? Many Nigerian women are convinced that the funds used for the distribution of condoms could have brought more benefits if they were used for the maternal and child health services or provision of food, good water, habitable environments and other health needs.

There is an obstinate insistence on the utilisation of contraceptive devices by the governmental health agencies in Nigeria, rather than on the moral principles and values. In regard to this matter, the Catholic moral values in contrast with the view of the Federal Ministry of Health, Abuja, affirms that "the conjugal act has its own total meaning; it engages the individual in such a way that the experience of communion and openness to life cannot be separated"[1067]. This position of the Catholic doctrine is based on the conviction that: "The love of a man and a woman must be understood in its fullest meaning, without dissociating the various aspects – spiritual, moral, physical, psychological – which comprises it. To ignore any one of these dimensions of love involves a serious risk to the unity of the person"[1068].

Humanae Vitae describes as evil "every action which, whether in anticipation of the conjugal act, or in its accomplishment, or in the development of its natural consequences, proposes, whether as an end or as a means, to render procreation impossible"[1069]. Hence, about the family planning model proposed in Nigeria, which promotes the use of contraceptives, the Catholic doctrine notes: "It is not authorised to promote demographic regulation by means contrary to the moral law"[1070]. In the same vein, the *Compendium of the Social Doctrine of the Church* affirms: "All

---

[1067] JOHN PAUL II, «Address to the Working Group on the Subject 'Scientific Bases of the Natural Regulation of Fertility and Associated Problems' 18 November 1994», n.3, in *Papal Addresses to the Pontifical Academy of Sciences 1917 – 2002 and to the Pontifical Academy of Social Sciences 1994 – 2002, The Pontifical Academy of Sciences, Vatican City 2003*, 364-366.

[1068] Ibid.

[1069] PAUL VI, «*Humanae Vitae*, Encyclical Letter On the Regulation of Birth», n. 14, (Vatican translation), Libreria Editrice Vaticana, Città del Vaticano 1968.

[1070] THE CATECHISM OF…, 2372, 547.

programmes of economic assistance aimed at financing campaigns of sterilization and contraception, as well as the subordination of economic assistance to such campaigns, are to be morally condemned as affronts to the dignity of the person and the family"[1071]. It is therefore obvious that the Catholic doctrine upholds only the "methods which strengthen respect for human dignity"[1072]. Instead of being obstinate with the promotion of contraceptives, the Catholic teaching thinks that "it is the duty of States and International organisations which recognise the principles of freedom of conscience to facilitate access to *methods which respect the ethical convictions of couples*"[1073]. The unremitting promotion and diffusion of contraceptives is a violent attack on the fundamental requirements and values of the family.

Some authors of Nigerian origin affirm that the most suitable family planning service is given through making available contraceptives. Therefore proffering solution to the public health challenges in a state in Nigeria they write: "Plateau state government should consider supplying more condoms, IUD and pills than any other method of family planning because most women prefer them"[1074]. Some other authors in line with the above position state: "the persistently high fertility in Nigeria despite family planning programmes in place suggests that there are yet undetermined factors associated with contraception that has been rendering previous strategies less effective"[1075]. Our dissertation does not accept contraception as the right method of family planning. It is not morally permissible, as such cannot be accepted as a method of family planning.

There are other authors that consider the use of contraceptives as the remedy to expansive population which according to them leads to the problem of food supply that does not match the population growth in some developing countries like Nigeria. Some authors cited by A. I. O.-Bello, O. L. Abodunrin and A. A. Adeomi, are convinced that "Nigeria is already facing

---

[1071] PONTIFICAL COUNCIL FOR JUSTICE AND PEACE, *Compendium of the…*, n. 234, 138.

[1072] JOHN PAUL II, «Address to the…», n.5, 364-366.

[1073] Ibid.

[1074] A. EMMANUEL – G. ACHEMA – O. OMALE, «Contraceptive choices of married market women in a north central state of Nigeria», *International Journal of Nursing and Health Science*, 1(2014), 41-45.

[1075] E. O. OLUWOLE – Y. A. KUYINU – O. O. GOODMAN – B. A. ODUGBEMI – M. R. AKINYINKA, «Factors Influencing the Uptake of Modern Family Planning Methods among Women of Reproductive Age in Rural Community in Lagos State», *International Journal of Tropical Disease & Health*, 11(2016), 1-11.

a population explosion with resultant effect that food production cannot match the growing population"[1076]. Others think that the birth rates in Nigeria today are higher than the world averages. Accordingly, they lament that Contraceptive Prevalence Rate (CPR) in Nigeria is embarrassingly very low. Citing the International women's health coalition, they affirm that in Nigeria, the CPR among married women aged 15-49 was 8% for modern methods and 12% for all methods. Ergo, they attribute the issues of population growth and food shortage to some factors, the most prominent among these according to them is low contraceptive usage[1077]. This position can be grouped with others that offer contraception as a solution.

The mentality of the Nigerian health system and some non-governmental organisation regarding the ongoing arguments recalls the question we asked in chapter three of this doctoral thesis[1078]. A Catholic prelate addressing this question reminds that each service rendered or whatever goods that are distributed in medicine, makes us forego doing other things in the same or other fields[1079]. Applying this to the distribution of condoms and other contraceptives, questions should be asked regarding whether it is necessary to make available such services? Is it worth it? What is the gain distributing condom when many children are dying of preventable diseases and others are dying because they drink dirty water and some die because they have no food to eat? Does what is being distributed fall under need or is it just a desire? Contraception cannot be a morally acceptable solution to population control and adequate food supply in Africa and particularly in Nigeria. Employing the appropriate moral principles means being ready to follow the right path towards solving some of these ethical problems. We propose the Catholic principles because they protect and rather than destroy the life of the human person.

[1076] Cfr. A. I. O.-BELLO – O. L. ABODUNRIN – A. A. ADEOMI, «Contraceptive Practice Among Women in Rural Communities in South-West Nigeria», *Global Journal of Medical Research*, 11(2011), 1-8.

[1077] Cfr. Ibid; Cfr. C. B. DURU – O. F. EMELUMADU – A. C. IWU – I. OHALE – C. C. AGUNWA – E. NWAIGBO – E. N. NDUKWU, «Prevalence, Pattern and Determinants of Contraceptive Use among Women of Reproductive Age (15-49) In Rural Communities in Imo State, Nigeria», *International Journal of Science and Healthcare Research*, 3(2018), ISSN: 2455-7587.

[1078] Cfr. This doctoral thesis, 3.4.5. What Kind of Health Care should be available to All?

[1079] Cfr. A. FISHER, «The ethics of …».

The Church in reaction to such above mentioned false solution teaches that:

> The answer to questions connected with population growth must instead be sought in simultaneous respect both of sexual morals and of social ethics, promoting greater justice and authentic solidarity so that dignity is given to life in all circumstances, starting with economic, social and cultural conditions[1080].

Rejecting contraception and using natural methods for regulating births according to the Catholic doctrine "means choosing to base interpersonal relations between spouses on mutual respect and total acceptance, with positive consequences also for bringing about a more human order in society"[1081]. The Church encourages recourse to periodic abstinence during the fertility period of the woman[1082]. We sustain there is a strong need to apply the Catholic principles in Nigeria because they proffer the right ways of protecting the dignity of human person. The Catholic doctrine has the view that "the practice of the natural methods of family planning helps couples to embrace the normative principles of their sexual activity, which flow from the very structure of their persons and their relationship"[1083]. The use of contraceptives represents an insensitive method through which the partner is considered only for pleasure. The natural method promotes openness and greater sensitivity of each partner towards the other and promotes interdependence, concern and respect for the partner's biological and psychological rhythms[1084]. Through the knowledge of human sexuality and the reproductive system, the married couples become aware of the spousal dimension of the body and God's plan for it. Such awareness helps them to understand better, the essential moral difference between the artificial methods that interrupt a process that is open to life and other methods – with a profound knowledge of the biological functioning of the body – affirm the inseparability of sexuality from the communion of persons and the gift of

---

[1080] Pontifical Council for Justice and Peace, *Compendium of the...*, n. 234, 138.

[1081] Ibid., n. 233, 137.

[1082] Cfr. Ibid.

[1083] John Paul II, «Address to the Working Group on the Subject 'Scientific Bases of the Natural Regulation of Fertility and Associated Problems' 18 November 1994», n. 3, in *Papal Addresses to...*

[1084] Cfr. Ibid., n. 4.

human life[1085]. The health capability approach we treated in chapter three admits it is important to help people (particularly women) to improve their ability to acquire correct health-related knowledge and have access to health-related resources and to make use of such knowledge to prevent the onset and exacerbation of morbidity. With an accurate knowledge in the field of human sexuality, they will be able to link knowledge of potential health advantages and disadvantages of some of their actions to the desirable values of health and health goals[1086].

The Catholic doctrine sustains that conjugal love implies a total involvement of all the elements of the person. It has personal unity as its aim. So, it is a total mutual giving that is open to fertility[1087]. The Catholic conception of conjugal act therefore excludes the use of contraceptives, which in some way ignores the equal personal dignity of the couple involved in the expression of love. The conjugal act is between two persons of equal personal dignity[1088], because of this, no partner should be seen as an object for pleasure. The use of contraceptives is often motivated by the idea of sex for pleasure and exclusively for pleasure, without any intention of accepting the eventual responsibilities. The Church's teaching makes it clear that "the fundamental task of marriage and family is to be at the service of life"[1089], and not to work against it. Refusing fertility and conception by using contraceptive devices turns married life away from that which represents its "supreme gift" the child[1090]. *Humanae Vitae* affirms that the teaching of the Magisterium concerning refusal of the use of contraceptives "is based on the inseparable connection, established by God, which man on his initiative may not break, between the unitive significance and the procreative significance which are both inherent to the marriage act"[1091]. Accordingly, the just mentioned Encyclical letter affirms: "By safeguarding both these essential aspects, the unitive and procreative, the conjugal act preserves in its fullness the sense of true mutual love and its orientation towards man's exalted vocation of parenthood"[1092].

[1085] Cfr. Ibid., n. 4.

[1086] J. P. RUGER, «Health Capability: Conceptualization…».

[1087] Cfr. THE CATECHISM OF…, n. 1643, 403.

[1088] Cfr. Ibid., 1645, 403.

[1089] Ibid., n. 1653, 405.

[1090] CONCILIO VATICANO II, *Gaudium et Spes…*, n. 50, 951.

[1091] PAUL VI, «*Humanae Vitae, Encyclical…*», n. 12.

[1092] Ibid., n. 12.

Some argue that contraception would help reduce abortions and death of women and adolescents. Contrary to this notion, concrete experience has proved that where the use of contraceptives is promoted with public funds like in Nigeria, there is a radical increase of abortions and deaths of women and young girls. The promotion of contraceptives increases the nightmare of sexual promiscuity, disrespect for women, family breakdown and the culture of death. The furtherance of contraceptives and related practices in Nigeria worsens the reproductive health situations especially of women and girls rather than improve it. This legitimates the application of the Church's Magisterium, which sustains that it is important to understand "the dignity of woman and her place in society, of the value of conjugal love in marriage and the relationship of conjugal acts to this love"[1093]. The sponsoring of the distribution of contraceptives in Nigeria as a solution to reproductive health issues means that the sponsors seem not to understand the important connection between these health issues with the human life and happiness; the dignity of the woman and her role in the society. The dignity of the woman has to be recognised because it has been there right from the creation of man. Highlighting this Pope John Paul II writes: "In creating the human race "male and female", God gives man and woman an equal personal dignity, endowing them with the inalienable rights and responsibilities proper to the human person"[1094]. The Roman Pontiff laments on the lack of cooperation in creating awareness; promoting and protecting the dignity of the woman; hence he remarks that:

> Unfortunately the Christian message about the dignity of women is contradicted by that persistent mentality which considers the human being not as a person but as a thing, as an object of trade, at the service of selfish interest and mere pleasure: the first victims of this mentality are women[1095].

[1093] Ibid., n. 2.

[1094] JOHN PAUL II, «*Familiaris Consortio*, Apostolic Exhortation, On the Role of the Christian Family in the Modern World», 1981, n. 22, in *The Post-Synodal Apostolic Exhortations of John Paul II*, J. M. MILLER (ed.), Our Sunday Visitor Publishing Division – Our Sunday Visitor Inc., Huntington, Indiana, 1998, 148-233.

[1095] Ibid., n. 24.

Evidently, such persistent mentality can be created where those who should protect the rights and dignity of every human person give wrong solutions, therefore exposing to danger that which they are supposed to protect. The civil authorities in most countries present unethical actions as solutions and model to be followed especially by the younger generation. The negative impact of such deviation was envisaged by Pope Paul VI in the Encyclical Letter *Humanae Vitae*:

> Another effect that gives cause for alarm is that a man who grows accustomed to the use of contraceptive methods may forget the reverence due to a woman, and, disregarding her physical and emotional equilibrium, reduce her to being a mere instrument for the satisfaction of his own desires, no longer considering her as his partner whom he should surround with care and affection[1096].

The magisterium of John Paul II emphasizes that "sexual expression of love as a specifically human act touches the very meaning of life and the dignity of the individuals involved"[1097].

The woman is not a sex toy. It is not right to see her as an object for sexual pleasure. As a result, human sexuality must not be limited to joy and pleasure. It goes beyond mere pleasure. It is therefore deductible that "sexuality, by means of which man and woman give themselves to one another through the acts which are proper and exclusive to spouses, is by no means something purely biological, but concerns the innermost being of the human person as such"[1098]. This total giving of themselves to one another as Pope John Paul II explains, "also corresponds to the demands of responsible fertility [...] by its nature it surpasses the purely biological order and involves a whole series of personal values"[1099]. It is not right to use the woman as an object for pleasure and it is condemnable to deceive or

---

[1096] PAUL VI, «*Humanae Vitae*, Encyclical...», n. 17.

[1097] JOHN PAUL II, Address to the Working Group on the Subject 'Scientific Bases of the Natural Regulation of Fertility and Associated Problems' 18 November 1994, n.3, in Papal Addresses to the Pontifical Academy of Sciences 1917 – 2002 and to the Pontifical Academy of Social Sciences 1994 – 2002, The Pontifical Academy of Sciences, Vatican City 2003 364-366.

[1098] JOHN PAUL II, «*Familiaris Consortio*, Apostolic...», n. 1.

[1099] Ibid., n. 11.

impose wrong and unethical methods like contraceptives and sterilization on the families. The Church's teaching frowns at such actions. Expressing the disapprovals of the Magisterium about the sponsoring of contraceptives by the civil authorities, Pope John Paul II avers:

> Thus the Church condemns as a grave offense against human dignity and justice all those activities of governments or other public authorities which attempt to limit in any way the freedom of couples in deciding about children. Consequently, any violence applied by such authorities in favour of contraception or, still worse, of sterilization and procured abortion, must be altogether condemned and forcefully rejected. Likewise to be denounced as gravely unjust are cases where, in international relations, economic help given for the advancement of peoples is made conditional on programs of contraception, sterilization and procured abortion[1100].

The political and economic leaders in Nigeria are urged to be docile to the principles of the Catholic teaching in order to render their services in a more appreciable manner. They are called to be at the service of life and not to suppress it.

There are views which consider the Nigerian female secondary school students as most vulnerable in terms of unintended pregnancies which often result in maternal morbidities and mortalities. According to those who uphold such position, to tackle this public health challenge, the girls should be provided with material to avoid unsafe sex and put them in the position to have appropriate family planning services (intending the provision of condom and other means of contraception)[1101]. The adolescents

---

[1100] Ibid., n. 30.

[1101] Cfr. A. Idowu – O. A. Aremu – F. Funmito – G. Popoola, «Knowledge, attitude and practice of contraception by female junior secondary school students in an urban community of Oyo-state, South west, Nigeria», *International Journal of Reproduction, Contraception, Obstetrics and Gynaecology*, 6(2017), 4759, in https://doi.org/10.18203/2320-1770.ijrcog20174983 [16-8-2018]; Cfr. U. C. Chima – T. O. Lawoyin – A. L. Llika – C. C. Nnebue, «Contraceptive knowledge and practice among secondary school students in military barracks in Nigeria», *Nigerian Journal of Clinical Practice*, 19(2016), 182-188; Cfr. E. O. Orji – O. A. Esimai, «Sexual behaviour and contraceptive use among secondary school students in Ilesa South West Nigeria», *Journal*

are often the victims of the horrors of wrong methods of approach to human sexuality. Because of curiosity or for the purpose of being like their peers; sometimes in the bid to do what others are doing or due to youthful exuberances, some adolescents indulge in sexual activities without actually knowing all that it entails. Therefore, in line with the Church's teaching, we think that the adolescents should be helped to acquire the capacity to develop "a right sense of values and achieve a serene and harmonious use of their mental and physical powers"[1102]. The adolescents should be protected by the civil authorities and their parents from "social communication which arouses men's baser passions and encourages low moral standards, as well as every obscenity in the written word and every form of indecency on the stage and screen"[1103]. This request of Pope Paul VI, made in 1968, is even more relevant today where the public without distinction is bombarded with pornographic images and statements everywhere in the world.

One of the most deceitful pieces of information used to convince the African youths and adolescents on the use of condom is that it protects from contacting HIV/AIDS. Since this represents a dreadful disease, adolescents and youths in Nigeria are swayed by any option that promises to guarantee "safe sex". But is this motive for distribution of condoms by

---

of *Obstetrics & Gynaecology*, 25(2005), 269-272; Cfr. T. ADETOKUNBO – A. OLUWAROTIMI – B. ABIOLA – A. ADENIYI – O. DELE – L. SHITU, «Contraceptive knowledge and usage amongst female secondary school students in Lagos, South West Nigeria», *Journal of Public Health Epidemiology*, 3(2011), 34-37; Cfr. I. C. ANOCHIE – E. E. KEPEME, «Prevalence of sexual activity and outcome among female students in Port Harcourt, Nigeria», *African Journal of Reproductive Health*, 5(2001), 63-67; Cfr. A. AJUWON – A. OLALEYA – B. FAROMOJU – O. LADIPO, «Sexual behaviour and experience of sexual coercion among secondary schools students in three states in North Eastern Nigeria», *BMC Public Health*, 6(2005), 310; Cfr. C. C. NNEBUE – U. CHIMA – C. B. DURU – A. L. LUKA – T. O. OLAOYIN, «Determinants of age at sexual initiation among Nigerian adolescents: a study of secondary school students in a Military Barrack in Nigeria», *The American Journal of Medical Science*, 4(2016),1-7; Cfr. B. O. IDONIJE – O. M. OLUBA – H. O. OTAMERE, «A study on knowledge, attitude and practice of contraception among secondary school students in Ekpoma, Nigeria», *Journal of Physics Conference Series*, 2(2011), 22-27; Cfr. C. O. ODIMEGWU, «Family planning attitude and use in Nigeria», *International perspective on sexual and reproductive health*, 25(1999), 86-91.

[1102] PAUL VI, «*Humanae Vitae*, Encyclical…», n. 21.

[1103] Ibid.

the Nigerian and non-Nigerian health and social agencies credible? In reference to this question, Alfonso Cardinal Lòpez Trujillo and Brain Clowes in their *"Case Against Condoms"* attest to the uncertainty of the claimed "condom safety". The Prelate warns about "safe sex" stating that:

> One cannot truly speak of objective and total protection by using the condom as a prophylactic, when it comes to the transmission not only of HIV/AIDS (Human Immunodeficiency Virus, which causes the Acquired Immune Deficiency Syndrome), but also of many other STDs (Sexually Transmitted Diseases)[1104].

The Catholic Bishops' Conferences around the world have denounced the distribution and purporting of condom it as a life-saving instrument, describing the motion as "safe-sex fallacy". The Church retains condom immoral because it goes against the human dignity. Still on the foregoing argument, Archbishop Ignatius Kaigama of the Catholic Archdiocese of Jos, Nigeria, recently appointed the Coadjutor of Abuja, Nigeria, while speaking at the 2014 Synod of Bishops emphatically stated that condoms and artificial contraceptives are not what Nigerians and the entire African continent need in terms of reproductive rights[1105].

Similarly, reacting to questions from journalists on his flight to Cameroon, Pope Benedict XVI acknowledged that "the problem of HIV/AIDS cannot be overcome with mere slogans [...] if Africans do not help one another, the scourge cannot be resolved by distributing condoms; quite the contrary, it worsens the problem"[1106]. The Church's description of condoms in terms of being "not a failsafe approach"[1107], is based on some scientific and non-scientific tests and proofs of condoms' deficiencies. These are classified as "condoms failures". Let us start with condoms failure and pregnancy. Concerning this failure, A. L. Trujillo and B.

[1104] A. L. TRUJILLO – B. CLOWES, *The Case Against Condom – The Scientific and Moral Basis for the Teaching of the Catholic Church on Preventing the Spread of Disease*, Human Life International, USA 2006, 3.

[1105] Cfr. J. J. MCELWEE, "African Archbishop Frankly Criticizes Western Attitude at Synod", National Catholic Reporter, October 8, 2014.

[1106] BENEDICT XVI, "Pope replies to Questions from Journalists", *Vatican Information Service*, March 17, 2009.

[1107] CATHOLIC BISHOPS' CONFERENCE OF THE PHILIPPINES, Pastoral Letter on AIDS *in the Compassion of Jesus*, January 23, 1993.

Clowes report that "the WHO explains that *perfect use* of the condom *does not* prevent pregnancy all the time"[1108]. The authors continue stating that "pregnancy in spite of condom use is well documented, with the Pearl index placed at around 15 failures per 100 women within the first year of use"[1109]. Following this deficiency of condoms, the authors rightly think condoms can also fail in protecting against HIV/AIDS. Citing an instance, they report that "some permeability and electric tests indicate that latex may allow passage of particles bigger than the HIV"[1110]. Condoms can allow passages due to holes and weak spots. These and some other instances demonstrate how condoms cannot perfectly assure "safe sex"; which is one of the major reasons for which the Federal Ministry of Health and other non-governmental agencies distribute condoms among the Nigerian youths and adolescents. The "safe sex fallacy" has created a lot of victims. The aforementioned Catholic Prelate maintains that instead of deceiving these young people, "the Ministries for Health should require labels for condoms, as they do in the case cigarettes, stating that the protection condoms provide is not total and that the risks are indeed significant"[1111]. This points out the right of adolescents and youths and others to "correct and complete information"[1112].

Cardinal Trujillo's solution is in synergy with our position because according to him "it is necessary to promote responsible sexual behavior that is inculcated by means of authentic sexual education that respects the dignity of man and woman, and does not consider others as mere instruments of pleasure and thus objects "to be used"[1113]. Since educating is an essential value of human life, parents should be involved in the education of their children. Such involvement does not start and end at home, because they "have the obligation to inquire about the methods

---

[1108] A. L. TRUJILLO – B. CLOWES, *The Case Against...*, 12. See also WHO, "Effectiveness of Male Latex Condoms in Protecting against Pregnancy and Sexually Transmitted Infections", in *Information Fact Sheet* number 243, June 2000.

[1109] Ibid.

[1110] Ibid., See also J. SUAUDEAU, Sesso sicuro in *Lexicon*, 795-817 and J. P. M. Lelkens, *AIDS:* il preservativo non preserva. Documentazioni di una truffa, in *Studi Cattolici*, 405(1994), Milano, 718 – 723.

[1111] Ibid., 4.

[1112] Ibid., 17.

[1113] A. L. TRUJILLO – B. CLOWES, *The Case Against...*, 3.

used for sexual education in educational institutions in order to verify that such an important and delicate topic is dealt with properly"[1114]. There is the need for projects, reformation of the health, political and economic sectors. Concrete efforts have to be made to restore the dignity of the Nigerian girl and woman. Sharing of condoms and other contraceptive devices cannot do this. Nigeria needs to adopt the Catholic approach which recognizes the dignity of the human person in all; especially the woman and her body and sustains the thesis of inalienable right to life from conception to natural death.

4.7.4. Ethical Issues concerning the practice of Abortion in Nigeria with Particular Reference to Dignity and Integrity of the Child and the Woman

There are two different laws for abortion in Nigeria: The Criminal Code of 1916 is in effect in the southern states. The Penal Code Law No. 18 of 1959 is in effect in the northern states. Both codes ban abortion in Nigeria and they apply similar criminal penalties for noncompliance in both regions. The major difference between the two Codes is that while the Criminal Code applies to anyone acting with the intent of procuring abortion, whether or not the woman is with child, the Penal Code applies to those cases where a woman is in fact with child. Abortion may be legally performed in Nigeria if it is necessary for saving the life of the pregnant woman. In February 1988, Nigeria adopted a population policy; new abortion policy, which take into consideration the idea that apart from saving the life of the pregnant woman, abortion, may be illicitly practiced in Nigeria to preserve physical health, and to preserve mental health. Abortion may also be performed for eugenic reasons[1115]. Thus, induced abortion is illegal in Nigeria unless it is practiced to save the life of the woman or to preserve her physical and mental health, or performed for eugenic reasons.

Defining abortion and its practice in Nigeria, O. J. Odia writes:

> Abortion, defined in this context as the deliberate termination of pregnancy, is illegal in Nigeria except when carried out to save the life of a pregnant woman. This is in agreement with the Nigerian code of medical ethics formulated by the MDCN and the views of

---

[1114] Pontifical Council for Justice and Peace, *Compendium of the…*, n. 243, 143.

[1115] Cfr. I. Okagbue, «Pregnancy termination and…».

various religious groups. Despite this firm stand against abortion by both the law, the MDCN and the various religious groups, there are hardly any prosecutions of persons in Nigeria that commit abortions. Many cases of illegal abortions occur in Nigeria[1116].

What the author describes as firm stand against abortion by the Nigerian law is seen in the same way by many Nigerians. This is because many believe that the Nigerian law, just like many laws of the countries in the Western World and some groups that declare to be for human life and the dignity of the human person, apparently prohibit actions against the life of the embryo, but provide shortcuts to crimes against the same human life and dignity of the human person. Instances abound in Nigeria. For example, the above-cited author narrates:

> In 1982, a termination of pregnancy bill was sponsored by the Nigerian Society of Obstetrics and Gynaecology in the national assembly. The Nigerian legislature failed to pass the bill due to overwhelming opposition by religious groups. The bill was intended to have permitted abortion, if two physicians certified that the continuation of pregnancy was harmful to the mother or the existing children in the family, and also if the baby had physical or mental abnormalities which would have resulted in it being seriously handicapped. Recently, the Governor of Imo State in the South East of Nigeria was accused of attempting to legalize abortion in the state under the guise of an apparently innocuous bill that would prohibit violence against persons. The bill was passed into law in 2012. However, there was an outcry by various religious and cultural groups, including the Association of Catholic Medical Practitioners of Nigeria. As a result, the Governor had to ask for the repeal of the law and gave a public apology. Despite these setbacks to the abortion law reforms in Nigeria, there are still advocacy groups fighting for the liberalization of the abortion law and the promotion of contraception, reproductive health and the training of service providers to ensure safe abortion in accordance with the law, and the improvement of post abortion care[1117].

[1116] O. J. ODIA, «The Relation Between Law, Religion, Culture and Medical Ethics in Nigeria», *Global Bioethics*, 25(2014), 164-169, in http://doi.org/10.1 080/11287462.2014.937949 [12-7-2018].

[1117] Ibid; Cfr. MITSUNAGA, T. M. – LARSEN, U. M. – OKONOFUA, F. E. «Risk

There are authors who affirm that "unsafe, induced abortion is one of the three major causes of maternal mortality in Nigeria"[1118]. Some people think that illegal abortion has continued to take place in Nigeria because of what they describe as unwanted pregnancy. For them unwanted pregnancy occurs because of the low knowledge and usage of contraceptives and pills among the adolescents and adult men and women in Nigeria. According to some of these authors "an estimated 1.25 million induced abortions occurred in Nigeria in 2012, equivalent to a rate of 33 abortions per 1,000 women aged 15–49"[1119]. The above statements reveal that the law or the legal ban alone is not enough. There is need to apply ethical principles that can rightly guide the people. The ethical principles, which can get to the conscience of the people to bring them to a change of mentality.

The egalitarian theory sustains that equitable distribution of health care services is a hallmark of justice. This egalitarian position disapproves the practice of abortion in Nigeria because, according to the same theory, the true sense of justice in health care is present where everyone's right to health and access to basic care are respected and ensured irrespective of one's social status. Abortion violates the fundamental and inalienable right to life of aborted human person. The dignity of the embryo and his right to health are not respected with the practice of abortion. There is the need to employ in Nigeria the Catholic moral principles that respects the sacredness of life and the dignity of every human person from conception to natural death. "Respecting the dignity of every human life means curing

---

factors for complications of induced abortions in Nigeria», *Journal of Women's Health*, 14(2005), 515–528. http://doi/10.1089/jwh.2005.14.515 [12-7-2018]; Cfr. OKOJIE, S. E., «Induced Illegal Abortion in Benin City, Nigeria», *International Journal of Gynecology & Obstetrics*, 14(1976), 571-521, in http://dx.doi.org/10.1002/j.1879-3479.1976.tb00098.x [13-7-2018]; Cfr. A. A. FAWOLE, – A. P. ABOYEJI, – T. M. AKANDE, «A Review of the Complications from Unsafe Abortions in Illorin, Nigeria», *Tropical Journal of Health Sciences*, 13(2006), 1-4, in http://dx.doi.org/10.4314/tjhc.v13i1.36699 [13-7-2018].

[1118] A. E. EHIGIEBA, – S. U. IGHEDOSA, – O. F. EMORE, – O. ONAFOWOKAN, «The Management Challenges of the Complications of Illegally Induced Abortions in Benin-City, Nigeria», *African Journals Online (AJOL)*. http://dx.doi.org/10.4314/smj2.v7i3.12878 [12-7-2018].

[1119] A. BANKOLE – I. F. ADEWOLE – R. HUSSAIN – O. AWOLUDE – S. SINGH – J. O. AKINYEMI, «The Incidence of Abortion in Nigeria», *International Perspectives on Sexual and Reproductive Health*, 4(2105), 170-181.

it of diseases and protecting it from destruction"[1120]. This implies that abortion, which destroys the unborn child, portrays the image of a society which neither respects the dignity of the unborn child nor protected his life. The right to life of all especially the vulnerable as the Catholic Church teaches must be defended and respected in every circumstance.

Understanding the term 'vulnerable' as that which applies to a person who could be harmed easily and cannot defend himself or herself or as one who needs special care and protection because of tender age or risk of being abused or harmed, we can correctly define the embryo as a vulnerable person. And we can correctly say that no one is more vulnerable than the human embryo. Thus, the Catholic moral tradition considers it imperative to defend, protect and respect the right to life and dignity of the human person from conception to natural death. The dignity of the human person does not cease to exist at any point of human life. For this reason the Church emphasizes that "the dignity of a person must be recognized in every human being from conception to natural death"[1121]. This affirmation opposes the motion that constitutional rights should be applied starting from birth and not from conception. The sacredness of life of the embryo is because life is a gift from God. His dignity as human person spurs from his relation with God. So abortion is an offence to God the creator and giver of life. Regarding this, Pope John Paul II remarks:

> When the sense of God is lost, there is also a tendency to lose the sense of man, of his dignity and his life; in turn, the systematic violation of the moral law, especially in the serious matter of respect for human life and its dignity, produces a kind of progressive darkening of the capacity to discern God's living and saving presence[1122].

The above statement of the Pope explains the gravity of this immoral act. Consequently, it is affirmed that "abortion and infanticide are abominable crimes"[1123]. A Catholic author, A. S. Moraczewski in line

---

[1120] J. THAM, «Human Dignity in…», 12-18.

[1121] CONGREGATION FOR THE DOCTRINE OF THE FAITH, *Instruction Dignitas Personae…*, n.1.

[1122] JOHN PAUL II, «*Evangelium vitae*, Encyclical Letter, (1995) On the Value of Human Life», n. 21, in J. M. MILLER (ed.), *The Encyclicals of…*

[1123] CONCILIO VATICANO II, *Gaudium et Spes* …, 51, 953-954.

with the Magisterium affirms: "In the moral order, an abortion can never be justified. There exists no condition which objectively can justify an abortion"[1124]. He further sustains that among the major reasons why the Catholic moral principles consistently and vigorously oppose abortion is that it is "unjust killing of a human person"[1125]. Pope John Paul II emphasizes the need to resist "the temptation to manipulate radically [...] with the risk of damaging human life even in the state of the embryo or the foetus, and of damaging the integrity and equilibrium of the human being"[1126]. The embryo is a human person and must be recognised as having the rights of the human person especially the inviolable rights every innocent being to life[1127]. The teaching authority of the Church hence, considers every procured abortion as immoral and gravely contrary to the moral law. It also condemns abortion willed either as an end or as a means[1128]. This simply implies that abortion is evil. The gravity of abortion is evident in the irreparable harm it inflicts on the innocent life of the unborn child, to the parents and the entire society[1129].

The Nigerian law condemns abortion but permits it for some reasons like when it is practiced to save the life of the woman, to preserve her physical and mental health and when it is performed for eugenic reasons. This is typical of many laws that usually open with the statement in favour of life especially of the conceived and within the same laws give room for violence against the right to life of the conceived. The reason for this inconsistency is often that of giving precedence to the life of the woman as if the life of the child is a "second class" life or an irrelevant and disposable material. This is an act of discrimination by the law which claims to be applicable in the same manner for all. The same law that proclaims

---

[1124] A. S. Moraczewski, «The Fetus and Human Embryo - Abortion», in E. J. Furton – P. J. Cataldo – A. S. Moraczewski (eds.), *Catholic Health Care…*, 73-77[2)].

[1125] Ibid.

[1126] John Paul II, «Address on the Occasion of the Fiftieth Anniversary of the Pontifical Academy of Sciences», 28 October 1986, n.8, in *Papal Addresses to the Pontifical Academy of Sciences 1917 – 2002 and to the Pontifical Academy of Social Sciences 1994 – 2002*, The Pontifical Academy of Sciences, Vatican City 2003. 280-288.

[1127] The Catechism of…, n. 2270, 528.

[1128] Cfr. Ibid., n. 2271, 529.

[1129] Cfr. Ibid., n. 2272, 529.

equality and should protect the vulnerable, does the contrary by promoting injustice and unfairness.

Most laws affirm that the embryo is a human person but without constitutional rights. This connotes a law that is inconsistent. It is unjust to respect and protect the life and dignity of the woman at the expense of that of the life of the child. "Respect for that dignity is owed to every human being because each one carries in an indelible way his own dignity and value"[1130]. The human embryo from the first instance of his life has the dignity proper to a person[1131]. The dignity of the human embryo is in no way inferior to that of the adults. We appreciate the just and right position of R. A. Aderemi that "a unique aspect of maternity nursing is that the nurse advocates for two individuals, the woman and the foetus"[1132]. This noble position should be applied why making reproductive health laws in Nigeria and every other nation.

Commenting on the awkward situation of legal inconsistency, Pope John Paul II writes:

> Really, what we have here is only the tragic caricature of legality; the democratic ideal, which is only truly such when it acknowledges and safeguards the dignity of every human person, is betrayed in its very foundations: "How is it still possible to speak of the dignity of every human person when the killing of the weakest and most innocent is permitted? In the name of what justice is the most unjust of discriminations practised: some individuals are held to be deserving of defence and others are denied that dignity?[1133]

This is really making mockery of the law and the people who hope on it for protection. There is the need to make unambiguous laws that are solemn and straightforward on the rights to life and dignity of the human person.

[1130] CONGREGATION FOR THE DOCTRINE OF THE FAITH, Instruction *Dignitas Personae…*, n.6.

[1131] Cfr. Ibid., n.5

[1132] R. A. ADEREMI, «Ethical Issues in Maternal and Child Health Nursing: Challenges Faced By Maternal and Child Health Nurses and Strategies for Decision Making», *International Journal of Medicine and Biomedical Research*, 5(2016), 67-76.

[1133] Cfr. JOHN PAUL II, «*Evangelium vitae*, Encyclical Letter, (1995) On the Value of Human Life», n. 20, in J. M. MILLER (ed.), *The Encyclicals of…*

The laws should be made in such a way that they cannot be interpreted by the stronger in their favour against the vulnerable unborn human persons. It is also very important to demonstrate the will to implement the laws that are rightly formulated.

The eugenic mentality accepts selective abortion, thus killing children affected with anomalies at the dawn of their lives. This is described by the Church's magisterium as a shameful and utterly reprehensible attitude[1134]. "Such discrimination is immoral and must therefore be considered legally unacceptable"[1135]. In addition, the fact that the conception of the child is called an unwanted pregnancy is already offensive language towards him or her. Distinguishing between wanted and unwanted babies is discriminating against the child tagged 'unwanted'. This form of discrimination violates the fundamental rights to life and dignity/integrity of the human person. For this, the Church considers abortion to be morally illicit. Abortion is a crime that constitutes serious moral disorder[1136].

The magisterium defines abortion as "the deliberate and direct killing, by whatever means it is carried out, of a human being in the initial phase of his or her existence, extending from conception to birth"[1137]. Permitting to kill the child for eugenic reason makes the Nigerian law inconsistent. The Nigerian law of abortion needs to be reviewed and reformulated. It cannot declare its defence for human life and at the same time permit one human person to kill another human person. The Catholic Church has as part of its doctrinal and pastoral mission to promote and exhort all people to protect and respect the dignity and the fundamental and inalienable right of every human being. To fulfil this duty there should be "courageous opposition to all those practices which result in grave and unjust discrimination against unborn human beings, who have the dignity of a person, created like others in the image of God"[1138].

The paradox of the legal inconsistency on the protection of the human life of the embryo is that almost every nation solemnly proclaim the

---

[1134] Cfr. Ibid., n.63.

[1135] CONGREGATION FOR THE DOCTRINE OF THE FAITH, *Instruction Dignitas Personae…*, n. 22.

[1136] PONTIFICAL COUNCIL FOR JUSTICE AND PEACE, *Compendium of the…*, n. 233, 137.

[1137] JOHN PAUL II, «*Evangelium vitae*, Encyclical Letter, (1995) On the Value of Human Life», n. 58, in J. M. MILLER (ed.), *The Encyclicals of…*

[1138] CONGREGATION FOR THE DOCTRINE OF THE FAITH, *Instruction Dignitas Personae…*, n. 37.

inviolable rights of the human person. The value of human life is celebrated and there are clear indications of a wide acceptance and an increasing moral sensitivity at the global level regarding the acknowledgement of the value of life and dignity of every human person. While the affirmations and proclamations grow stronger on papers of declarations etc., the tragic repudiation on the other hand contradict them in practice. For this Pope John Paul II asks:

> How can these repeated affirmations of principle be reconciled with the continual increase and widespread justification of attacks on human life? How can we reconcile these declarations with the refusal to accept those who are weak and needy, or elderly, or those who have just been conceived? These attacks go directly against respect for life and they represent a direct threat to the entire culture of human rights[1139].

The experience of many Nigerian women and especially young girls push them into practicing abortion:

> For many girls, the risk associated with abortions are outweighed by the fear generated from an unplanned pregnancy: fears of parental disapproval, abandonment by a boyfriend or husband, financial and emotional responsibilities of childbearing, expulsion from school or inability to secure husbands if they have a child out of wedlock[1140].

For this, the solutions provided by most authors who have treated the issue of abortion in Nigeria show their inclination to giving more opportunities to those who want to practice abortion. Instead of them highlighting the moral implications, they argue on the fears surrounding the act. For instance, there some Nigerian authors who claim that:

[1139] JOHN PAUL II, «*Evangelium vitae*, Encyclical Letter, (1995) On the Value of Human Life», n. 18, in J. M. MILLER (ed.), *The Encyclicals of…*

[1140] V. T. ADEKANMBI – S. T. ADEDOKUN – S. T.-PHILLIPS – O. A. UTHMAN – A. CLARKE, «Predictors of differences in health services utilization for children in Nigeria communities», *Preventive Medicine*, 96(2017), 67-72, in http://dx.doi. org/10.1016/j.ypmed.2016.12.035. [7-8-2018].

Solving the problem of unsafe abortion in Nigeria, however, requires a pragmatic approach using public measures. Primarily through education of the girl-child and educational programmes to sensitize the community about the dangers of unsafe abortion, tackling the unmet needs for contraception, the use of better techniques for abortion where the law permits and improving providers skills, secondarily, by availability of post-abortion care[1141].

This is the line of thought sustained by those whose link the increased rate of abortion practice in Nigeria to the legal restriction of abortion in the country[1142]. Some authors rightly agree that abortion is a preventable cause of maternal deaths in Nigeria. But some ethical problems arise from how they want to prevent abortion. According to these authors:

Barriers to the use of contraception in Nigeria include the lack of access to information and services about effective contraception; socio-cultural and religious beliefs that prevent women and men from seeking available contraceptives; and

---

[1141] Ibid.

[1142] Cfr. F. E. OKONOFUA, Abortion, in F. E. OKONOFUA – K. ODUNSI, (eds.), *Contemporary Obstetrics and Gynaecology for developing countries*, Women's health and Action Research Centre 2003, 179-201; Cfr. L. B. HADDAD – N. M. NOUR, «Unsafe abortion: Unnecessary Maternal Mortality», *Reviews in Obstetrics and Gynecology*, 2(2009), 122-126; Cfr. F. E. OKONOFUA, «Unwanted pregnancy, unsafe abortion among Adolescents», *Tropical Journal of Obstetrics & Gynaecology*, 19(2002), 515-517; Cfr. F. E. OKONOFUA – S. O. SHITTU – F. ORONSAYE – D. OGUNSAKIN – S. OGBOMWAN – A. ZAYYAN, «Attitudes and practices of private medical providers towards family planning and abortion services in Nigeria», *Acta Obstetetricia Gynecologica Scandinavica*, 84(2005), 270-280; Cfr. M. E. IKEANYI – C. A. OKONKWO, «Complicated illegal induced abortions at a tertiary health institution in Nigeria», *Pakistan Journal Medical Sciences*, 30(2014), 1398-1402; Cfr. WORLD HEALTH ORGANIZATION, Unsafe abortion: *Global and Regional Estimates of the Incidence of Unsafe Abortion and Associated Mortality in 2003*, Geneva, WORLD HEALTH ORGANIZATION, http://www.who.int/reproductivehealth/publications/unsafeabortion_2003/ua_estimates03.pdf. [9-8-2018]; Cfr. WORLD HEALTH ORGANIZATION, The prevention and management of unsafe abortion, *Report of a Technical Working Group*, in http://whqlibdoc.who.int/hq1992/WHO_MSM_92.5.pdf. [9-8-2018].

services delivery systems that have limited capacity and abortion-related mortality[1143].

In the same vein, other Nigerians scholars and international health agencies think that:

Effective contraception should be promoted for women at risk of unwanted pregnancies, especially unmarried adolescents and highly parous married women. Such interventions must seek to provide appropriate information and services for contraceptive delivery and to eliminate barriers that currently limit women's and men's access to contraception in developing countries[1144].

[1143] E. I. AKPANEKPO – E. D. UMOESSIEN – E. I. FRANK, «Unsafe Abortion and Maternal Mortality in Nigeria: A Review», *Pan-African Journal of Medicine*, 1(2017)1-6.

[1144] Ibid; Cfr. O. P. ADEFUYE – A. O. S.-ODU – A. O. OLATUNJI – M. A. LAMINA – T. O. OLADAPO, «Maternal deaths from induced abortion», *Tropical Journal of Obstetetrics Gynaecology*, 20(2003), 101-104; Cfr. O. E. AKANDE, «Reducing morbidity from unsafe abortion in Nigeria», *Archives of Ibadan Med*, 2(2001), 11-13; Cfr. O. B. FASUBAA – S. T. AKINDELE – A. ADELEKAN – H. OKWUOKENYE, «A politico-medical perspective of induced abortion in a semi-urban community of Ile-Ife, Nigeria», *Journal of Obstetetrics and Gynaecology*, 22(2002), 51-57; Cfr. F. E. OKONOFUA – U. ONWUDIEGWU – A. ODUNSIN, «Illegal induced abortion, A study of 74 cases in Ile-Ife, Nigeria», *Tropical Doctor*, 22(1992), 75-78; Cfr. O. M. ODUJINRIN, «Sexual activity, contraceptive practice and abortion among adolescents in Lagos, Nigeria», *International Journal of Gynaecology and Obstetrics*, 34(1991), 361-366; Cfr. E. ARCHIBONG, «Illegal induced abortion – a continuing problem in Nigeria», *International Journal of Gynaecology and Obsetetrics*, 34(1991), 261-262; Cfr. O. C. EZECHI – O. B. FASUBAA – F. O. DARE, «Abortion related deaths in South Western Nigeria», *Nigerian Journal of Medicine*, 8(1999), 112-114; Cfr. ID., «Contraceptive promotion and utilization, Solution to problem of illegally induced abortion in countries with restrictive law», *Nigerian Quarterly Journal of Hospital Medicine* 9(1999), 167-168; Cfr. O. B. FASUBAA – S. T. AKINDELE – O. C. EZECHI, «Illegal induces abortion in Nigeria, An examination of its consequences and policy implications for social welfare and health policy makers», *Journal of Human Ecology*, 14(2003), 433-443; Cfr. M. I. IBRAHIM – R. U. OKORO, «Profile of contraceptive acceptors in UDUTH, Sokoto, Nigeria», *Nigerian Medical Practioner*, 13(1997), 9-13; Cfr. E. I. AKPANEKPO – E. D. UMOESSIEN – E. I. FRANK, «Unsafe Abortion and ...».

Obviously, the solution offered here is not morally acceptable because access to services for contraceptives is not morally justifiable. Instead of making available condoms and other contraceptives devices, the adolescents should be given proper sex education which helps them to discover the immense value sex and the dignity of their body and the importance of self-control. Sexual intercourse is exclusively for married couples who have no authority to exercise it arbitrarily. For example married couples have the duty of avoiding every intervention that separates the conjugal act from its correspondent procreative consequence. We think that the right thing to do is to guide the girls, mothers and families through educational programmes on the ethical implications of abortion. This will be aimed at discouraging abortion because of the harm it causes to the life and dignity of the human person of both the mother and the unborn child. Meeting the needs for contraception, providing better techniques for abortion and improving the skills of the providers of abortion as the above mentioned authors suggested will only help to encourage "the culture of death". The right way to follow is to make effort to nip in the bud the unjust and immoral acts of contraception and abortion.

Abortion as well as contraceptives are insistently offered as help to the developing countries. But this help has been revealed as "pseudo-charity". A false charity/solidarity that represents threat to life, is exposed by the following detailed comment of Pope John Paul II:

> Another present-day phenomenon, frequently used to justify threats and attacks against life, is the demographic question. This question arises in different ways in different parts of the world. In the rich and developed countries, there is a disturbing decline or collapse of the birth rate. The poorer countries, on the other hand, generally have a high rate of population growth, difficult to sustain in the context of low economic and social development, and especially where there is extreme underdevelopment. In the face of over- population in the poorer countries, instead of forms of global intervention at the international level-serious family and social policies, programmes of cultural development and of fair production and distribution of resources-anti-birth policies continue to be enacted. Contraception, sterilization and abortion are certainly part of the reason why in some cases there is a sharp decline in the birth rate. It is not difficult to be tempted to use the same

methods and attacks against life also where there is a situation of "demographic explosion". The Pharaoh of old, haunted by the presence and increase of the children of Israel, submitted them to every kind of oppression and ordered that every male child born of the Hebrew women was to be killed (cf. Ex 1:7-22). Today not a few of the powerful of the earth act in the same way. They too are haunted by the current demographic growth, and fear that the most prolific and poorest peoples represent a threat for the well-being and peace of their own countries. Consequently, rather than wishing to face and solve these serious problems with respect for the dignity of individuals and families and for every person's inviolable right to life, they prefer to promote and impose by whatever means a massive programme of birth control. Even the economic help which they would be ready to give is unjustly made conditional on the acceptance of an anti-birth policy[1145].

This may not be far from the motive for the presence of numerous foreign abortion and contraceptive projects introduced by some social health agencies operating in Nigeria. The principle of subsidiarity invites the better off countries to help the poorer ones in what they cannot do and not to substitute their better moral standard, with a weak morality. Actions such as those described by Pope John Paul II are delicts that militate against the common good and the dignity of the human person. It is also a betrayal of the principles of solidarity and subsidiarity.

A report on the abortion practice in Nigeria shows that is on the increase every year:

> The first national study to examine the incidence of abortion estimated that in 1996, about 610,000 abortions, or 25 per 1,000 women aged 15-44, occurred in Nigeria. A decade later, another study noted that if the abortion rate had not changed since 1996, then 760,000 abortions would have occurred in 2006, given the increase in Nigeria's population during this period[1146].

[1145] JOHN PAUL II, «*Evangelium vitae*, Encyclical Letter, (1995) On the Value of Human Life», nn. 16-17, in J. M. MILLER (ed.), *The Encyclicals of...*

[1146] A. BANKOLE – I. F. ADEWOLE – R. HUSSAIN – O. AWOLUDE – S. SINGH – J. O. AKINYEMI, «The Incidence of ...»; Cfr. S. K. HENSHAW – S, SINGH – B. A. O-.ADENIRAN – I. F. ADEWOLE – N. IWERE, «The incidence of induced

Abortion and contraception are immoral; as such, they are wrong means of family planning. Where there is poverty, the Catholic social teaching invites all who can, in the spirit of the principle of solidarity to help the poor and the vulnerable. The foreign aids should have poverty alleviation as their objective and not the promotion of contraceptives, sterilization and abortion. Some Nigerian authors have the intention of convincing the religious groups to accept the ethics that promote contraceptives and abortion. They argue that in Nigeria people's

> Religious beliefs govern the ethics and morality of their private lives [...] and (inter) personal conduct [...] Nigerian faiths – Islam and Christianity, which in concert with the Nigerian adult-oriented culture, condemns premarital sex, especially young people's attempts to manage its unintended outcomes through self-medication and/or patronage of CPs and PMVs[1147].

According to one of the authors who want the religious groups to accept the secular views:

> Religious groups that have profound bias for contraception and abortion related issues should be encouraged to come on board through building their capacity to teach their adherents about the correct and effective use of whatever contraceptive method they choose in order to reduce the incidence of unwanted pregnancy[1148].

---

abortion in Nigeria, International Family Planning Perspectives», 24(1998), 156-164; Cfr. G. SEDGH – A. BANKOLE – B. O-. ADENIRAN – I. F. ADEWOLE – S. SINGH – R. HUSSAIN, «Unwanted pregnancy and associated factors among Nigerian women», *International Family Planning Perspectives*, 32(2006), 175-184.

[1147] A. D. OKONKWO – U. P. OKONKWO, «Patent medicine vendors...»; Cfr. C. O. IZUGBARA, «Representations of sexual abstinence among rural Nigerian adolescent males», *Sexuality Research and Social Policy*, 4(2007), 74-87; ID., «The Socio-cultural context of adolescents' notions of sex and sexuality in rural Southeastern Nigeria», *Sexualities*, 8(2005), 600-617; D. J. SMITH, «Imagining HIV/AIDS: Morality and perception of personal risk in Nigeria», *Medical Anthropology*, 22(2003),343-372; ID., «Youth, sin and sex in Nigeria: Christianity and HIV/AIDS-related beliefs and behaviour among rural-urban migrants», *Culture, Health, & Sex*, 6(2004), 425-437.

[1148] E. D. ADINMA, «Unsafe Abortion and its Ethical, Sexual and Reproductive Rights Implications», *West African Journal of Medicine*, 30(2011), 245-249; Cfr.

The strong abortion/contraceptive mentality in Nigeria justifies our insistence on applying the Catholic principles to enlighten the various ethical views in Nigeria so that they can choose what is good, right and just for the Nigerian women and children. The Nigerian woman needs solutions to her low status; she needs education; she needs work; poverty alleviation; she needs solutions to her health and health care needs; she needs good health facilities; infrastructures; steady power supply and all that are recommended by the Catholic principles of the common good and dignity of human person; to live a more fulfilled and dignified life. These are what the Nigerian women need for themselves and for their children and not contraceptives and abortion. We are reminded that we all are responsible for all.

For the foregoing argument, the respect for the dignity of the human person is of paramount importance. This is why the Church insists that human sexual and reproductive health care are issues that cannot be ignored because "they concern matters intimately connected with the life and happiness of human beings"[1149]. What the Church teaches about sexual and reproductive health is in accordance with that natural moral law. Establishing this relationship between the Church's teaching and natural moral law Pope Paul VI argues:

> The fact is, as experience shows, that new life is not the result of each and every act of sexual intercourse. God has wisely ordered laws of nature and the incidence of fertility in such a way that successive births are already naturally spaced through the inherent operation of these laws. The Church, nevertheless, in urging men to the observance of the precepts of the natural law, which it interprets by its constant doctrine, teaches that each and every marital act must of necessity retain its intrinsic relationship to the procreation of human life[1150].

J. I. B. Adinma – E. D. Adinma, «The Sexual and Reproductive Rights of Women in Nigeria», *Ebonyi Medical Journal*, 2(2003), 35-38; Cfr. J. I. B. Adinma, «An overview of the global policy consensus on Women Sexual and Reproductive Rights: The Nigerian Perspective», *Tropical Journal of Obstetrics & Gynaecology*, 19(2002), 10-12.

[1149] Paul VI, «*Humanae Vitae*, Encyclical…», n. 1.

[1150] Ibid., n. 11.

In the Catholic moral tradition, "we see that there is no contradiction between the affirmation of dignity and affirmation of the sacredness of human life"[1151]. It is therefore contradictory for any law or theory to affirm that rights to reproductive health and dignity of the Nigerian woman implies abortion; the killing of the unborn child. The Catholic doctrine condemns abortion because it violates the principle of the sacredness of life which holds from conception till natural end of a person's life. Morally speaking, neither contraception nor abortion can be permissible because they are "specifically different evils: the former contradicts the full truth of the sexual act as the proper expression of conjugal love, while the latter destroys the life of a human being". Accepting anyone of them implies going contrary to the will of God because contraception "is opposed to the virtue of chastity in marriage", while abortion "is opposed to the virtue of justice and directly violates the divine commandment "You shall not kill"[1152].

4.7.5. Major Consequences of the Failures and Debacles of the Nigeria Health Care System Borne by Children and Mothers

The poor performances, failures and indifferent attitudes in the Nigerian Health care system have many grave consequences suffered by women and children. The general health indicators of Nigeria as we have seen in the first chapter of this work, legitimate our proposal of the application of the Catholic principles of distributive justice, because millions of Nigerians especially women and children need liberation from lives without any sense of the dignity of the human person. We chose the following aspects of the Nigerian health indicators: Infant/Child morbidity and mortality and Maternal mortality, because of our sensibility towards these classes (women and children) that are majorly discriminated against, marginalized, ignored, denied of their rights to health and access to care. They are often abandoned to die in their various vulnerable states. We propose the respect of the principles of justice epitomized in the

---

[1151] CONGREGATION FOR THE DOCTRINE OF THE FAITH – *Instruction* Dignitas personae *on Certain Bioethical Questions* in E. J. FURTON – P. J. CATALDO – A. S. MORACZEWSKI (eds.), *Catholic Health Care…*, 411-423[2].

[1152] JOHN PAUL II, «*Evangelium vitae*, Encyclical Letter, (1995) On the Value of Human Life», nn. 13, in J. M. MILLER (ed.), *The Encyclicals of…*

Catholic social teaching as possible instruments for resolving the problem of mortalities among infants/child and mothers caused by inappropriate handling of their health issues.

– Children

The major health indicators as we have treated in chapter one, include life expectancy at birth male/female; maternal mortality ratio and other maternal health indictors; infant and child mortalities (Under 5 mortality rate) and immunisation coverage. In this part of our work, we will treat dedicate our attention to infant and child mortalities showing how the application of the Catholic principles of justice can help to ameliorate the negative situations in these areas. Clear consequences of the indifferent attitude and the insufficient performances of the government reflect in the high rate of infant/child mortalities in Nigeria. This is contained in the statements that "childhood mortality has remained a major challenge to public health amongst families in Nigeria"[1153]. In some cases, the government endeavours to make accessible the health care services to the children and their mothers but does not succeed because of some factors. The first Presidential summit on health care in Nigeria pledged to be committed in realizing the following maternal and child health targets and results: reducing infant and under-five mortality; reducing the prevalence of underweight children under-five; reducing the prevalence of malaria in children under the age of five and achieving universal access to reproductive health. The actual health indicators and major causes of child deaths in Nigeria show that only an insignificant part of the pledges made during the aforementioned first summit has been realized and just in few zones of the country. The problem is that most of the pledges, policies, programmes and decision in Nigeria remain on papers and are not translated into action.

A study on the access to quality child primary health care (PHC) services in Cross River State, in the south-southern part of Nigeria, by J. E. Ehiri, A. E. Oyo-Ita, E. C. Anyanwu, M. M. Meremikwu and M. B.

[1153] S. Yaya – M. Ekholuenetale – G. Tudeme – S. Vaibhav – G. Bishwajit – B. Kadio, «Prevalance and determinants of childhood mortality in Nigeria», *BMC Public Health*, 17(2017), 1, in https://doi.org/10.1186/s12889-017-4420-7 [14-8-2018].

Ikpeme, applauds the effort of the governor to provide primary health care especially to children in some areas of the country. According to the study:

> PHC facilities were adequately equipped to the extent of providing immunization services and management of diarrhoea [...] Many of the health workers (68.3%) had adequate training on immunization, and their knowledge scores on immunization issues (62%) was higher than in other aspects[1154].

This study at the same time reports that in Cross River State, the government's effort to protect the life of the poor, weak and vulnerable is efficient. Nevertheless, the study points out that the Primary Health Care facilities were not adequately equipped for management of acute respiratory infections (ARI) and that there is no adequate supply of essential drugs[1155].

In Nigeria, it is usual to see health care facilities widely dispersed. For this reason, many patients are constrained to travel long distances in order to utilize them. This problem is particularly heightened for those in the rural areas because the modern health care facilities are located in the cities. Therefore, most rural dwellers have to face the problems of poor transportation systems and road infrastructures in order to reach the places where the facilities are located. The outcome for the children with their mothers is nothing to write home about. "For instance, children born or raised in communities that lack a health care facility are likely to suffer poorer health outcomes compared to those children from communities where good health facilities are available"[1156]. What we have seen so far makes more evident our reason for thinking that Nigeria needs a health care system with Catholic orientation. We make this proposal because:

> Catholic health care [...] is rooted in a commitment to promote and defend human dignity; this is the foundation of its concern to respect the sacredness of every human life from the moment of conception till death. The first right of the human person, the

---

[1154] J. E. EHIRI – A. E. O.-ITA, E. C. ANYANWU, M. M. MEREMIKWU AND M. B. IKPEME, «Quality of Child health services in primary health care facilities in south-east Nigeria», *Child: Care, Health and Development,* 31(2005), 31,181-191.

[1155] Cfr. Ibid.

[1156] S. A. ADEDINI – C. ODIMEGWU – E. N. IMASIKU – D. N. ONONOKPONO – L. IBISOMI, «Regional Variations in Infant and Child Mortality in Nigeria: A Multilevel Analysis», *Journal of Biosocial Science,*47(2015), 165-187.

> right to life, entails a right to the means for proper development
> of life, such as adequate health care[1157].

The direct exposition of the major health indicators of Nigeria presented in chapter one of this dissertation shows that the performance of the Nigerian health sector is not in line with the standard of the principles of justice seen in the light of the Catholic principles. For further exposition, D. Eboh reveals that "one in 5 children born in Nigeria die before the age of 5, a much higher incidence than many other low-income countries. This under-5 mortality rate has virtually stagnated over the past 10 years while most countries have seen declines"[1158]. In the same vein, some other authors indicate that Under-5 mortality rates (MRs) vary from 83/1,000 live births (LB) in the south-west to 201/1,000 LB in the north-west[1159].

The foregoing arguments warrant moral questions concerning how seriously the Nigerian government is taking the issue at stake and how much it is respecting the fundamental rights of the human person of the Nigerian child. Some above-mentioned authors think that generally, only a little effort is made by the Nigerian authorities to respect the rights to life and health of the vulnerable. Referring to the child and maternal health indicators, they claim that "these indicators are driven by the fact that for the majority of women and children, life-saving, high quality **PHC** and referral services are unavailable"[1160]. J. Adinma thinks that an appropriate knowledge and application of bioethics is very necessary to save the life of the Nigerian Child. Furthermore, basic knowledge of bioethics is a necessary requirement for the application of ethics to perinatal medicine. Such application is very important in Nigeria. The current trend in perinatal medicine confronts problems posed to infant survival by neonatal prematurity and other diseases that require new-born intensive care[1161].

[1157] UNITED STATES CONFERENCE OF CATHOLIC BISHOPS, *Ethical and Religious Directives for Catholic Health Services*, USCCB, Washington, D.C., 2018[6], part 1, Introduction; JOHN XXIII, «*Pacem in Terris*, Encyclical Letter of on Establishing Universal Peace, in Truth, Justice, Charity, and Liberty, (1963)», n. 11, in C. CARLEN (ed.), *The Papal Encyclicals…*

[1158] D. EBOH, *Strategic Concept for…*, 21.

[1159] Cfr. G. TIMOTHY – O. IRINOYE – U. YUNUSA – A. DALHATU – S. AHMED – A. SUBERU, «Balancing Demand and …».

[1160] Ibid.

[1161] Cfr. J. ADINMA, «Ethics in Perinatal Medicine», *Nigerian Journal of Paediatrics*,

The application of bioethics in all aspects of perinatal medicine, the author affirms, will undoubtedly improve the quality of care for obstetric patients and their new-born infants[1162].

The rights to life is a fundamental one and should always be protected by making available the necessary life-saving services and by eliminating those services that encourage the suppression of human life. The Catholic Prelates of England and Wales indicating how the human life should be treated from the medical point of view write:

> New ethical challenges in the field of medical treatment will not be satisfactorily resolved unless the foundations of medical ethics are securely rooted in respect for human life at all its stages. Everything involving the use or disposal of human life, as a means to another end, must be categorically rejected[1163].

The position of these Bishops to oppose every activity that militate against the right to life of every human person is in line with the entire Catholic Magisterium.

The Catholic principle of common good indicates that the authorities should provide the social conditions the members of the society need to, as groups and individuals, to achieve their fulfillment more fully and more easily[1164]. This implies the duty of the Nigerian civil authority to make accessible to each citizen what is needed to lead a truly human life[1165]. When the life-saving services and the standard primary health care and referral services are not available and as well not accessible to women and children in Nigeria, the government cannot claim to be doing her duty in accordance with the principle of common good. Whether they are infant, children, and women, weak, poor or vulnerable, the truth that the social doctrine of the Catholic Church affirms is that "the roots of human rights are to be found in the dignity that belongs to each human being"[1166]. This dignity as the Universal Church teaches is inherent in the nature of human life and it is equal in every person[1167].

43(2016), 221, in https://doi.org/10.4314/njp.v43i3.12 [16-8-2018].

[1162] Cfr. Ibid.

[1163] CATHOLIC BISHOPS OF ENGLAND AND WALES, «*The Common Good...*», n. 19.

[1164] Cfr. THE CATECHISM OF..., n. 1906, 457.

[1165] Cfr. Ibid., n. 1908, 457.

[1166] PONTIFICAL COUNCIL FOR JUSTICE AND PEACE, *Compendium of the...*, n. 153, 85.

[1167] Ibid.

Similarly, in one of its statements, the Catholic Bishops' Conference of Nigeria expresses its concern about the way many poor Nigerians are treated, stating that they are "committed to the life and dignity of every human person and common good"[1168]. The Bishops declare their stance affirming: "We insist on the sacredness and dignity of human life being created in the image and likeness of God"[1169]. They also declare with firmness that "life is a precious gift from God. This gift must be respected"[1170]. The under-five deaths occur most often in Nigeria due to preventable diseases such as malaria, measles, respiratory infections, and diarrhoea[1171]. This indicates that the decent minimum primary health care interventions for child survival are not sufficiently provided. The ability to access most life-saving basic healthcare services, which are parts of common good, by many poor Nigerians is hampered most often by the lack of respect for the life and dignity of the human person. With this, one can say that the Nigerian government is acting in a way contrary to its identity, because the common good is the reason for existence of the civil authority[1172]. Therefore, in its efforts to achieve the common good, the public authorities are obliged to respect the fundamental and inalienable rights of the human person[1173]. The inalienable right to life and the right to health are inseparable rights of every child, including the Nigerian child.

Often, insufficient efforts are made by those responsible to obtain clean and hygienic delivery practices, but these are necessary conditions required to improve the health outcomes of all infants irrespective of where they are born, whether at home or in a health care facility. This causes unnecessary morbidity and mortality for the defenceless Nigerian children. The issue at stake here is that of human life. Human life is prominent among those

---

[1168] CATHOLIC BISHOPS CONFERENCE OF NIGERIA, «Time to end death penalty», *Statement by the Catholic Bishops Conference of Nigeria (CBCN)*, in https://www. cbcn-ng.org/docs/g14.pdf [20-4-2018].

[1169] Ibid.

[1170] Ibid.

[1171] G. TIMOTHY – O. IRINOYE – U. YUNUSA – A. DALHATU – S. AHMED – A. SUBERU, «Balancing Demand and …».

[1172] Cfr. JOHN XXIII, «*Pacem in Terris*, Encyclical Letter of on Establishing Universal Peace, in Truth, Justice, Charity, and Liberty, (1963)», n. 54, in C. CARLEN (ed.), *The Papal Encyclicals…*

[1173] Cfr. THE CATECHISM OF…, n. 1907, 457.

rights that are defined as "universal, inviolable, and inalienable"[1174]. Such are universal since they are present in all human beings, including infant, women and children, without exception. Inviolable, hence inherent in human persons and in human dignity, so imperatively necessary to be respected by all people. Inalienable because it cannot be denied legitimately and any derivation of any form should be considered a violation of their nature[1175]. This description of the characteristics of the right to life as the highest human value, and its close companion, the right to health, shows how grave any offence against them should be considered. More so, because the right to life is the condition for the exercise of all other rights[1176]. Without respecting or protecting the right to life, it would be absurd to claim of fostering other rights. Thus, regarding the unacceptably high rate of maternal death and new born and child morbidity and mortality, caused especially by the scandalous dysfunctional primary health care in Nigeria, we suggest that there be innovations aimed at providing enduring health care services to better their health conditions and survival ratio. For this to happen, it is evident that there should be intervention and systematic changes in the Nigerian health systems and especially in the distribution of health care resources. The application of the principles of the Catholic social teaching that sustains the dignity of every human person especially the most vulnerable, women and children consequently is indispensable.

The right to life is an alienable right of the person from conception till death. Therefore, the child should be accorded with this right, from the very beginning of his or her life that is from conceptions. Affirming this, Pope John Paul II's Encyclical *Centesimus Annus* clearly states: "the right to life, an integral part of which is the right of the child to develop in the mother's womb from the moment of conception"[1177]. The health and life of the child from conception are very important values, despite the fact that they cannot speak for themselves or do anything for themselves. The principle of solidarity entails that we provide for them all that they need to grow and to live a fulfilled life as the common good demand. We all

---

[1174] PONTIFICAL COUNCIL FOR JUSTICE AND PEACE, *Compendium of the…*, n. 153, 85.

[1175] Cfr. Ibid.

[1176] Cfr. Ibid., n. 155, 86.

[1177] JOHN PAUL II, «*Centesimus Annus*, Encyclical Letter on The Hundredth Anniverssary of *Rerum Novarum*, (1991) », n. 47, in J. M. MILLER (ed.), *The Encyclicals of…*

have this moral obligation and failure to fulfill it may characterize us as being inhuman, uncharitable and immoral. The Church's social teaching admits that: "Concern for the health of its citizens require that society helps in the attainment of living-conditions that allow them to grow and reach maturity"[1178].

— Mothers

The experiences of mothers are not different from those of their children in the Nigerian health care system. The experience of childbirth for most Nigerian women, unlike in most parts of the world where it is accompanied with joyful expectation, is characterized by anxiety, uncertainty, suffering and tragedy that often end up in death[1179]. Some authors after a proper comparative study of the experiences of most Nigerian mothers and their counterparts all over the world, have identified the maternal and child outcomes in Nigeria as the worst in the world[1180]. The United Nation Inter-Agency estimates risk of maternal death in Nigeria at 1 in 8. This ugly situation is caused mostly by lack of adequate health care facilities, lack of transportation to hospitals, clinics and maternal care homes, inability of the women and their families to pay for services, hospital detention and lack of will by the authorities to apply the already formulated policies and plans. Authors identify some of the factors affecting women willingness to pay for maternal, neonatal and child health services as lack of income and employment, illiteracy and poor access to maternal and child health facilities. With these factors, a great deal of women especially in the villages is vulnerable to more poverty and maternal deaths[1181]. It is obvious here that poverty plays a key role in exposing the Nigerian women and children to numerous health risks and causes of death. In addition, there is lack of interest of those in charge to look into the issues of the poor and the

---

1178 THE CATECHISM OF…, n. 2288, 532.

1179 L. O. OLUSEGUN − T. R. IBE − M. M. IKOROK, «Curbing maternal and child…».

1180 H. V. DOCTOR − R. BAIRAGI - S. E. FINDLE − S. HELLERINGER − T. DAHIRU, «Northern Nigeria Maternal…».

1181 M. B., YAHYA − T., PUMPAIBOOL, «Factors Affecting Women Willingness to Pay for Maternal, Neonatal and Child Health Services (MNCH) in Gombe State, Nigeria», *Journal of Women's Health Care*, 6(2017), 404, in http://dx.doi.org/10.4172/2167-0420.1000404 [13-7-2018].

vulnerable. In some cases, there is clear resistance among some populations to modern health care, due to religious beliefs and holding tenaciously to their cultural practices.

Among the causes of death of mothers as we have seen, there is deprivation of their right to health care and access to care. This confirms the aforementioned concerning maldistribution of public good due to lack of respect for life and dignity of the human person among some administrators of common good in Nigeria. A significant number of pregnant women in Nigeria do not have access to these essential "life-saving" health care services. This means that the indissolubly linked right to life and right to health are violated. The principles of solidarity instead makes it imperative to guarantee the availability and accessibility of such goods and services especially for people in conditions such as that of the expectant mothers. Instead of allocating money and creating services for contraception, abortion, sterilization and all practices that infringe on the right of the women and their children, the government should use the resources to save the lives of numerous pregnant women yearning for safe motherhood in Nigeria. Health care centres are meant to save life and not to suppress it. More so, among the rural settlers, there are some life-threatening situations because most women have babies whilst malnourished, in poor hygienic conditions and with no access to medical treatment.

We have established that everyone has the right to health and right to life and this is undoubtedly being made evident by reason. The idea is sustained by the social teaching of Pope John XXIII which affirms that "in human society to one man's right there corresponds a duty in all other persons: the duty, namely, of acknowledging and respecting the right in question"[1182], the government has the duty of acknowledging and respecting these fundamental rights of the Nigerian mothers. The duty however is not only that of the government but also of the entire society. The social teaching of the Church concerning this discloses that the common good involves all members of society, thus everyone without exemption has the duty according to his or her possibilities, to contribute to its attainment[1183]. The notion of the common good is enshrined in the

---

[1182] JOHN XXIII, «*Pacem in Terris*, Encyclical Letter of on Establishing Universal Peace, in Truth, Justice, Charity, and Liberty, (1963)», n. 55, in C. CARLEN (ed.), *The Papal Encyclicals*....

[1183] Cfr. PONTIFICAL COUNCIL FOR JUSTICE AND PEACE, *Compendium of the...*, n.

statement of the Catholic Bishops' Conference of Nigeria which urges the Nigerian government and all citizens to cooperate in protecting and defending the dignity of every Nigerian and to reach out in charity and solidarity to help those in need "wherever they are and so sustain our God-given human dignity"[1184]. Health is a common good; therefore, the health of the Nigerian mothers and their children is the responsibility of the entire Nigerian community. The responsibility of the common good the Church teaches, falls on individual persons as well as the state. The state however has the responsibility to lead by example because, common good is the reason that the political authority exists[1185].

4.8. Distribution of Health Care Resources: Applying the Principles in Practice

4.8.1. Can We avoid rationing in Health Care?

Health care allocation refers to the policies, programmes and practices involved in the distribution of the available resources among the citizens. Health care allocation is an ethical issue; it needs to be governed by ethical principles. Distribution is ubiquitous in every health care system. "Because of the scarcity of health care resources, rationing is also inevitable [...] two relevant, basic moral ideas are the maximization of the benefits from the use of health care resources and the fairness of the distribution of those benefits"[1186]. For G. Bognar and I. Hirose therefore, rationing is inevitable. In the same vein, many authors sustain that distribution of health care resources is unavoidable and that it must be done in fairness, respecting the ethical principles. A. Fisher accepts the necessity of allocation of health care resources but raises important questions on how to go about it: "The basic question in healthcare allocation is therefore not whether we should ration or prioritize but how we should do so given that this is inevitable. On what basis should we decide? How do we know when the resources are inappropriately

---

167, 94.

[1184] CATHOLIC BISHOPS CONFERENCE OF NIGERIA, «Time to end...».

[1185] Cfr. Ibid., n. 168, 95.

[1186] G. BOGNAR – I. HIROSE, *The Ethics of Health Care Rationing – An Introduction*, Routledge, London and New York 2014, 25-26.

distributed?"[1187]. The issue raised by A. Fisher aptly underline the points that create ethical problems like inequalities, unfair distribution, discrimination etc., during the distribution of health care resources.

The question on "how", that is, the criteria for decisions concerning health care allocation is very important. Allocation of health care resources "includes the controlled allocation of things such as subsidies for medicines, operating costs for hospitals, places on waiting lists, organs for transplantation, or funds for public health programs and medical research"[1188]. Similarly, A. Fisher lists the health resources, which include: "budgets, hospitals, beds, equipments, the time and energies of health professionals, drugs, procedures, organs-for-transplant and the like"[1189]. What are included as health resources differ from country to country depending on the exigencies of the population, their social and economic condition and the resources available. However, Fisher reiterates the big problem that is faced by every health system in the distribution of resources. According to him, "the crux of the question is usually how we should allocate finite healthcare resources"[1190]. On the question: Why is the allocation of health care is unavoidable? A. Fisher thinks it is "unavoidable because of the finitude of human life and health, technology, institutions, and natural resources"[1191]. He further explains the inevitability of healthcare allocation based on the simple fact that "not everyone can have every possible healthcare service. Nor would this necessarily be desirable even where it is practicable"[1192].

The issue of "opportunity costs" according to the author reminds us that "for everything we choose to do in medicine we forego doing certain other things"[1193]. The ethical views of A. Fisher on why health care allocation is unavoidable are clear and in accordance with the position of this dissertation. As Fisher rightly pointed out, because of our finite human nature, we do not have all we need. Even the richest country does not have all it takes to satisfy the health care needs of every single member of the country. More so, all health care services are usually not available for everyone. Even

---

[1187] A. FISHER, «The ethics of…».

[1188] G. BOGNAR – I. HIROSE, *The Ethics of…*, 25-26.

[1189] A. FISHER, «The ethics of…».

[1190] Ibid.

[1191] A. FISHER, «The ethics of…».

[1192] Ibid.

[1193] Ibid.

when certain services are possible, there is the need to consider what we are foregoing in other sectors by embarking on such services. For example, if attending to certain needs of a member of the family puts the lives of the rest at risk, by leaving them without the necessary things to survive, the question that must be asked is whether it is ethically right to go ahead giving that particular service to that sick member of the family. The same thing is applicable at the level of the society in relation to the administration of the common good. Health care allocation is obviously unavoidable but how it is done determines whether it satisfies moral standards or not; whether it is fair or unjust. As we have demonstrated above, the application of the Catholic principles can help to confront the numerous moral dilemmas faced during the distribution of resources.

4.8.2. Identifying Justice and Fairness in Health Care

In the distribution of resources there are always the issues of maximization and fairness which are considered to fall into different categories of the normative concepts: *deontic* concepts which include "right" and "wrong" "fair" and unfair" and *axiological* concepts which includes "good" and "bad", "benefit" and "harm"[1194]. Regarding the relationship of the deontic and axiological concepts, utilitarian ethics provides us with two approaches that are deontology and consequentialism. The deontological theories retain that there is no form of dependence of deontic concepts on the axiological concepts in defining the rightness or wrongness of an act. This implies that the rightness or wrongness of an act is determined independently of the goodness or badness of its consequences. On the other hand, the consequentialists' theories hold that the rightness or the wrongness of an act is defined considering its consequences. So for the deontological approaches, it is clear that right and wrong are a different matter which could be that of individual rights or that of fairness. However, this according to some authors does not mean that for the deotonlogical approach the issues of goodness or badness of consequences is irrelevant.

G. Bognar and I. Hirose, reveal that the most contemporary deontologists agree that the goodness of the consequences of an act is one of the important factors that could affect the definition of its ethical status[1195].

[1194] G. Bognar – I. Hirose, *The Ethics of…*, 24.
[1195] Cfr. Ibid.

For the consequetialists therefore: "the allocation of health care resources should aim at the best consequences – to achieve the best health outcomes [...] deontic concepts, such as fairness, can be given a consequentialist justification"[1196]. It is important to note that what is fair and just does not solely depend on the consequence. The means or how the consequence is arrived at is very important. A good or positive consequence obtained through a negative means cannot be ethically permissible. A positive end cannot justify a negative means. This is true also because the end does not mean what comes at the end, but that which motivates, nurtures and guides the action.

In the light of some principles of distributive justice, what is fair or just in health care is that which carries along everyone, especially the vulnerable. This, according to the social teachings of the Catholic Church, implies that the individual, whether he or she is poor, sick, weak or vulnerable should be considered as the origin, the subject and object of every social organisation[1197]. The human rights-based approaches: Universality, Availability, Accessibility, Acceptability, Quality, Equality and non-discrimination are features of a fair or just health care. These features help us to identify what is fair and just in health care because in accordance with some principles of distributive justice, guided by the Catholic principles, they assist to eliminate all inequalities and unhealthy discriminations, guarantee a universal access of quality health care services. For the Catholic teaching, when the dignity of the human person is defended with utmost care, it is easy to notice justice and fairness. John Paul II simply explains this position thus:

> The Magisterium has not ceased, in season and out of season, to recall the essential principles of her social teaching: man always has priority over the socio-economic systems in which he participates; human realities are for man, who has a central place within society and cannot be considered a mere element: he has an inalienable natural dignity[1198].

[1196] Ibid., 25.

[1197] Cfr. CONCILIO VATICANO II, *Gauduim et Spes*, n. 25, § 1.

[1198] JOHN PAUL II, «Address to Plenary Session on the Subject 'The Study of the Tension Between Human Equality and Social Inequalities from the Perspective of the Various Social Sciences'», n.4, in *Papal Addresses to...*; Cfr. ID., «*Centesimus Annus*, Encyclical Letter on The Hundredth Anniversary

The Catholic principles of dignity/integrity of the human person, preferential option for the most vulnerable, common good/solidarity and subsidiarity are clear indicators and features of what is right or just in health care: the human person should be at the center of all decisions. Policies, programmes and practices based on these principles will always guarantee a fair distribution of resources and hence an ethical health care system. When health care is depersonalized, logically it will be guided by egoism, lacks charity and the ethics of care, thus it ignores the weak, the poor and the vulnerable. It is obvious that such health care cannot be described as being fair or just.

4.8.3. What is the Difference Between Health Care Needs and other Social Needs?

To identify health care needs, it is important to understand the meaning of the word health. The origin of the 'word' health can be traced to the old English word 'hoelth' that means wholeness or being whole, sound or well. This definition is in line with the list of the rights to health care in the Catholic teaching, which is more extensive because it includes food, shelter, clothing, housing, transportation, education and access to basic health care[1199]. More so, the Catholic teaching sees the human person as a unified totality, in the profound unity of body and soul, thus, sustaining all those aspects that together help a person to live a more dignified life. In other words, to arrive at identifying health care needs, it is important to consider the person in his or her totality: physical, emotional, social, intellectual, and spiritual[1200]. "Healthcare needs are requirements for health secured by healthcare. Nevertheless, health is not the only good and healthcare is not the only activity that secures health"[1201]. That means to say that health requires other conditions that are described as health needs[1202]. Without such conditions, it will be difficult to talk about a good or complete state of health. B. A. Lanre-Abass' idea makes the above argument more appreciable:

---

of *Rerum Novarum*, (1991) », n. 13, in J. M. MILLER (ed.), *The Encyclicals of…*; CONCILIO VATICANO II, *Gauduim et Spes*, n. 84, § 2.

[1199] PONTIFICAL COUNCIL FOR JUSTICE AND PEACE, *Compendium of the…*, n. 164, 93-94.

[1200] Cfr. P. GATELY – A. BECK – D. A. JONES, *Healthcare Allocation &…*, 50.

[1201] Ibid., 51.

[1202] Ibid.

> Health needs must not be subordinated to human needs. Without a sufficiency of health, we cannot satisfy any of the other needs such as material goods and security. Ethics concerns the needs and values of human persons. Health is a vital human needs; nothing is more human, more personal and must always be one of the main concerns of any human community[1203].

The identification of health care needs can be easier if we are able to distinguish them from health needs. This distinction has to be made without separation of the two needs. The health needs are those needs that cannot be ignored if health care needs must be satisfied. The following are some health needs: "adequate food and shelter, hygiene and sanitation, reasonable conditions of work, social care and also education"[1204]. Attention must be given to health needs in order to address health care needs. Neglects of health needs while pursuing health care needs can lead to long futile efforts. Distinction should be made between the two needs without separation or creating contrast between them. In fact, a good number of authors believe that "inequalities in health (life expectancy, morbidity) are determined more by wider inequalities in society (income, housing and education) than they are by an unequal access to healthcare"[1205].

To further identify health care needs, it is necessary to distinguish them from wants. Health care needs are clear in the cases of emergencies or cases where, if a person does not receive medical treatments, he or she risks dying or suffering severe injury[1206]. The above health care needs are distinguishable from wants, which are mere desires for medical treatments that are not necessary and are avoidable. It is however true that in some cases it is not easy to make this distinction, especially where a person does not risk death or suffer ulterior serious injury but needs the treatment to improve his or her quality of life[1207]. Procedure is another element, which reveals the difficulty in distinguishing health care needs from wants, especially when the efficacy is contested. For the Catholic health care ethics, procedures that are unjust or unethical cannot be included under

---

[1203] B. A. L.-ABASS, «Poverty and maternal ...».

[1204] Ibid.

[1205] P. GATELY – A. BECK – D. A. JONES, *Healthcare Allocation &...*, 50.

[1206] Cfr. Ibid.

[1207] Cfr. Ibid.

health care needs. For example, elective abortion is not a health care need[1208].

Health care needs can also be identified by distinguishing health care from social care. Health care from the Catholic perspective include "medical care and basic nursing care but is distinguished from social care"[1209]. Health care has to do with "the good of life and physical and mental health"[1210] that can be obtained through medicine and surgery. Social care includes "support and care of a non-medical kind aimed towards helping people flourish in the social environment"[1211].

4.8.4. Who Should guarantee fair distribution Health Care Resources?

The state has the responsibility of ensuring that health care allocation is done in justice and fairness. The *Catechism of the Catholic Church* in this regard teaches: "It is the role of the state to defend and promote the common good of civil society, its citizens and intermediate bodies"[1212]. Health as earlier mentioned is considered part of the common good by the social doctrine of the Church. This reveals the duty of the state to apply the right principles of justice in health care resource distribution. The fundamental principle of equality of every human person is necessary for the state to carry out this responsibility in a worthy manner. Adhering to the four Catholic principles is a very important step to take in order to do a fair health care allocation. "The government also has a role in ensuring that all citizens have access to affordable medical care"[1213]. The Catholic teaching affirms that common good implies that everyone should enjoy the public goods. For this teaching, the common good is the reason for the existence of the civil authorities, hence it is the duty of the government to lead in the march towards the realization of the common good.

The *Compendium of the social doctrine of the Church* highlights that responsibility towards the common good is not exclusively for the civil authorities. Thus, the Church teaches that the common good involves all members of the society, reaffirming that "no one is exempt from cooperating,

---

[1208] Cfr. Ibid.

[1209] Ibid., 52.

[1210] Ibid.

[1211] Ibid.

[1212] CATECHISM OF THE…, n. 1910, 458.

[1213] P. GATELY – A. BECK – D. A. JONES, *Healthcare Allocation &…*, 54.

according to each one's possibility"[1214]. The Church reminds every citizen of the importance of participation in the realization of the common good stating that: "Participation is a duty to be fulfilled consciously by all, with responsibility and with a view to the common good"[1215]. Such obligation according to the Church's social vision "is inherent in the dignity of the human person"[1216].

Whatever we spend unnecessarily on health care on one person deprives another something in terms of health care needs and other needs. This indicates that individuals have responsibility for fair distribution of health care resources. Such duty is manifested in the responsibility of every adult to take care of his health. Participation implies assuming such personal responsibility and being faithful to it for the good of others and the society[1217]. Neglecting what I should do to avoid ill health or involving myself and insisting in a behaviour (like insisting in smoking of tobacco against doctor's advice) can lead to an unfair distribution of health care resources. This is very clear in the statement that "if people neglect their health, they will require healthcare which is taken away from others"[1218]. This is also applicable to the responsibility of adults toward children. Helping children to lead a healthy lifestyle is a way of carrying out our responsibility for fair health care allocation. Explaining further on this point the above cited Catholic authors remark:

> The dignity of the human person in the Catholic teaching implies both rights and responsibilities. If health is primarily a responsibility of individual, then it is reasonable for a system to incentivise responsible behaviour and to disincentives irresponsible behaviour [...] Many public health interventions mix incentives and disincentives, for example by increasing the tax on cigarettes and reducing the places where it is possible to smoke[1219].

Inviting or helping people to avoid unhealthy lifestyles, which may cause health problems, helps in a fair administration of health care resources.

[1214] Pontifical Council for Justice and Peace, *Compendium of the...*, n. 166, 94.

[1215] Ibid.

[1216] The Catechism of..., n. 1913, 458.

[1217] Ibid., n. 1914, 458.

[1218] P. Gately – A. Beck – D. A. Jones, *Healthcare Allocation &...*, 52.

[1219] Ibid., 54.

The Catholic teaching also encourages people to renounce some of their rights in terms of health care or some of the extraordinary Medicare to enable others to enjoy from what they have renounced. This according to the universal church is not only good but also licit. The principle of solidarity has a role to play here because according the Catholic social teaching; this principle "requires each person as a member of the human community, to play an active part in the destiny of society and to feel responsible for the well-being of all"[1220].

4.8.5. How do we know when the Resources are Appropriately Distributed?

To give a precise indication, we can say that we have no doubts to base our arguments on the Catholic principles of distributive justice, without denying that the secular principles, theories and approaches have their values. However, we maintain that their foundations are not without faults. Some of their parts can be acceptable only in the light of the Catholic principles: dignity/integrity of the human person, preferential option for the most vulnerable, common good/solidarity and subsidiarity. The secular principles mentioned above have their strong points as well as weak points. The Catholic principles contains all their strong points without any trace of their limits. According to the social teaching of the Church, fair distribution concentrates on allocating to each according to need, prioritising those in greatest need. In this regard, "the key requirement is to ration fairly and to respect the human dignity of every person, especially the most vulnerable"[1221]. In addition, John Paul II mentions one of the qualities of fair management of the common good. According to him:

> The moral goodness of all progress is measured by its genuine benefit to man, considered in relation to his twofold corporeal and spiritual dimension; as a result, justice is done to what man is; if the good were not linked to man, who must be its beneficiary, it might be feared that humanity were heading for its own destruction[1222].

[1220] JOHN PAUL II, «Address to the…», n. 6, 405-410.
[1221] P. GATELY – A. BECK – D. A. JONES, *Healthcare Allocation &…*, 59.
[1222] JOHN PAUL II, «Address to the…», n.5, 358-363.

The Catholic principle of preferential option for the poor and the vulnerable invites the society not to trample the needy because of their socio-economic and health conditions. Special attention should be given to them, respecting their dignity as human persons. Only when this is observed, can we talk of appropriate distribution of the public good. The Catholic principles support an equal distribution, access and utilization of health care. They urge that the right to life, right to health and the dignity of the human person be respected and protected. For the Catholic reflection, an appropriate distribution of health care resources is one done paying attention to the "claim that every human being has intrinsic, equal and inalienable dignity or worth, deserving uncompromising reverence and respect"[1223]. The resources are appropriately distributed when the allocation is done in accordance with the principle of common good, focusing on the dignity of every human person. In reference to this, the United States Conference of Catholic Bishops cite instances of an appropriate distribution of resources: "The common good is realized when economic, political and social conditions ensure protection for the fundamental rights of all individuals and enable all to fulfil their common purpose and reach their common goals"[1224]. Applying this to health care the American Bishops comment:

> A just health care system will be concerned both with promoting equality of care–to assure that the right of each person to basic health care is respected–and with promoting the good health of all in the community. The responsible health care resources allocation can be accomplished best in dialogue with people from all levels of society, in accordance with the principle of subsidiarity and with respect for the moral principles that guide institution and persons[1225].

The resources certainly are appropriately distributed where the decisions are made justly. Making just decisions means applying the right principles of distributive justice that are not contrary to the dignity of every human person. For the utilitarian principle, happiness of the majority and the economic gain are preferred to the dignity of the vulnerable person;

[1223] P. GATELY – A. BECK – D. A. JONES, *Healthcare Allocation &...*, 30.
[1224] UNITED STATES CONFERENCE OF CATHOLIC BISHOPS, «Ethical and Religious...».
[1225] Ibid.

therefore, it does not suit a fair distribution of health care resources. Price is for things while dignity is for the human person. A theory or approach that inverts this, should be considered unjust and unethical; such principle cannot lead to an appropriate distribution of health care resources. The social teaching of the Church has been consistent in proposing the moral principles that provide the moral criteria for decisions and actions and present the integral conception of man and his intrinsic dignity[1226]. The person-centered approach is a significant characteristic of a system that intends to realize a fair or appropriate distribution of health care resources. The Catholic vision of fair distribution is such which remarks that "no model of economic growth which neglects social justice or marginalises human groups is sustainable in the long term, even from the purely economic point of view"[1227].

The above Church's teaching is in conformity with the call by John Paul II to ensure that activities in the area of health regulation and market law be subject to solidarity. This step according to him will save individuals and societies from being sacrificed by economic changes and protect them from the upheavals caused by the deregulation of the market[1228]. In addition, the Pope invites all men and women "to leave their selfishness and show each other greater solidarity"[1229]. These ways indicated by the Roman Pontiff can lead to a just and fair distribution of health care resources.

4.8.6. Health Care Financing and Expenditures in Nigeria confronted with the Social Teaching of the Church

How do we apply what we have considered hitherto on the principles in practice to the Nigerian health care system? Regarding the appropriate distribution of resources, we can say that most of the problems of health care distribution in Nigeria boil down to the issues of health care financing

---

[1226] Cfr. JOHN PAUL II, «*Centesimus Annus*, Encyclical Letter on The Hundredth Anniversary of *Rerum Novarum*, (1991) », n. 11, in J. M. MILLER (ed.), *The Encyclicals of...*

[1227] ID., «Address to Plenary Session on the Subject 'The Study of the Tension Between Human Equality and Social Inequalities from the Perspective of the Various Social Sciences', 25 November 1994», n. 6, in *Papal Addresses to...*

[1228] ID., «Address to the plenary Session on the Subject 'Intergenerational Solidarity', 11 April 2002», n. 5, in *Papal Addresses to...*

[1229] Ibid.

and expenditures. By way of definition, health care financing is the method of generating, allocating and utilizing funds for health care[1230]. The most commonly used mechanisms for generating funds in Nigeria are tax-based financing, out-of-pocket payments, donor funding, and health insurance (social and community)[1231]. It is on record that Nigeria's health expenditure is relatively low, compared with other African countries[1232]. The irony of this is that Nigeria is richly endowed and has more human and other resources than these countries. B. O. Olakunde affirms that "the success of the different health financing methods can be measured by the overall effect on equity of access and health outcomes"[1233]. Unfortunately, this success is not known to Nigerians and the Nigerian health care system. T. O. Oyewale and T. R. Mavundla, cited some public documents to prove how the Nigerian government has failed women in terms of health care. According to them:

> The poor transportation system and low public expenditure on health worsen the exclusion of women from maternal health services in Nigeria. According to the Health Reform Foundation of Nigeria [HERFON] 2006:201, the general expenditure on health by the Nigerian government over the period of 1998 to 2002 was 20% of the Total Health Expenditure. In 2003, public health expenditure in Nigeria was less than $8 per capita compared with the $34 recommended globally for low-income countries (FMOH 2004:2). Private health expenditure accounted for 69% of the Total Health Expenditure in Nigeria (HERFON 2006:201). It is therefore not surprising that maternal mortality in Nigeria remains a concern (WHO 2017:17)[1234].

It is unethical to exclude anyone, especially the vulnerable groups from health care because health is a resource for everyday life and it is essential

---

[1230] Cfr. B. O. OLAKUNDE, Public healthcare financing…

[1231] Cfr. Ibid.

[1232] M. I. OLATUBI – O. O. OYEDIRAN – I. O. ADUBI – O. C. OGIDAN, «Health Care Expenditure in Nigeria and National Productivity: A Review», *South Asian Journal of Social Studies and Economics*, 1(2018), 1-7.

[1233] B. O. OLAKUNDE, Public healthcare financing…

[1234] Cfr. T. O. OYEWALE – T. R. MAVUNDLA, «Socioeconomic factors contributing to exclusion of women from maternal health benefit in Abuja, Nigeria», *Curationis*, 38(2015), 1-11.

to wellbeing and economic development. Health is fundamental to people's ability to enjoy and value every other aspect of life[1235].

Realizing a formidable health care financing system has continued to be a herculean task for Nigeria because the civil authorities have failed to realize as the Catholic Church teaches that their duty is that of stewardship of the public good. In addition, that this duty must be carried out with transparency, justice and fairness. Factors that contribute to the failure to achieve a successful health financing system in Nigeria include: poor institutional capacity, corruption, unstable economy and inefficiency of the political leaders. The Nigerian government generates revenue through taxation, but the country's major source of the bulk of the revenue as we mentioned in chapters one and two is the gas and oil market. The proceeds of this market, as we have seen in the first two chapters of this work, are not properly used for the people. Consequently, for the health care financing in Nigeria, the most commonly used means is out-of-pocket payments. The National Health Insurance Scheme covers very few Nigerians. The budgetary allocation for health is very low, not more 6%. With this, Nigeria has remained far below the 15% signed by the governments of African countries including Nigeria in the Abuja declaration.

The above-mentioned situations reveals why it is very important for the Nigerian government to consider the Catholic principles proposed by this dissertation. We think this is necessary because the failure in achieving a formidable health care financing in Nigeria depends on a system of operation and other factors contrary to the principles of the social teaching of the Catholic Church. For instance, poor institutional capacity, corruption and inefficiency of the political leaders owing to dishonesty, selfishness, embezzlement and appropriation of public funds are all contrary to the requirements of the principle common good, founded on the principle of the dignity of the human person. Nigeria ranks among the poorest countries in the world, with about 70% of the population living below US$1 per day. Nevertheless, out-of-pocket payments represent over two thirds of its health expenditure[1236]. In a country where out-of-pocket spending is the major means of health care financing and most of its

---

[1235] Cfr. O. B. AKPOMUVIE, «Poverty, Access to Health Care Services and Human Capital Development in Nigeria», *African Research Review*, 4(2010), in https:// doi.org/10.4314/afrrev.v4i3.60149 [16-8-2018].

[1236] Cfr. WORLD HEALTH ORGANIZATION, «Primary Care Systems…».

population is poor, it means that majority of its citizen are denied access to health care and means of living with dignity. Hence, health care financing in Nigeria, one can say does not take into consideration and does not satisfy the requirements for the respect for the dignity of the human person. The moral tradition of the Catholic Church therefore reminds that:

> The human person, must always be understood in his unrepeatable and inviolable uniqueness [...] This entails above all the requirement not only of simple *respect* on the part of others, especially political and social institutions and their leaders with regard to every man and woman on the earth, but even more, this means that the primary commitment of each person towards others, and particularly of these same institutions, must be for the promotion and integral development of the person[1237].

The Church in besides underlines the necessity to "consider every neighbour without exception as another self, taking into account first of all his life and the means necessary for living it with dignity"[1238], especially the means of health care needs. The Magisterium emphasizes that: "Respect for human dignity can in no way be separated from obedience to this principle"[1239], that is; being our brother's keeper. The Nigerian leaders and everyone involved in the administration of the health care funds should always remember that the funds are made for the human person and not the other way around. Regarding this, the Catholic doctrine instructs: "Every political, economic, social scientific and cultural programme must be inspired by the awareness of the primacy of each human being over society"[1240].

The foregoing arguments suggest that Nigeria should reconsider the long tradition of allocating more money to arms and war instruments, in the name of security, and turn to giving sufficient funds to the health care sector. The budgetary allocation for arms and ammunitions that foster the "culture of death" should not outweigh what is allocated to the health care sector which should promote the "culture of life". Furthermore, we invite the Western World that produce and sell these destructive products

---

[1237] PONTIFICAL COUNCIL FOR JUSTICE AND PEACE, *Compendium of the...*, n. 131, 73.

[1238] CONCILIO VATICANO II, *Gaudium et Spes...*, n. 27, 895.

[1239] Ibid., n. 133, 74.

[1240] PONTIFICAL COUNCIL FOR JUSTICE AND PEACE, *Compendium of the...*, n. 132, 74.

to the African political leaders, to look for a way of discouraging them from patronizing excessively this business activity which brings no benefits but rather, work against and destroy the people's interest. Rather, they should be urged to give more funds to the activities that promote and increase the means of living with dignity for their citizens, as the Catholic social doctrine advises. Health is a part of common good. The civil societies should consider this in their decision on health and other policies[1241]. Pope John Paul II epitomizes such advice stating that: "We are all really responsible for all"[1242].

The Nigerian leaders we think can be exhorted to do better with the view of the common good, applying with the right vision, policies and programmes formulated and intended as means of resolving the health care financing problems in Nigeria. However, the current health outcomes in Nigeria demonstrate that it is not enough to make laws, policies, and plans and establish strategies for the heath sector, there is the need for agents to know how to apply them with justice and fairness. The Catholic principles of distributive justice according to the present dissertation are virtuous agents that can help in their implementation; towards the realization of the set objectives; the good of the individual and the good of the society. Common good is important in the Christian ethics because it lies in human fulfilment, thus, in the end for measuring the moral goodness of an action[1243]. Considering the actions and outputs of the Nigerian political leaders in the light of the principle of common good, which sustain human fulfilment, we can say that their actions are not morally good and consequences logically resemble the actions.

This is so because many Nigerians remain unfulfilled and most have lost hope of being fulfilled owing to the bizarre comportments and reactions of the authorities, which are contrary to justice and the principle of common good. "The requirement of justice implies that respect for the dignity and worth of each person is a necessary component of the common good of society"[1244]. To act in accordance with justice means to

---

[1241] PONTIFICIO CONSIGLIO PER GLI OPERATORI SANITARI, *Nuova Carta degli…*, 114.

[1242] JOHN PAUL II, «*Sollicitudo Rei Socialis*, Encyclical Letter, (1987), for the twentieth anniversary of *Populorum Progressio*», n. 38, in J. M. MILLER (ed.), *The Encyclicals of…*

[1243] Cfr. D. M. GALLAGHER, «The Common Good», in E. J. FURTON – P. J. CATALDO – A. S. MORACZEWSKI (eds.), *Catholic Health Care Ethics…*, 29-31.

[1244] Ibid.

distribute the common good in a manner that not only the rich, but also every member of the society enjoys it. Results of some studies on Nigeria reveal that "income level of the people affects their health status and the poor are more strongly affected by public spending on health care relative to the non-poor"[1245]. R. K. Edeme emphasizes on the necessity of Public health expenditure arguing that it "is very important for decision makers to know the amount of government-funding on health care, the effectiveness of health care programs and the level of efficiency of this public health expenditure on achieving improvements in health outcomes"[1246]. Other Nigerian authors similarly observe that:

> In recent time Nigeria's health indicators have either stagnated or worsened despite the federal government's acclaimed efforts to improve health care delivery [...] It therefore becomes imperative to ask if governance has an impact on the effectiveness of health expenditure in Nigeria[1247].

Health is a part of the common good. Therefore, sharing health care goods with the criterion that permits only a few to get a share of it is unjust. In the same way, the concentration of the health care funds for the facilities in the urban areas, ignoring the rural areas where the higher population; the weakest and the poorest members of the society reside is neither just nor fair.

To arrive at a health care funding done in justice and in fairness, the *Catechism of the Catholic Church* enjoins that "much care should be taken to promote institutions that improve the conditions of human life"[1248]. This implies that ministries of health, hospitals, clinics, community health centres and other health care institutions should be the focus of

---

[1245] R. K. Edeme, «Public health Expenditure and Health Outcome in Nigeria», *African Journal of Biomedical and Life Sciences*, 5(2017), 96-102, in https://doi.org/10.11648/j.ajbls.20170505.13 [21-8-2018]; Cfr. A. Eneji, «Health care Expenditure, Health Status and National Productivity in Nigeria (1999-2012)», *Journal of Economics and International Finance*, 5(2013), 258-272, in https://doi.org/10.5897/JEIF2013.0523 [21-0-2018].

[1246] R. K. Edeme, «Public health expenditure ...».

[1247] M. I. Olatubi – O. O. Oyediran – I. O. Adubi – O. C. Ogidan, «Health Care Expenditure ...».

[1248] The Catechism of..., n.1916, 459.

the budgetary allocation (in a manner that is just) and efforts should be made to see that the sum allocated to health care is used for the purpose for which it is disbursed. It is incumbent on those who exercise authority to do this and by so doing; they can encourage others who, following their footsteps can put themselves generously at the service of others[1249]. As well, the Catholic social doctrine reminds that the common good is principally but not exclusively the responsibility of the civil authority. Every member of the society has the responsibility, each according to his or her capacity, to contribute to the realization of the common good. We are all invited to be responsible for all. The principle of subsidiarity clearly underlines this, affirming that permitting people to participate by giving what they can, is a way of respecting their dignity as human persons.

As we have seen in the present sector of this chapter, Nigeria is a country richly endowed with natural and human resources. However, it is difficult to see the impact of this endowment on the lives of its citizens. Many ask questions concerning health care services. For example, there are those who ask whether Nigeria does not provide the decent minimum health care to all its citizens because it is a poor country or because the political leaders are not willing to do so?

4.8.7. Does Nigeria provide Insufficient Standard of Health Care because it is Poor, so cannot, or it can but does not?

The question above makes reference to the faithful management of the common good. Nigeria is a rich country with many poor citizens. Commenting this paradox of poverty in the midst of plenty, K. Asoga-Allen writes:

> The abundant resources the nation is endowed with has been cornered and are being cornered by less than one percent (1%) of Nigerians while the Nigerian masses wallow in the ocean of poverty and penury [...] Every Nigerian today is the provider of his security and social amenities like electricity, water and so on[1250].

[1249] Cfr. Ibid., n.1917, 459.

[1250] K. A.-ALLEN, *Nigerian Democracy and Democratic Experience. A Historical, Political, Economic, Social and Religious Analysis*, Kayode Asoga-Allen, Great Britain 2016, 4-5.

Pope Francis in a letter to the Nigerian Catholic Bishops noted the important position of Nigeria and its economic growth. The Pope recalls that "Nigeria, known as the "African giant", with its more than 160 million inhabitants, is set to play a primary role, not only in Africa but in the world at large. It has experienced robust growth"[1251]. The correct description of Nigeria by the Pope is the irony that is responsible for the disappointment written all over the faces of numerous Nigerians who are poor citizens of a wealthy nation. This is one of the obvious incongruities of Nigeria. Pope Francis in accordance to the Church's social teaching invited the bishops to continue to sustain projects that "serve the weakest and the excluded"[1252].

Most Nigerians are denied the basic health care which is an essential element, and so, are constrained to provide for themselves that which should be the duty of the government to provide according to the principle of common good sustained by the social teaching of the Catholic Church. Due to the lack of concern for the good of all individuals by the government and the society, the situations of real and unique human persons who are suffering under the intolerable burden of poverty has noticeably worsened. Additionally, under the present administration, both the federal and the state levels, millions of Nigerians are living under the tragedies of total indigence and need. They are deprived of hope because there is little sign of concern for justice and the common good by most of the political leaders. John Paul II, addressing such unjust conditions of human persons affirms:

> Looking at all the various sectors - the production and distribution of foodstuffs, hygiene, health and housing, availability of drinking water, working conditions (especially for women), life expectancy and other economic and social indicators - the general picture is a disappointing one [...] The word "gap" returns spontaneously to mind[1253].

Reducing this gap is very important to make Nigeria a better home and to save many who are dying without any hope for rescue.

[1251] FRANCIS, «*Letter to the Catholic Bishops' Conference of Nigeria*, Vatican, 2 March 2015», in https://www.cbcn-ng.org/docs/g19.pdf [20-4-2018].

[1252] Ibid.

[1253] JOHN PAUL II, «*Sollicitudo Rei Socialis*, Encyclical Letter, (1987), for the twentieth anniversary of *Populorum Progressio*», n. 14, in J. M. MILLER (ed.), *The Encyclicals of...*

The situation till date in Nigeria is such that most people with notable difficulties provide the essential health care needs for themselves. It is unjust for the government to abandon its duty of the common good of all citizens, especially the poor and the vulnerable. It will be wrong to think that the right thing is for the people to take care of their public needs all alone. The individuals can participate in the production of some of their public needs, but not without the aid of the government. The government has the particular duty of creating occasions that will enable the citizens to do what they can do for themselves. The paradox of having a very high rate of poverty and insufficient provision of minimum decent health care in a country such as Nigeria, richly bequeathed with natural goods, is affirmed by K. Asoga-Allen: "Experience has shown that no matter the economic resources available in a state, if there are no honest leaders or individuals who are willing to harness the resources for the common good of all citizens, the nation would remain poor"[1254]. It is against this background that the State, as the Church teaches should remember that its duty is that of stewardship of the people's resources and that this duty has to be carried out always with a view to the common good[1255]. This implies transparency, accountability and a profound sense of justice and fairness. Such conditions if respected, can help Nigeria to rebuild a public ethics based on the dignity of the human person, solidarity and concrete cooperation geared towards the good of every individual especially the good of the weakest and the neediest[1256].

There is always a logical connection between living in poverty amid affluence and inefficiency on the part of those responsible for the administration of common good. Concerning this, an already cited author reminds that: "During the second Republic in Nigeria (1979-1983), the politicians impoverished the nation by diverting the nations resources to their personal uses [...] The level of poverty among the masses during this regime and open display of wealth by politicians led to military coup"[1257].

The attitudes of misuse and dishonest appropriation of the common good have continued till date and the negative impacts are high on the health sector. Pope John Paul II sustains that it is right and just to judge the

---

[1254] K. A.-ALLEN, *Nigerian Democracy and...*, 54-55.

[1255] PONTIFICAL COUNCIL FOR JUSTICE AND PEACE, *Compendium of the...*, n. 412, 232.

[1256] Cfr. Ibid. n., 420, 236.

[1257] K. A.-ALLEN, *Nigerian Democracy and...*, 58.

role of the political leaders by their interest or "willingness to contribute widely and generously to the common good"[1258]. Contributing widely and generously to the good of all and that of every individual is the hallmark of a good governance. The Nigerian political authorities are invited to imbibe these qualities in order to ameliorate the lives of many Nigerians who are dying because of the very poor performance of the health sector in the country. The basic healthcare needs especially of women and children in Nigeria are far from being met because there is often lack of will to give attention to them. The Nigerian political elites and the entire society have to change their mentalities, because so far, what is obtainable in Nigeria as far as health care indicators are concerned is unsatisfactory and very far below standard.

Highlights by L. A. Amaghionyeodiwe of the impacts of unwillingness to be committed to the common good in Nigeria, reveals that despite the increase in most components of health care spending in Nigeria, there is no notable improvement on both the health status of the average Nigerian and the condition of health infrastructure. He further reveals that, there is a big gap between the health status of the poor and the rich and that the poor are more affected by diversion of public spending on health care than the rich[1259]. This shows that the problem is not really whether there are enough resources, but that many mothers, children and many other Nigerians die because of how the resources are distributed. Most of the resources do not reach the public who are the true recipients. This has continued to cost the lives of many vulnerable in the country. D. Eboh reveals that: "There is evidence that trends in death rate and low life expectancy in Nigeria will continue to rise due to inefficient healthcare management and delivery system"[1260].

The above statement indicates how the health problems are persisting because the political leaders have not shown enough interest in addressing the problems the people. Correspondingly, the *Compendium of the Social Doctrine of the Church* teaches that "those with political responsibilities must

---

[1258] JOHN PAUL II, «*Sollicitudo Rei Socialis*, Encyclical Letter, (1987), for the twentieth anniversary of *Populorum Progressio*», n. 24, in J. M. MILLER (ed.), *The Encyclicals of...*

[1259] Cfr. L. A. AMAGHIONYEODIWE, «Government health care spending and the poor: evidence from Nigeria», *International Journal of Social Economics*, 36(2009), 220-236.

[1260] D. EBOH, *Strategic Concept for...*, 21.

not forget or underestimate the moral dimension of political representation, which consists in the commitment to share fully in the destiny of the people and to seek solutions to social problems"[1261]. One of the reasons for this moral degradation which is contrary to the respect of human rights is political corruption. This is one of the biggest problems of Nigeria: *corruption*, which has been eloquently condemned by the social teaching of the Catholic Church.

Conclusion

Chapter four is the most essential part of this dissertation. Within this chapter, we have done an exposition of the Catholic principles of distributive justices: dignity/integrity of the human person, common good and solidarity, preferential option for the most vulnerable and subsidiarity, using texts and documents on the Church's social teachings and Catholic moral tradition. The Catholic principles have enabled us to have an ethical focus on the social realities of Nigeria which were presented in chapters one and two with the aid of many authors, particularly of Nigerian origin. A critical analysis of these Nigerian phenomena in this fourth chapter has demonstrated how Catholic principles are the most preferred for the attainment of a just health care system in Nigeria. Referring to our previous points, the Catholic principles contain all the positive features of the principles, theories and approaches of distributive justice in the secular sphere, without possessing any of their deficiencies.

Respect for the human person underlies the principles of the common good, preferential option for the poor and the most vulnerable, solidarity and subsidiarity. The common good cannot be achieved without particular concern for distributive justice. The society and the state in particular are hence obliged to defend and promote common good[1262]. The Nigerian government has the responsibility to create health and other conditions to enable every member of the society to enjoy the common good. Thus, the civil authorities in Nigeria should consistently observe the principles of subsidiarity and solidarity in order to establish the common good and to be committed to authentic integral human development inspired by the

---

[1261] PONTIFICAL COUNCIL FOR JUSTICE AND PEACE, *Compendium of the…*, n. 410, 231.
[1262] FRANCIS, «*Laudato Sì*, Lettera…», n. 157, 120.

human values of charity and truth[1263]. The civil authority can only do this if it has regard for justice and respect for human rights and the dignity of the human person especially, those of the poor and the vulnerable as the Church teaches.

Pope Benedict XVI underlines the intrinsic interconnectedness that exist between the Catholic principles. Without this synergy, any of these principles may not fully realize that for which it is intended and applied, especially in health care. In his encyclical *Catritas in Veritate* the Roman Pontiff writes: "The principle of subsidiarity must remain closely linked to the principle of solidarity and vice versa, since the former without the latter gives way to paternalist social assistance that is demeaning to those in need"[1264]. The Pope's statement highlights the relationship of complementarities that exist among the Catholic principles. This means that it is better to apply at the same time more than one of the four principles in every case of the distribution of health care resources and other activities in the health sector in Nigeria in order to obtain an ethical health care system. Any division, separation or contrariness created among these principles can lead to derailment, which may cause serious harm to the lives, health and dignity of the human persons. Therefore, it is evident that a proper application of the Catholic principles is needed to improve the lives of Nigerians. Lack of consideration of these ethical principles has inflicted harms on the citizens of Nigeria. Such harms we have already seen in the use of contraceptives, sterilization, abortion, female genital mutilation, medical detention and other mistreats of human life and dignity caused by corruption and political inefficiency in Nigeria.

The individualism and relativism typified in the egoistic model of life that govern some of the health care laws, policies, programs, practices and activities globally and other individual and social activities today, make most people think that they are not responsible for other people's health and life. They prefer to think they owe nothing to anyone except to themselves. For this, we call for a change of attitude and we insist that reformation is very important to save the image of health care in Nigeria. This change can be realized by embarking on a new trajectory of thinking. The new trajectory of thinking can be identified in the application of the Catholic principles, together with the principles and theories of distributive

---

[1263] Cfr. POPE BENEDICT XVI, «*Caritas in Veritate...*», n.67, 109-111.
[1264] Ibid., n. 58, 97.

justice that demonstrate synergies with them in the allocation of health care resources. Where injustice abound and people are deprived of basic human rights, like the right to basic health, the principles of distributive justice contained in the Catholic approach to health care are logically inevitable[1265].

We believe the application of the Catholic principles to Nigeria's health, political and economic systems can help to develop an ethical health care system; a system that respects the right to health and the dignity of every human person. We propose the Catholic approach because it indicates how to avoid the unjust practices that create societies, which focus on maximizing benefits and utility "by denying access to health care for some of its sickest and most vulnerable populations"[1266]. Health care is necessary and suitable for the proper development and maintenance of life. Provision of health care, respecting the right to health and the dignity of the human person is a matter of justice. When justice is neglected and no longer dwells in social relationships, life itself is endangered[1267]. This is evident in the inequality between individuals and between the urban and rural areas in Nigeria; in the course of the distribution of health care and other resources. This as we have demonstrated in our work has led to the premature death of many of the poorest and the weakest[1268] in Nigeria.

Therefore, it is essential in every case not to abandon or deny anyone access to and utilization of health care. Priority should be given to providing everyone with the basic care, shelter, nutrition, hydration and nursing care where needed. Finitude of health care resources warrants rationing. Nevertheless, limits in resources and on treatment do not and should not at anytime equate to limits on care. The sickest and the most vulnerable members of the society must not be abandoned at anytime. All these we believe can be obtained with the adoption of the Catholic, person centered, approach to health care in Nigeria. The Catholic principles contain the main features of an ethical health system: universality, availability, accessibility, acceptability, quality, equality and non-discrimination. We are convinced that for any health system to be considered "a just health system", it must guarantee the presence of these attributes.

[1265] FRANCIS, «*Laudato Sì*, Lettera…», n. 158, 120-121.

[1266] T. L. BEAUCHAMP – J. F. CHILDRESS, *Principles of Biomedical…*, 231.

[1267] FRANCIS, «*Laudato Sì*, Lettera…», n. 70, 53-54.

[1268] Ibid., n. 48, 35.

General Conclusion

With this dissertation, we have set the goal of studying the Nigerian health care system to apply Catholic social teaching and its personalist principles. At this point we can take a general glance of our work. At the beginning, this dissertation offered a straightforward account of Nigeria from the geographical, socio-cultural, economic, political and historical perspectives, identifying some vital factors that influence the life of Nigerians. We specifically examined Nigeria's key health indicators and the major causes of death and main pathologies in Nigeria. Both gave a picture of failures and debacles of the health care system and political leadership. The problems emerging from the first chapter are clear indications that much still needs to be done to meet the requirements of the Sustainable Development Goals (SDGs) adopted by the world powers in September 2015 to ameliorate the lives of people living in the less prieviledged countries. Poverty alleviation and improving the health situation of the people being amongst the 17 SDGs, are the core issues of the Nigerian populace.

The areas of sexual reproductive health in this work revealed that the way this question is interpreted and practiced needs to be re-evaluated and improved upon, in order to respect the integrity/dignity of the child (unborn and born), the woman and the adolescents. The insufficient performance of the health system, as seen in all of the above-mentioned issues, is perceived as alarming by many Nigerians. Nonetheless Nigeria efficiently tackled the problem of the Ebola outbreak, a deadly disease which sowed panic within the public health communities all around the world[1269]. The Nigerian "spectacular success story"[1270], is a sign that all hope is not lost in its health care system.

We also analysed the Nigerian health system. Within this context, we briefly highlighted the definition of health system by the World Health Organization (WHO). The brief history of the Nigerian health care system disclosed the Christian origin and evolution of health care in Nigeria. This section revealed that the Catholic missionaries who operated in the area of health care were solely inspired by the Christian charity which promotes respect for the dignity of the human person, with special attention to the poor and the vulnerable.

The consideration of the origin of the health care system in Nigeria was followed by an analysis of laws, bills, policies, plans and strategies available for the administration of the Nigerian health care system. The Nigerian health care system has continued to look for answers to the health problems we considered in chapter one, by formulating and establishing the national health policy geared towards the realization of millennium development goals (MDGs). Other strategies and approaches also emerged to ameliorate the health situation of Nigerians. Our study revealed that, despite the promising health policies, Nigeria has failed to render efficient health care services. This failure has inflicted much suffering on the citizens and many have died because of it.

The nature, structure and administration of the Nigerian health care system studied in this dissertation showed that it is organized according to the three-level system of government in Nigeria: federal, state and local levels of government. The three tiers of government, in an ascending order, are each responsible for the administration of a sector of the health system: local government for the primary health care, the state government for the secondary health care and the federal government for the tertiary health care. Results show that primary health care receives only the crumbs from the higher arms of government. This, as we have seen, hampers the efforts of the grassroots level health care services. Our dissertation criticized this

---

[1269] WORLD HEALTH ORGANIZATION, «One year into.

[1270] Cfr. Ibid., WORLD HEALTH ORGANIZATION, «WHO declares end…»; FEDERAL MINISTRY OF HEALTH, «Status of Ebola…».

attitude because, regarding the distribution of health care resources, we cannot talk of giving the decent minimum health care through acts of charity or surges in human compassion, because it is demanded by justice. It is a basic necessity for every human person.

We examined how the theories of distributive justice from the secular perspective are applied to some issues of unending debates regarding rights to health care and how society reacts to these rights. Again, we saw the criteria applied by society in carrying out the duty of distribution of health care resources, and precisely which ethical principles society applies in health care allocation. With regard to this, our thesis retained in chapter three that it is important to understand the concept of distributive justice for a proper examination of the principles, theories and approaches of distributive justice applied to health care allocation.

Some of these theories and approaches of distributive justice which include, procedural, libertarian, utilitarian, egalitarian and Rawls theory, often do not represent ideal justice when it comes to the distribution of health care resources. In Nigeria one can hardly see great theoretical debates about the principles of justice as they have, for examples, in the USA, however, with the implementation of the health policies and some practices in Nigeria, there is a practical application of some of these theories and approaches. For instance, by implication, libertarian approach is utilized in Nigeria where out-of-pocket spending and private health system (market forces) are prominent among the ways of ensuring health care services. Hospital or medical detention is widely practiced in some Nigerian Hospitals and clinics because discriminatory approaches like libertarian and utilitarian models are implicitly employed in the distribution of health care resources.

Additionally, the egalitarian approach, Rawls theory of justice and need principles are understood in the functions of the National health policy, the National Health Insurance Scheme and other policies meant to realize Universal Health Coverage. Regarding this, the problem in Nigeria is based mostly on political commitment and the will to correctly implement existing health policies.

As we have aptly confirmed through this dissertation, the most diffused theories and approaches of distributive justice, have their strong points, but they also have strong limits. Their weak points distinguish them from the main features of an ethical health care system which comprise non-discrimination, availability, accessibility, acceptability, quality, accountability and universality. These features are in accordance with the person-centred Catholic principles studied in chapter four.

The foregoing argument shows how the core sector of this dissertation is the fourth chapter, where we had an ethical approach to the problems inherent to the distribution of health care resources in Nigeria with the aim of proposing an ethical health system. Critical analysis of the failures in the Nigerian health care system revealed lack of consideration of health as a common good as one of the motives for the default. The unpleasant results of administrative breakdown are infant, child and maternal morbidity and mortalities, inequality in health, with other consequences we studied under health and social justice. These negative developments are borne by the poorest and the most vulnerable. Likewise, some pragmatic ethical questions were addressed in the light of the Catholic moral principles. Such questions include: Is rationing unavoidable in health care? How can we identify what is fair or just in health care? How can we identify health care needs? Who has responsibility for fair health care allocation? How do we know when the resources are appropriately distributed? Gross difficulties regarding health care financing and expenditures in Nigeria prompted another important question: Does Nigeria provide an insufficient standard of health care because it is poor, so cannot provide the funding, or, it is capable of providing a sufficient standard of health care but it does not? The answers provided in this work indicated that the reasons for the insufficient provision of standard health are not dissimilar to those of economic debacles due to administrative inefficacy.

Comparatively, the first chapter of this dissertation remarked that the mismanagement of public funds, according to our consideration, stands as an obstacle to the realization of common good in Nigeria. Over $16 billion of oil revenues were selfishly taken by some civil authorities between 1979 and 1983. The same chapter also noted that a Minister of the Federal Republic of Nigeria, Alhaji Umaru Dikko, was alleged to have maladministered about N4 billion meant for the importation of food[1271]. Inquiries regarding such matters revealed that the burden of corruption of political leaders are borne by the population and that "the price of corruption is paid by using monies intended for the legitimate use of society"[1272]. Instances of such corrupt practices abound in Nigeria.

[1271] Cfr. M. M. OGBEIDI, «Political Leadership and…».

[1272] PONTIFICAL COUNCIL FOR JUSTICE AND PEACE, «*The Fight against…*».

Corruption at any level of government constitutes a hindrance to political activities and forces the citizens to mistrust public institutions[1273]. The inability on the part of government to deal effectively with poverty has been, to a large extent, due to corruption maintained by the Catholic social teaching as a great enemy of the common good.

Corruption and poor governance are among the factors that have plunged Nigeria into extreme levels of poverty and the far-reaching effects of low standard living, denial of health care and other essential social resources, causing the unnecessary deaths of mothers and children[1274]. It is important to reiterate that the decisions and actions of the administrators on health and other social goods have inevitable consequences on real persons. To that effect, the Church warns that: "the person cannot be a means for carrying out economic, social or political projects imposed by some authority"[1275]. Nigeria's key health indicators and major causes of death and main pathologies in Nigeria we saw in chapter one clearly confirmed this. As a result, it is necessary to affirm that the distribution of these resources "must be governed by the principles proper to distributive justice, and implied here is access to health care by all members of society"[1276].

Similarly, chapter two showed evidences of brilliant health polices of Nigeria which are not translated into practice for the benefit of the citizens. Where these policies are implemented, they do not contribute to the development of the health system because of some Nigerian factors like insufficient health facilities, improper remuneration, poor sustainable health care financing, government spending on health that is often very much below standard, high out-of-pocket expenditure in health, corruption and mismanagement[1277]. There is no response to the basic health care and social needs which are requisites for reaching fulfilments both as individuals and as groups. The common good is the reason why the civil authority exists[1278]. Hence public authorities are bound to respect and

---

[1273] Cfr. ID., *Compendium of the...*, n. 411, 231.

[1274] Cfr. L. O. OLUSEGUN – T. R. IBE – M. M. IKOROK, «Curbing maternal and...».

[1275] PONTIFICAL COUNCIL FOR JUSTICE AND PEACE, *Compendium of the...*, n. 133, 74.

[1276] D. M. GALLAGHER, «The Common Good...».

[1277] Cfr. G. TIMOTHY – O. IRINOYE – U. YUNUSA – A. DALHATU – S. AHMED – A. SUBERU, «Balancing Demand and...».

[1278] Cfr. JOHN XXIII, «*Pacem in Terris*, Encyclical Letter of on Establishing Universal Peace, in Truth, Justice, Charity, and Liberty, (1963)», n. 54, in C. CARLEN (ed.), *The Papal Encyclicals...*

protect the rights and dignity of every human person[1279]. Accordingly, adopting the approach of transparent stewardship is necessary in order to serve the people well.

A report study already cited in this dissertation disclosed there is a significant deficit in well-equipped and staffed health care facilities in Nigeria[1280]. Nigeria is bestowed with great economic and human resources, but the truth is there is no evidence that points to the existence of this wealth when one observes the conditions of most Nigerians. One of the major issues in administrative inadequacy according to A. Fisher is about 'how' the available resources are distributed. So for him the 'crux' of the matter is relative to the 'how'[1281] and not often to the quantity. Even in the case of limited resources, the truth remains that a basic minimum of health and material good is needed by human beings in order to live fulfilled lives, both materially and spiritually. Similarly, a United Nations report affirms that besides the level of resources, the civil authorities must make efforts to meet the rights of the citizens by taking immediate steps within their means[1282]. Health is a common good and the right to the common use of goods according to John Paul II is the primary principle of the entire ethical and social order[1283]. Common good belongs to the human person. The human person is the origin of social life. The human person is the subject, foundation and goal of social life[1284].

In the same fashion, the principle of subsidiarity sustains that there is no way the dignity of the human person can be protected where the family, groups, associations and local territorial realities are ignored[1285]. This implies

---

[1279] Cfr. THE CATECHISM OF..., n. 1907, 457.

[1280] Cfr. NIGERIAN HEALTH SECTOR, *Market Study Report...*, 20.

[1281] Cfr. A. FISHER., «The ethics of...».

[1282] UNITED NATIONS HUMAN RIGHTS, OFFICE OF THE HIGH COMMISSIONER, *Special Rapporteur on...*

[1283] Cfr. JOHN PAUL II, «Address to the Plenary Session and to the Study Week on the Subject 'Cosmology and Fundamental Physics' with Members of Two Working Groups who had Discussed 'Perspectives of Immunisation in Parasitic Diseases' and 'Statements on the Consequences of the Use of Nuclear Weapons' 3 October 1981», n. 4, in *Papal Addresses to...*

[1284] Cfr. PONTIFICAL COUNCIL FOR JUSTICE AND PEACE, *Compendium of the...*, n. 106, 61-62; Cfr. PIUS XII, Radio Message of 24 December 1944, 5: *AAS* 37 (1945), 12.

[1285] Cfr. Ibid., n. 185, 104-105.

that it will be in most cases difficult to help people without their participation. Such approach does not promote, instead it violates the dignity of the human person. Respecting the dignity of the human person according to the principle of subsidiarity means helping those in need in what they cannot do without absorbing them. This is one very reason for describing this principle as the most effective antidote against any form of paternalistic assistance[1286].

Allowing the people to participate means giving them the possibility to do what is inherent to the dignity of the human person[1287]. Procedural justice follows the same line by admitting that involvement of all parties in decision-making and in carrying out agreements is a necessary condition for a just society. Also *acceptability* demands that laws, policies and programmes must be in the best interest of the people. This is very important because it is only through the acknowledgement of the dignity of the human person that common and personal growth of everyone is possible[1288]. In reality, this path is not often followed in Nigeria. The low funding and *laissez-faire* attitude to the community health has been identified as one of the major threats to human life in Nigeria. In connection with this, we stress the importance of an adequate budget for this level of the health sector. Equally, the Catholic social principles affirm that it is a matter of justice to give opportunity to smaller communities in participating and contributing to the common good. Helping the less privileged without suppressing their liberty and dignity of human person is a way of being just and fair.

Related to the foregoing is the issue of unequal and inequitable distribution of health care and other social resources. Some authors affirm the basic truth that there is inequality in financing health care in Nigeria[1289]. Also, the persistence of gross inequality in Nigeria between the rich and the poor, the urban and rural areas has drawn the attention of the Catholic Bishops Conference of Nigeria which has condemned the situation, warning that it creates fertile ground for violence[1290]. Thus, the call for equity in health which strives to curb the avoidable gap in health and its determinants[1291]. Equity in health is connected to the features of

---

[1286] Cfr. BENEDICT XVI, «*Caritas in Veritate…*», n. 57, 96.

[1287] Cfr. THE CATECHISM OF…, nn. 1913-1917, 458-459.

[1288] Cfr. PONTIFICAL COUNCIL FOR JUSTICE AND PEACE, *Compendium of the…*, n. 145, 80.

[1289] Cfr. A. O. LAWANSON – O. S. OPELOYERU, «Equity in healthcare…».

[1290] Cfr. CATHOLIC BISHOPS CONFERENCE OF NIGERIA, «Our Dignity, Our…».

[1291] Cfr. Ibid.

a just health system inherent to the Catholic principles. Identically, the egalitarian approach which stands for equal opportunities is pragmatically closer to the aforementioned features because it gives opportunity to the poor to receive equal health care, in the same way as the rich. Correspondingly, the Catholic approach recommends the necessity of creating economic and social balances[1292]. Such a move is needed now more than ever in Nigeria.

Dissimilarly, libertarian and utilitarian principles do not support pro-poor principles because, according to many, they discriminate against the poorest, the weakest and the sickest. Such theories are not distant from the motive for hospital detention and similar unjust practices in Nigeria. We stand with the motion that faults hospital detention, because it is unjust and causes menace to the life of women and children[1293]. Such practice is a sign of a health care system devoid of the Catholic principles which promote charity as a fundamental human value of life in society[1294]. The Nigerian government ought to do more in tackling the problem of poverty. Most Nigerians, as our dissertation has revealed, are denied their right to health care because they are poor and out-of-pocket spending is the primary method of assuring access to health care services in the country. Payment rather than need is the first criterion for receiving health care in most Nigerian hospitals. Such trend is the reason poverty is prominent among the barriers to access to health care in Nigeria. Money seems to count more than the health or life of the sick. It is very unfortunate to talk of out-of-pocket spending on basic health care in a country where more than half of its population live on less than $1 a day and are unable to afford the high cost of health care[1295].

[1292] Cfr. JOHN PAUL II, «Address to the plenary Session on the Subject 'Intergenerational Solidarity', 11 April 2002», n. 3, in *Papal Addresses to the Pontifical Academy of Sciences 1917 – 2002 and to the Pontifical Academy of Social Sciences 1994 – 2002, The Pontifical Academy of Sciences*, Vatican City 2003, 435-437.

[1293] Cfr. D. DEVAKUMAR – R. YATES, «Medical Hostages: Detention...»; Cfr. R. YATES, «Women and children...».

[1294] Cfr. JOHN PAUL II, «Address to Plenary Session on the Subject 'The Study of the Tension Between Human Equality and Social Inequalities from the Perspective of the Various Social Sciences', 25 November 1994», n.9, in *Papal Addresses to...*

[1295] Cfr. M. O. WELCOME, «The Nigerian health...».

Everyone, including the poorest and the most vulnerable, has dignity and the rights to health, shelter, drinking water and education. Regarding this, John Paul II teaches: "no one can legitimately deprive another person, whoever they may be, of these rights, since this would do violence to their nature"[1296]. This affirmation, according to the Catholic social teaching is because "the ultimate source of human rights is not found in the mere will of human beings, in the reality of the State, in public powers, but in man himself and in God his creator"[1297]. By the same token, we reiterate that it is unjust to deny anyone decent minimum health care. Such harsh treatment against the poorest and the weakest are clear indications of a society that understands contrariwise the ethics-related tenet that the order of things must be subordinate to the order of persons[1298]. These remarks are signals of grave procedural problems. Nevertheless, we believe this dissertation can help reawaken the hope of Nigerians, because the condition of the Nigerian health care system is not beyond reversal.

A proper application of the Catholic principles observes the intrinsic interconnectedness among them. Practically, there is no way one can think of applying any of the principles while supporting practices like hospital detention, contraceptives, sterilization, abortion, female genital mutilation, discrimination based on social worthiness and other unjust practices that maim and destroy the human person. This doctoral dissertation calls for a new trajectory of thinking which should be translated into acting morally by respecting the dignity of the human person. Such application is inevitable for justice to reign because it is a question of justice to respect the right and dignity of the human person. Whenever justice is neglected or relegated to the background in social relationships life itself is at risk[1299]. Right to life is inseparable from the right to health. These rights "are inherent in the human person and in human dignity"[1300]. We hope to offer help through this academic exercise.

We are conscious of the fact that what we are proposing may not be easily accepted in a pluralistic society such as Nigeria where there are

---

[1296] JOHN PAUL II, Message for the 1999 World day of Peace, 3: *AAS* 91(1999), 379.

[1297] Cfr. PONTIFICAL COUNCIL FOR JUSTICE AND PEACE, *Compendium of the…*, n. 153, 85.

[1298] Cfr. THE CATECHISM OF…, n.1912, 458.

[1299] FRANCIS, «*Laudato Sì*, Lettera…», n. 70, 53-54.

[1300] PONTIFICAL COUNCIL FOR JUSTICE AND PEACE, *Compendium of the…*, n. 153, 85.

divergent views on principal issues concerning lifestyle, and these views in most cases turn into unhealthy oppositions. Our appeal may be judged with prejudice as a move to 'catholicize' the Nigerian health system. However, we are courageously proposing the Catholic principles because we are convinced that the basic tenets of Catholic personalist social doctrine does not offend the rights of any individual conscience.

We also know that some ideas of the social teaching of the Catholic church are contained in the African ethics. According to the Social doctrine of the Church, man "is not a solitary being, but a social being, and unless he relates himself to others, he can neither live nor develop his potential"[1301]. It is also affirmed by the Church that:

> A society that wishes and intends to remain at the service of the human being at every level is a society that has the common good — the good of all people and of the whole person [...]—as its primary goal. The human person cannot find fulfilment in himself, that is, apart from the fact that he exists "with" others and "for" others[1302].

Such conceptions of the common good and solidarity are fundamental moral principles of the African ethics of care. They are deeply considered in the African cultures and traditions where everyone tends to contribute something for the good of all, especially for the wellbeing of the weak[1303]. The African societies are essentially communalistic and the African ethics is profoundly communal in outlook[1304 1305].

Africans believe that the life of the individual is fully realized only in the community. The individual cannot exist alone, he can only exist corporately. African culture strongly supports the idea of social solidarity, brotherhood and mutual well-being. In Africa it is unusual to suffer alone, just as it unusual to rejoice alone. This reflects what the common good implies:

[1301] PONTIFICAL COUNCIL FOR JUSTICE AND PEACE, *Compendium of the...*, n. 110, 63.

[1302] Ibid. n. 165, 93.

[1303] Cfr. V. UCHENDU, *The Igbos of South East Nigeria*, London, Rinehart & Winston 1965, 34.

[1304] Cfr. J. OMOREGBE, *Ethics A Systematic and Historical Study*, Joja Educational Publishers, Lagos 1989, 140.

[1305] K. WIREDU, Morality and Religion in Akan Thought, in H. Odera, D. Wasola (eds.), *Philosophy and Cultures*, Book Wise Publishers, Nairobi 1983, 7.

> The common good does not consist in the simple sum of the
> particular goods of each subject of a social entity. Belonging
> to everyone and to each person, it is and remains "common",
> because it is indivisible and because only together is it possible to
> attain it, increase it and safeguard its effectiveness, with regard
> also to the future[1306].

The communalistic African ethics which is identified in the Catholic principles of common and good and solidarity is an indication that well-meaning Nigerians can accept our proposals without difficulty.

Furthermore, the person-centred principles of the Catholic social teaching go beyond religious, political, cultural and other differences, because the personalist principle is a universal concept and it is objective. Universality and indivisibility are qualities, according to John Paul II that make just principles suitable for any culture[1307]. The quality of being 'a person' unites all in the Catholic social doctrine. For this reason, we believe the person-centred principles of the Catholic moral teaching are not, and should not be perceived as an imposition of the Catholic or foreign doctrines on non-Catholics and non-Christians. What the Catholic Church teaches in the area of medicine is in a profound dialogue with the world of science and medicine. So, good health and the Catholic health care ethics are never at odds.

Again, we believe our proposal will surmount all hindrances in Nigeria because the core of the Catholic principles are known to the Constitution of the Federal Republic of Nigeria. Chapter IV of the Nigerian Constitution that treats Fundamental rights, art. 33(1), for example, indicates that every person has the right to life and no individual shall be deprived intentionally of their life[1308]. In addition, art. 34(1) provides that every person is entitled to respect for the dignity of their person[1309]. Therefore, the application of the Catholic principles which are person-centred and sustain the sacredness of human life, should not be alien to Nigerians who are ready to abide by the Constitution.

[1306] PONTIFICAL COUNCIL FOR JUSTICE AND PEACE, *Compendium of the...*, n.164, 93.

[1307] JOHN PAUL II, Message for the 1998 World Day of Peace, 2 *AAS* 90 (1998), 149.

[1308] Cfr. *Constitution of the Federal Republic of Nigeria* [Nigeria], Act n. 24, 5 May 1999, in http://www.refworld.org/docid/44e344fa4.html [16-05-2018].

[1309] Cfr. Ibid., n. 34.

Our work made a brief comparative study of the Catholic principles of justice and Islamic idea of distributive justice, seeing their similarities and differences. The result shows that Muslims who apply a correct interpretation of the Islamic doctrine of the principles of distributive justice would not hesitate to accept the ethical considerations and proposals by this dissertation.

The present dissertation is inspired by the Catholic social teaching; thus, it hopes to offer support to the Catholic Bishops Conference of Nigeria because it is part of its duty to defend justice, guide the priests and the hospital chaplains and educate the health care workers. It is our wish to see an Ethical and Religious Directives for Catholic Health Care Services in Nigeria, spurred by this doctoral dissertation. Equally, the present thesis wishes to serve as an opportunity to the health care providers in Nigeria to increase their knowledge of the Catholic teachings in order to answer questions on health care issues and to make ethical decisions in clinical activities. Thus, our intention is in synergy with a noteworthy affirmation by E. D. Pellegrino: "All Catholic health care professionals share the responsibility to give witness to Church teachings on bioethical questions in their work and daily lives"[1310]. Finally, the personalist approach proposed in this dissertation is articulated for the non-Catholic health workforce and politicians, especially all those who seek the truth with sincerity. This is possible because the human person is a concept that unites all human beings. The human person is the same everywhere in the world and health care and other social conditions necessary to live a dignified life are rights that legitimately belong to human beings by virtue of possessing a human nature[1311].

[1310] E. D. Pellegrino, «Foreward», in E. J. Furton – P. J. Cataldo – A. S. Moraczewski (eds.), *Catholic Health Care Ethics. A Manual for Practitioners*, The National Catholic Bioethics Centre, Philadelphia 2009², xv-xvi.

[1311] Cfr. D. A. Scrandis, «Jacques Maritain on the Rights of Man and the Common Good» in *The National Catholic Bioethics Quarterly*, E. J. Furton (ed.), Philadelphia, 17(2017), 615-621.

Recommendations

The following are recommendations to the Nigerian government in achieving a just distribution of health care and other social resources:

1. The Nigerian government is invited to consider the Catholic principles of distributive justice as a suggestion for national health policy. The basic values of Social doctrine of the Church: human person, common good and solidarity, are known to Africans and the communal mentality is typical of African societies. Therefore, the proposed principles can easily be linked to the Nigerian values.

2. Political leadership should eschew theft and corruption and imbibe the culture of justice, fairness, altruism and transparent stewardship.

3. The Nigerian government should reconsider the habit of allocating more funds to arms and war instruments, knowing full well that sound health care financing system can improve the socio-economic situation of Nigeria more than high expenditures on arms and ammunitions. Priority should be given to the health sector because a nation with healthy citizens is a wealthy nation.

4. The government should not leave health care in the hands of market forces alone, especially where they do not respect the dignity of the weakest members of society. This should be done

remembering that "A nation's greatness is measured by how it treats its weakest members".

5. The administrator of social goods in Nigeria should consider community-based interventions by passaging from "do-for" to "do-with" to improve the Health and social life of the rural dwellers. The rural areas should not be neglected because 55% of the Nigerian Population lives in these geographical zones.

6. The law or the legal ban on issues regarding right to life should be strong and clear.

7. The government should implement law and also apply ethical principles in its effort to protect the vulnerable. Laws are not enough because people's consciences are easily reached by moral approaches.

8. Both Government and the public health authorities should remember in their duty to protect the vulnerable, that no one is more vulnerable than the human embryo.

9. The Nigerian woman should be empowered through education, and provided with health and other social goods as opposed to making contraceptives accessible and giving her the legal right to kill her child. "Women constitute half of Nigeria's population [...] Women should be provided with maximum opportunity so that they could play their role in growth of GDP"[1312]

10. The Nigerian government should give proper attention to youth empowerment programmes.

11. The Federal Ministry of Health should make policies for correct moral sex education for adolescents and halt distribution of condoms as sexual reproductive rights.

12. The family must play a major role in educating adolescents and youths in handling sexual and reproductive issues.

13. Schools should be encouraged to create awareness in sexual and reproductive health. Schools are good channels of communication because the age for first sexual experience for adolescents in Nigeria is 15 years.

[1312] R. C. OKOYEUZU – O. P. EGBO – J. U. J. ONWUMERE, «Shaping the Nigerian Economy: The Role of Women» *Acta Universitatis Danubius Œconomia*, 4(2012), 15-24.

Bibliography

1. Ecclesiastical Magisterium

CONCILIO VATICANO II, *Gauduim et Spes*, Libreria Editrice Vaticana, Città del Vaticano 1998.

THE CATECHISM OF THE CATHOLIC CHURCH, *Paulines Publications-Africa*, Nairobi, Kenya 1995.

2. Popes

LEO XIII, «*Rerum Novarum, Encyclical Letter on Capital and Labour, (1891)*», in C. CARLEN (ed.), *The Papal Encyclicals 1878-1903*, The Pierian Press, United States of America 1981, 241-261.

PIUS XI, «*Quadragesimo Anno, Encylical Letter on Reconstruction of the Social Order, (1931)*», in C. CARLEN (ed.), *The Papal Encyclicals 1903-1939*, The Pierian Press, United States of America 1981, 415-443.

PIUS XII, *Radio Message of 24 December 1944*, 5: AAS 37 (1945), 12.

JOHN XXIII, «*Pacem in Terris, Encyclical Letter of on Establishing Universal Peace, in Truth, Justice, Charity, and Liberty, (1963)*», in C. CARLEN (ed.), *The Papal Encyclicals 1958-1981*, The Pierian Press, United States of America 1981, 107-129.

PAUL VI, «*Populorum Progressio, Encyclical letter (1967)*», in HTTP://W2.VATICAN. VA/CONTENT/PAUL-VI/EN/ENCYCLICALS/DOCUMENTS/HF_P-VI_ENC_26031967_POPULORUM.HTML [11-12-2019].

——————————, «*Address to the Plenary Session and to the Study on the Subject 'The Econometric Approach to Development Planning' 13 October 1963*», in Papal Addresses to the Pontifical Academy of Sciences 1917 – 2002 and to the Pontifical Academy of Social Sciences 1994 – 2002, The Pontifical Academy of Sciences, Vatican City 2003, 180-182.

——————————, «*Sharing in the Suffering of Mankind*», November 6th 1968, in The Teachings of Pope Paul VI (29-12-1967 – 18-12-1968).

——————————, «*Octogesima Adveniens, Apostolic Letter, On the Occasion of the Eightieth Anniversary of the Encyclical "Rerum Novarum"*», in http:// w2.vatican.va/content/paul-vi/en/apost_letters/documents/hf_p-vi_apl_19710514_octogesima-adveniens.html [10-02-2018].

——————————, «*Humanae Vitae, Encyclical Letter On the Regulation of Birth*», (Vatican translation), Libreria Editrice Vaticana, Città del Vaticano 1968.

JOHN PAUL II, «*Redemptor Hominis, Encyclical letter (1967)* », in J. M. MILLER (ed.), The Encyclicals of John Paul II, Our Sunday Visitor Publishing Division – Our Sunday Visitor Inc., Huntington, Indiana 1996, 31-96.

——————————, «*Address to the Plenary Session and to the Study Week on the Subject Cosmology and Fundamental Physics' with Members of Two Working Groups who had Discussed 'Perspectives of Immunisation in Parasitic Diseases' and 'Statements on the Consequences of the Use of Nuclear Weapons'*» 3 October 1981, in Papal Addresses to the Pontifical Academy of Sciences 1917 – 2002 and to the Pontifical Academy of Social Sciences 1994 – 2002, The Pontifical Academy of Sciences, Vatican City 2003. 249-252.

——————————, «*Laborem Exercens, Encyclical Letter on Human Work, (1981)* », in J. M. MILLER (ed.), The Encyclicals of John Paul II, Our Sunday Visitor Publishing Division – Our Sunday Visitor Inc., Huntington, Indiana 1996, 165-214.

——————————, «*Familiaris Consortio, Apostolic Exhortation, On the Role of the Christian Family in the Modern World*», 1981, in J. M. MILLER (ed.), The Post-Synodal Apostolic Exhortations of John Paul II, Our Sunday Visitor Publishing Division – Our Sunday Visitor Inc., Huntington, Indiana, 1998, 148-233.

——————————, «*Address on the Occasion of the Fiftieth Anniversary of the Pontifical Academy of Sciences*», 28 October 1986, in Papal Addresses *to the Pontifical Academy of Sciences 1917 – 2002 and to the Pontifical Academy of Social Sciences 1994 – 2002, The Pontifical Academy of Sciences, Vatican City 2003. 280-288.*

—————, *«Sollicitudo Rei Socialis, Encyclical Letter, (1987), for the twentieth anniversary of Populorum Progressio», in J. M. MILLER (ed.), The Encyclicals of John Paul II, Our Sunday Visitor Publishing Division – Our Sunday Visitor Inc., Huntington, Indiana 1996, 425-477.*

—————, *«Address to the Study Week on the Subject 'Science for Development in a Solidarity Framework' 27 October 1989», in Papal Addresses to the Pontifical Academy of Sciences 1917 – 2002 and to the Pontifical Academy of Social Sciences 1994 – 2002, The Pontifical Academy of Sciences, Vatican City 2003, 306-310*

—————, *«Address to the Study Week on the Subject 'Resources and Population' 22 November 1991», in Papal Addresses to the Pontifical Academy of Sciences 1917 – 2002 and to the Pontifical Academy of Social Sciences 1994 – 2002, The Pontifical Academy of Sciences, Vatican City 2003, 331-335.*

—————, *Veritatis splendor Encyclical Letter Regarding Certain Fundamental Questions of the Church's Moral Teaching (1993), in J. M. MILLER (ed.), The Encyclicals of John Paul II, Our Sunday Visitor Publishing Division – Our Sunday Visitor Inc., Huntington, Indiana 1996, 673-771.*

—————, *«Centesimus Annus, Encyclical Letter on The Hundredth Anniverssary of Rerum Novarum, (1991)», in J. M. MILLER (ed.), The Encyclicals of John Paul II, Our Sunday Visitor Publishing Division – Our Sunday Visitor Inc., Huntington, Indiana 1996, 587-650.*

—————, *«Address to the International Congress on Assistance to the Dying», March 17, 1992, in Medicina e Morale, 42(1992), 419-422.*

—————, *«Address to the Plenary Session on the Subject 'Human Genome; Alternative Energy Sources for Developing Countries; the Fundamental Principles of Mathematics; and Artificial Intelligence, 28 October 1994», in Papal Addresses to the Pontifical Academy of Sciences 1917 – 2002 and to the Pontifical Academy of Social Sciences 1994 – 2002, The Pontifical Academy of Sciences, Vatican City 2003, 358-363.*

—————, *«Address to the Working Group on the Subject 'Scientific Bases of the Natural Regulation of Fertility and Associated Problems' 18 November 1994», in Papal Addresses to the Pontifical Academy of Sciences 1917 – 2002 and to the Pontifical Academy of Social Sciences 1994 – 2002, The Pontifical Academy of Sciences, Vatican City 2003, 364-366.*

__________, «*Address to Plenary Session on the Subject 'The Study of the Tension Between Human Equality and Social Inequalities from the Perspective of the Various Social Sciences', 25 November 1994*», in *Papal Addresses to the Pontifical Academy of Sciences 1917 – 2002 and to the Pontifical Academy of Social Sciences 1994 – 2002*, 405-410

__________, «*Evangelium vitae, Encyclical Letter, (1995) On the Value of Human Life*, in *J. M. Miller (ed.), The Encyclicals of John Paul II*, Our Sunday Visitor Publishing Division – Our Sunday Visitor Inc., Huntington, Indiana 1996.

__________, *Message for the 1998 World Day of Peace, 2: AAS 90 (1998), 149.*

__________, *Message for the 1999 World day of Peace, 3: AAS 91(1999), 379.*

__________, «*Address to the Plenary Session on the Subject 'Democracy – Reality and Responsibility', 23 February 2000*», in *Papal Addresses to the Pontifical Academy of Sciences 1917 – 2002 and to the Pontifical Academy of Social Sciences 1994 – 2002*, 427-430.

__________, «*Address to the plenary Session on the Subject 'Intergenerational Solidarity', 11 April 2002*», in *Papal Addresses to the Pontifical Academy of Sciences 1917 – 2002 and to the Pontifical Academy of Social Sciences 1994 – 2002*, 435-437.

Benedict XVI, *Caritas in Veritate, Lettera Enciclica, Sullo Sviluppo Umano Integrale nella Carità e nella Verità*, Libreria Editrice Vaticana, Città del Vaticano 2009.

__________, «*Pope replies to Questions from Journalists*», *Vatican Information Service*, March 17, 2009.

Francis, «*Laudato Sì Lettera Enciclica Sulla Cura della Casa Comune*», Paoline Editoriale Libri, Milano 2015.

__________, «*Letter to the Catholic Bishops' Conference of Nigeria*», Vatican, 2 March 2015, in *https://www.cbcn-ng.org/docs/g19.pdf* [20-4-2018].

__________, *Unite to care*, «*Address to the International Conference on Regenerative Medicine, April 28, 2018*», in *The National Catholic Bioethics Quarterly*, 18(2018), The National Catholic Bioethics Center, Philadelphia, 503-505.

3. **Vatican Dicasteries**

Congregation for the Doctrine of the Faith, *Instruction Dignitas Personae, On certain Bioethical questions*, Veritas Publications, Dublin, Ireland 2009.

__________, «*Instruction Dignitas personae on Certain Bioethical Questions*», in E. J. FURTON – P. J. CATALDO – A. S. MORACZEWSKI (eds.) *Catholic Health Care Ethics. A Manual for Practitioners*, The National Catholic Bioethics Center, Philadelphia 2009².

PONTIFICAL COUNCIL FOR JUSTICE AND PEACE, *Compendium of the Social Doctrine of the Church*, Libreria Editrice Vaticano, Citta Del Vaticano 2010.

PONTIFICIO CONSIGLIO PER GLI OPERATORI SANITARI, *Nuova Carta degli Operatori Sanitari*, Libreria Editrice Vaticana, Città del Vaticano 2016.

PONTIFICAL COUNCIL FOR JUSTICE AND PEACE, *The Fight Against Corruption*, in *http://www.vatican.va/roman_curia/pontifical_councils/justpeace/documents/rc_pc_justpeace_doc_20060921_lotta-corruzione_en.html* [22-04-2018].

4. **Episcopal Conferences**

CATHOLIC BISHOPS CONFERENCE OF NIGERIA, «*Time to end death penalty*», Statement by the Catholic Bishops Conference of Nigeria (CBCN), 28 June 2013, in *https://www.cbcn-ng.org/docs/g14.pdf* [20-4-2018].

__________, «*Our Stand on Marriage, Family and Human Society*», Statement by the Catholic Bishops Conference of Nigeria (CBCN), in *https://www.cbcn-ng.org/docs/g20.pdf* [17-5-2018].

__________, «*Our Dignity, Our Nation and Our Citizenship*», Statement by the Catholic Bishops Conference of Nigeria (CBCN), in *https://www.cbcn-ng.org/docs/g26.pdf* [20-6-2018].

__________, «*Nigeria: Citizenship Rights and Duties*», A Communiqué at the End of the First Plenary Meeting of the Catholic Bishops' Conference of Nigeria (CBCN) at Daughters of Divine Love Retreat and Conference Centre (DRACC), Abuja, 4-10 March, 2107, in *https://www.cbcn-ng.org/docs/g26.pdf* [20-6-2018].

__________, *On the Recurrent Wave of Violence and the Cheapening of Human Lives in Different Parts of Our Country*, A Statement by the Catholic Bishops Conference of Nigeria (CBCN), 16 January, 2108 [14-4-2018].

CATHOLIC BISHOPS OF ENGLAND AND WALES, «*The Common Good and the Catholic Church's Teaching*», 1996, in *http://www.catholicsocialteaching.org.uk/wp-content/uploads/2010/10/THE-COMMON-GOOD-AND-THE-CATHOLIC-CHURCH_1996.pdf* [20-04-2018].

CONFERENZA EPISCOPALE ITALIANA, *Ufficio Nazionale per la pastorale della salute, XXVI Giornata Mondiale del Malato, 11 febbraio 2018*.

UNITED STATES CONFERENCE OF CATHOLIC BISHOPS, *Ethical and Religious Directives for Catholic Health Services (2009)[5] in* E. J. FURTON – P. J. CATALDO – A. S. MORACZEWSKI *(eds.) Catholic Health Care Ethics. A Manual for Practitioners, The National Catholic Bioethics Center, Philadelphia 2009[2]*.

———————————, *Ethical and Religious Directives for Catholic Health Services, USCCB, Washington, D.C., 2011[4], part 1, introduction*.

———————————, *Ethical and Religious Directives for Catholic Health Services, USCCB, Washington, D.C., 2018[6], part 1, Introduction*.

CATHOLIC BISHOPS' CONFERENCE OF THE PHILIPPINES, *Pastoral Letter on AIDS In the Compassion of Jesus, January 23, 1993*.

5. Ethics, Healthcare and Medicine in Nigeria (Nigerian authors)

ABDULMALIK, J. – KOLA, L. – FADAHUNSI, W. – ADEBAYO, K. – YASAMY, M. T. – MUSA, E. – GUREJE, O. *«Country Contextualization of the Mental Health Gap Action Programme Intervention Guide: A Case Study from Nigeria», PLoS Medicine, 10(2013), e1001501, in https://doi.org/10.1371/journal.pmed.1001501[23-11-2017]*.

ABDULRAHEEM, I. S. – OLAPIPO, A. R. – AMODU, M. O., *«Primary health care services in Nigeria: Critical issues and strategies for enhancing the use by the rural communities», Journal of Public Health Epidemiology, 4(2012) 5-13*.

ABDULRAHEEM, I. S. – PARAKOYI, D. B., *«Factors affecting mothers' healthcare-seeking behaviour for childhood illness in a rural Nigerian setting», Early Child Development Care, 179(2009), 671-683*.

ABIODUN, O. A. – SOTUNSA, J. – JAGUN, O. – FATUROTI, B. – ANI, F. – JOHN, I. – TAIWO, A. – TAIWO, O., *«Prevention of unintended pregnancies in Nigeria ; the effect of socio-demographic characteristics on the knowledge and use of emergency contraceptives among female university students», International Journal of Reproduction, Contraception, Obstetrics and Gynecology, 4(2015), 755-764, in https://doi.org/10.18203/2320-1770.ijrcog20150087 [17-8-2018]*.

ABIODUN, O. A. – O.-ABIODUN, O. O., *«The determinants of choice of health facility in Sagamu, South-west, Nigeria», Scholars Journal of Applied Medical Science, 2(2014), 274-282*.

ABUBAKAR, I. – ILIYASU, Z. – KABIR, M. – UZOHO, C. C. – ABDULKADIR, M.B., «Knowledge, attitude and practice of female genital cutting among antenatal patients in Amino Kano Teaching Hospital, Kano», Nigerian Journal of Medicine, 13(2004), 250-253.

ABOSEDE, O. A. – CAMPBELL, P. C. – OLUFUNLAYO, T. – SHOLEYE, O. O., «Establishing A Sustainable Ward Health System In Nigeria: Are Key Implementers Well Informed?» Journal of Community Medicine & Health Education, 2(2012), in https://doi.org/10.4172/2161-0711.1000164 [12-9-2016].

ADAM, V. Y. – AWUNOR, N. S., «Perceptions and factors affecting utilization of health services in rural community Southern Nigeria», Journal of Medicine and Biomedical Research, 13(2014), 117-124.

ADAMU, A. L. – ALIYU, M. H. – GALADANCI, N. A. – MUSA, B. M. – GADANYA, M. A. – GAJIDA, A. U. – AMOLE, T. G. – BELLO, I. W. – GAMBO, S. – ABUBAKAR, I., «Deaths during tuberculosis treatment among paediatric patients in a large tertiary hospital in Nigeria», PLoS One, 12(2017):e0183270, in https://doi.org/10.1371/journal.pone.0183270 [20-12-2017].

ADAMU, A. L. – GADANYA, M. A. – ABUBAKAR, I. S. – JIBO, A. M. – BELLO, M. M. – GAJIDA, A. U. – BABASHANI, M. M. – ABUBAKAR, I., «High mortality among tuberculosis patients on treatment in Nigeria: a retrospective cohort study», BMC Infectious Diseases, 17(2017), in https://doi.org/10.1186/s12879-017-2249-4 [12-9-2017].

ADEBAYO, A. M. – ASUZU, M. C., «Utilisation of a community-based health facility in a low-income urban community in Ibadan, Nigeria», African Journal of Primary Health Care & Family Medicine, 7(2015), 735, in https://doi.org/10.4102/phcfm.v7i1.735 [2-8-2018].

ADEFUYE, O. P. – S.-ODU, A. O. – OLATUNJI, A. O. – LAMINA, M. A. – OLADAPO, T. O., «Maternal deaths from induced abortion», Tropical Journal of Obstetrics Gynaecology, 20(2003), 101-104.

ADEDINI, S. A. – ODIMEGWU, C. – IMASIKU, E. N. – ONONOKPONO, D. N. – IBISOMI, L., «Regional Variations in Infant and Child Mortality in Nigeria: A Multilevel Analysis», Journal of Biosocial Science, 47(2015), 165-187, in https://doi.org/10.1017/s0021932013000734 [7-8-2017].

ADEDOKUN, S. T. – ADEKANMBI, V.T. – UTHAM, O. A. – LILFORD, R. J., «Contextual factors associated with health care service utilization for children with acute childhood illness in Nigeria», PLoS ONE, 12(2017), e0173578, in https://doi.org/10.1371/journal.pone.0173578 [3-8-2018].

ADEKANMBI, V. T. – ADEDOKUN, S. T. – T.-PHILLIPS, S. – UTHMAN, O. A. – CLARKE, A., «Predictors of differences in health services utilization for children in Nigeria communities», Preventive Medicine, 96(2017), 67-72, in http:// dx.doi.org/10.1016/j.ypmed.2016.12.035 [7-8-2018].

ADEKUN, L. A. – ODUWOLE, M. – ORONSANYA, F. – GBOGBAODE, A. O. – ALIYU, N. – ADEKUNLE, W. – SADIQ, G. – SUTTON, I. – TAIWO, M., «Trends in female circumcision between 1933 and 2003 in Osun and Ogun State, Nigeria: a cohort analysis», African Journal of Reproductive Health, 10(2006), 48-56.

ADELOYE, D. – DAVID, R. A. – OLAOGUN, A. A. – AUTA, A. – ADESOKAN, A. – GADANYA, M. – OPELE, J. K. – OWAGBEMI, O. – ISEOLORUNKANMI, A., «Health workforce and governance: the crisis in Nigeria, Human Resources for Health», 15(2017), 32. https://doi.org/10.1186/s12960-017-0205-4 [30-7-2018].

ADEPOJU, E. G. – ONAJOLE, A. T. – OREAGBA, L. O. – ODEYEMI, K. A. – OGUNNOWO, B. O. – OLAYEMI, S. O., «Health education and caregivers' management of malaria among under five in Ede North L. G. A, Osun State of Nigeria», The Nigerian Medical Practitioner, 48(2005), 72-81.

ADEREMI, R. A., «Ethical Issues in Maternal and Child Health Nursing: Challenges Faced By Maternal and Child Health Nurses and Strategies for Decision Making», International Journal of Medicine and Biomedical Research, 5(2016), 67-76.

ADETOKUNBO, T. – OLUWAROTIMI, A. – ABIOLA, B. – ADENIYI, A. – DELE, O. – SHITU, L., «Contraceptive knowledge and usage amongst female secondary school students in Lagos, South West Nigeria», Journal of Public Health Epidemiology, 3(2011), 34-37.

ADETORO, O. O. – AGAH, A., «The implications of childbearing in postpubertal girls in Sokoto, Nigeria», International of Gynaecology and Obstetrics, 27(1988), 73-77.

ADEWALE, I. F., «Trends in postabortal mortality and morbidity in Ibadan, Nigeria», International Journal of Gynaecology & Obstetrics, 38(1992), 115-118.

ADEYEMI, A. S. – ADEKUNLE, D. A. – KOMOLAFE, J. O., «Pattern of contraceptive choice among the married women attending the family planning clinic of a tertiary health institution», Nigerian Journal of Medicine, 17(2008), 67-68.

ADIKA, V. O. – BALARABE, S. – AGADA, J. J. – NNEOMA, N., «Mothers Perceived Cause and Health Seeking Behaviour of Childhood Measles in Bayelsa, Nigeria», Journal of Research in Nursing and Midwifery, 2(2013), 6-12.

ADINMA, E., «Unsafe Abortion and its Ethical, Sexual and Reproductive Rights Implications», West African Journal of Medicine, 30(2011), 245-249.

ADINMA, J. I. B., «Ethics in Perinatal Medicine», Nigerian Journal of Paediatrics, 43(2016), 221, in https://doi.org/10.4314/njp.v43i3.12 [16-8-2018].

——————, «Adolescent sexuality, contraception and reproductive rights», MediZik Journal, 1(1999), 13-24.

——————, «An overview of the global policy consensus on Women Sexual and Reproductive Rights: The Nigerian Perspective», Tropical Journal of Obstetrics and Gynaecology, 19(2002), 10-12.

——————, «Bioethics in Obstetrics», in https://doi.org/10.5772/28758 [22-8-2018].

ADINMA, J. I. B. – AGBAI, A. O., «Practice and perceptions of female genital mutilation among Nigerian Igbo women, Journal of Gynaecology & Obstetrics», 19(1999), 44-48.

ADINMA, J. I. B. – ADINMA, E., «Impact of reproductive health on socio-economic development: a case study of Nigeria», African Journal of Reproductive Health, 15(2011), 7-12.

——————, «Ethical considerations in women's sexual and reproductive health care», Nigerian Journal of Clinical Practice, 12(2009), 92-98.

——————, «The Sexual and Reproductive Rights of Women in Nigeria», Ebonyi Medical Journal, 2(2003), 35-38.

ADISA, R. – FAKEYE, T., «Assessment of the knowledge of community pharmacists regarding common phytopharmaceuticals sold in southwestern Nigeria», Tropical Journal of Pharmaceutical Research, 5(2006), 619-625.

ADIUKWU, M. U., «Sales practices of patent medicine sellers in Nigeria», Health Policy Planning, 11(1996), 202-205.

ADIKWU, M. U. – OKOYE, K. C., «Patient factors militating against the laws governing prescriptions-only medicines in Nigeria», Nigerian Journal of Pharmacy, 23(1992), 7-11.

AFOLABI, A. O., «Factors influencing the pattern of self-medication in an adult Nigerian population», Annals of African Medicine, 7(2008), 120-127.

AHMAD, K., «Drug company sued over research trial in Nigeria», Lancet, 358(2001), 815, in https://doi.org/10/1016/S0140-6736(01)06011-1 [14-0-2018].

AIGBIREMOLEM, A. O. – ALENOGHENA, I. – EBOREIME, E. – ABEJEGAH, C., «Primary Health Care in Nigeria: From Conceptualization to Implementation», Journal of Medical and Applied Biosciences, 6(2014), 35-43.

AJAYI, A. I. – ADENIYI, O. V. – AKPAN, W., «Maternal health care visits as predictors of contraceptive use among childbearing women in a medically underserved state in Nigeria», *Journal of Health, Population and Nutrition*, 37(2018), 19, in *https://doi.org/10.1186/s41043-018-0150-4* [17-8-2018].

AJUWON, A. – OLALEYA, A. – FAROMOJU, B. – LADIPO, O., «Sexual behaviour and experience of sexual coercion among secondary schools students in three states in North Eastern Nigeria», *BMC Public Health*, 6(2005), 310.

AJUWON, A. J. – OLLEY, B. O. – A.-JIMOH, I. – AKINTOLA, O., «Experience of sexual coercion among adolescents in Ibadan, Nigeria», *African J Reproductive Health*, 5(2001), 120-131.

AJUWON, A. J. – McFARLAND, W. – HUDES, S. – ADEDAPO, S. – OKIKIOLU, T. – LURIE, P., «Risk-related behaviour, sexual coercion and implication for prevention strategies among female apprentices tailors in Ibadan, Nigeria», *AIDS & Behaviour*, 6(2002), 233-241.

AKANBI, M. O. – UKOLI, C. O. – ERHABOR, G. E. – AKAMBI, F. O. – GORDON, S. B., «The burden of respiratory disease in Nigeria», *African Journal of Respiratory Medicine*, 8(2013), 10-17.

AKANDE, O. E., «Reducing morbidity from unsafe abortion in Nigeria», *Archives of Ibadan Medicine*, 2(2001), 11-13.

AKANDE, T. M., «Referral system in Nigeria: study of a tertiary health facility», *Annals of African Medicine*, 3(2004), 130-133.

AKESODE, F. A., «Factors affecting the use of primary health care clinics for children», *Journal of Epidemiology and Community Health*, 36(1982), 310-314.

AKOGUN, O. B. – JOHN, K. K., «Illness-related Practices for the Management of Childhood Malaria among Bwatiye People of North-eastern Nigeria», *Malaria Journal* 4(2015), 4-13, in *https://doi.org/10.1186/1475-2875-4-13* [3-09-2018].

AKINLOYE, O. – TRUTER, E. J., «A review of management of infertility in Nigeria: framing the ethics of a national health policy», *International Journal of Women's Health*, 3(2011), 265-275, in *http://dx.doi.org/10.2147/IJWH.S20501* [22-8-2018].

AKINTOLA, S. O. – EGBOKHARE, O. O., «Parenthood: Is the law in Nigeria fit for assisted reproductive technology?», *Indian Journal of Medical Ethics*, 3(2018), ISSN:0975-5691, in *https://doi.org/10.20529/IJME.2018.012* [24-8-2018].

AKINTOLA, S. O. –F. OKONFUA, O. O., *Female and Male Infertility in Nigeria*, Karolinska University, Press, 2005.

AKINLOYE., O., – TRUTER, E. J., «A review of management of infertility in Nigeria: framing the ethics of a national health policy», *International Journal of*

Women's Health, 3(2011), 265-275, in <u>http://dx.doi.org/10.2147/IJWH.S20501</u> [22-8-2018].

AKINGBADE, O., «Perspectives on Community Tuberculosis Care in Nigeria», *International Journal of Tropical Disease & Health*, 16(2016), 1-13, in <u>https://doi.org/10.9734/ijtdh/2016/23447</u> [10-3-2017].

AKINYEMI, F. – BIGIRIMANA, F.,«A Spatial Analysis of Poverty in Kigali, Rwanda using indicators of household living standard», *Rwanda Journal*, 26(2012), in <u>https://doi.org/10.4314/rj.v26i1.1</u> [16-10-2017].

AKPANEKPO, E. I. – UMOESSIEN, E. D. – FRANK, E. I., «Unsafe Abortion and Maternal Mortality in Nigeria: A Review», *Pan-African Journal of Medicine*, 1(2017)1-6.

AKPATA, E. S., «Oral health in Nigeria», *International Dental Journal*, 54 (2004), 361-366, in <u>https://doi.org/10.1111/j.1875-595x.2004.tb00012.x</u> [15-9-2017].

AKPOMUVIE, O. B., Poverty, «Access to Health Care Services and Human Capital Development in Nigeria», *African Research Review*, 4(2010), in <u>https://doi.org/10.4314/afrrev.v4i3.60149</u> [16-8-2018].

ALENOGHENA, I. O. – ISAH, E. C. – ISARA, A. R. – AMEH, S. S. – ADAM, V. Y., «Uptake of Family Planning Services Among Women of Reproductive Age in Edo North Senatorial District, Edo State», Nigeria, *Sub-Sahara African Journal of Medicine*, 2(2015),154, in <u>https://doi.org/10.4103/2384-5147.172433</u> [17-8-2018].

ALI, A. D., «Leadership and Socio-Economic Challenges in Nigeria, Singaporean Journal of Business Economics and Management Studies», 1(2013), 1-8, in <u>https://doi.org/10.12816/0003789</u> [20-10-2017].

ALUBO, O., «The Promise and limits of private medicine: health policy dilemmas in Nigeria», *Health Policy Plan*, 16(2001), 667-676.

———, «Adolescent reproductive health practices in Nigeria», *African Journal of Reproductive Health*, 5(2001), 109-119.

AMAGHIONYEODIME, A. L., «Determinants of the choice of health care providers in Nigeria», *Health Care Management Science*, 11(2008), 215-217.

AMAGHIONYEODIWE, L. A., «Government health care spending and the poor: evidence from Nigeria», *International Journal of Social Economics*, 36(2009), 220-236, in <u>https://doi.org/10.1108/03068290910932729</u> [12-8-2017].

AMORAN, O. E., «Impact of health education intervention on malaria prevention practices among nursing mothers in rural communities in Nigeria», *Nigerian Medical Journal*, 54(2013), 115-122, in <u>https://doi/10.4103/0300-1652.110046</u> [29-7-2018].

ANAND, P.,«Capabilities and health», *Journal of Medical Ethics*, 31(2005), 299-303. https://doi.org/10.1136/jme.2004.008706 [10-2-2018].

ANTAI, D. «Rural-urban inequities in childhood immunisation in Nigeria: The role of community contexts», *African Journal of Primary Health Care & Family Medicine*, 3(2011), 238, in https://doi.org/10.4102/phcfm.v3i1.238 [23-8-2017].

ANOCHIE, I. C. – KEPEME, E. E., «Prevalence of sexual activity and outcome among female students in Port Harcourt, Nigeria», *African Journal of Reproductive Health*, 5(2001), 63-67.

ARAOYE, M. O. – FAKEYE, O. O., «Sexuality and contraception among Nigerian adolescents and youths», *African Journal of Reproductive Health*, 2(1998), 142-150.

ARCHIBONG, E., «Illegal induced abortion – a continuing problem in Nigeria», *International Journal of Gynaecology and Obstetrics*, 34(1991), 261-262.

A.-RAHMAN, L. O. – MUSA, O. I. – OSHAGBEMI, G. K., «Community-based study of circumcision practices in Nigeria», *Annals of Tropical Medicine and Public Health*, 5(2012), 231-235.

AREGBESHOLA, B. S., (2016). «Institutional corruption, health-sector reforms, and health status in Nigeria», *THE LANCET*, 388(2016), 757, in https://doi.org/10.1016/s0140-6736(16)31365-4 [22-11-2017].

AREGBESHOLA, B. S. – KHAN, S. M., «Factors affecting the uptake of malaria prevention strategies among pregnant women in Nigeria: evidence from 2013 Nigeria demographic and health survey», in https://doi.org/10.1007/s10389-017-0877-1 [22-11-2017].

__________, «Primary Health Care in Nigeria: 24 Years after Olikoye Ransome-Kuti's Leadership», *Frontier Public Health*, 5 (2017), 48, in https://doi.org/10.3389/fpubh.2017.00048 [22-11-2017].

AREMU, L. O. GATs and Nigeria's National Health Policy: The Issue for Negotiation, *LAP LAMBERT Academic Publishing*, Saarbrucken, Germany 2017.

ASKEW, I. D., «Planning and Implementing Community Participation in Health Programmes», in R. AKHTAR (ed.) *Health Care Patterns and Planning in Developing Countries*, Greenwood Press, New York 1991, 3-19.

ASUQUO, E. – ORAZULIKE, N. – ONYEKWERE, E. – EKENOBI, A. – ORAGE, J., «Unintended Pregnancy among Married Antenatal Clinic Attendees in a Tertiary Institution in Nigeria», *British Journal of Medical Research*, 19(2017), 1-11.

ASUZU, M. C. «The necessity for a health system's reform in Nigeria», *Journal of Community Medicine & Primary Health Care*, 16(2004), 1-3.

AUTA, A., «Demographic Factors Associated with Insecticide Treated Net among Nigerian Women and Children», North American Journal of Medical Sciences, 4(2012), 40-49, in https://doi.org/10.4103/1947-2714.92903 [10-9-2016].

AVIDIME, S. – A.-AKAI, L. – MOHAMMED, A. Z. – EJEMBI, C. – ADAJI, S. – SHITTU, O., «Fertility Intentions, Contraceptive Awareness and Contraceptive Use among Women in Three Communities in Northern Nigeria», African Journal of Reproductive Health, 14(2010), 65-70.

AWODELE, O. – ADEWOYE, A. A. – OPARAH, A. C., «Assessment of medical waste management in seven hospitals in Lagos, Nigeria», BMC Public Health, 16(2016), 269, in https://doi.org/10.1186/s12889-016-2916-1 [30-7-2018].

AWOLEYE, O. J. – THRON, C., «Improving access to malaria rapid diagnostic test in Niger State, Nigeria: an assessment of implementation up to 2013», Malaria Research and Treatment, 2(2016), 1-13, in https://doi/10.1155/2016/7436265 [12-7-2018].

AWOSIKA, L. «Health insurance and managed care in Nigeria», Annals of Ibadan Postgraduate Medicine, 3(2007), 40-51.

AWOSUSI, A. – FOLARANMI, T. – YATES, R., «Nigeria's new government and public financing for universal health coverage», The Lancet Global Health, 3(2015), e514-e515, in http://dx.doi.org/10.1016/S2214-109X(15)00088-1 [23-11-2017].

AYANLEYE, O. A., «Women and Reproductive Health Rights in Nigeria», International Journal of Sustainable Development, 6(2013), 127-140.

ANYIKA, E. N., «Challenges of implementing sustainable health care delivery in Nigeria under environmental uncertainty», Journal of Hospital Administration, 3(2014), 113-126.

—————, «Regulatory uncertainties in the pharmaceutical sector: perceptions among Nigerian pharmacists and policy implications for decision making», Journal of Hospital Administration, 5(2016), 48-55, in https://doi/10.5430/jha.v5n3p48 [28-7-2018].

BAKARE, A. S. – OLUBOKUN, S., «Health care expenditure and economic growth in Nigeria: An empirical study», Journal of Emerging Trends in Economic Management Science, 2(2011), 83-87.

BRAVEMAN, P., – GRUSKIN, S., «Poverty, equity, human rights and health», Bulletin of the World Health Organization, 81(2003), 539-545.

BANKOLE, A. – ADEWOLE, I. F. – HUSSAIN, R. – AWOLUDE, O. – SINGH, S. – AKINYEMI, J. O., «The Incidence of Abortion in Nigeria», International Perspectives on Sexual and Reproductive Health, 4(2105), 170-181.

BBAALE, E., «*Immunization status and child survival in Uganda*», African Journal of Economic Review, 3(2015), 1-20, in https://doi.org/10.3329/jhpn.v31i1.14756 [20-3-2017].

BINGEL, D. D., «*An ethical examination of the challenges of in-vitro fertilisation in Nigeria*», International Letters of Social Sciences, 14(2013), 20-25.

BRIEGER, W. R. – OSAMOR, P. E. – SALAMI, K. S. – OLADEPO, O. – OTUSANYA, S. A., «*Observations of patent medicine vendor and customer interaction in urban and rural areas of Oyo State*», Nigeria, Health Policy Planning, 2004, 19(2004), 177-182.

BRIEGER, W. R. – RAMAKRISHNA, J. – ADENIYI, J. D., «*Self-treatment in rural Nigeria, a community health education diagnosis*», Hygiene International Journal of Health Education, 5(1986), 41-46.

BRIEGER, W. R. – SALAKO, L. A. – UMEH, R. E. – AGOMO, P. U. – AFOLABI, B. M. – ADENEYE, A. K., «*Promoting pre-packaged drugs for prompt and appriopriate treatment of febrile illness in rural Nigerian Communities*», International Quarterly of Community Health Education, 21(2002), 19-40.

CHIDERA, E., «*What Factors Influence the Persistence of Female Genital Mutilation in Nigeria? A Systematic Review*», Journal of Tropical Diseases & Public Health, 6(2018), 256, in https://doi.org/10.4172/2473-3350.1000256 [5-4-2018].

CHIMA, U. C. – LAWOYIN, T. O. – LLIKA, A. L. – NNEBUE, C. C., «*Contraceptive knowledge and practice among secondary school students in military barracks in Nigeria*», Nigerian Journal of Clinical Practice, 19(2016), 182-188.

CHIGBU, C. – ONYEBUCHI, A. K. – ONWUDIWE, E. N. – IWUJI, S. E., «*Denial of women's rights to contraception in south-eastern Nigeria*», International Journal of gynaecology and obstetrics, 121(2013), 154-156.

CHUBIKE, N. E., «*Evaluation of National Insurance Scheme [NHIS] awareness by civil servants in Enugu and Abakiliki*», International Journal of Medicine and Medical Sciences, 5(2013), 356-358.

CHUKUDEBELU, W. O. – OZUMBA, B. C., «*Maternal mortality in Anambra State of Nigeria*», International Journal of Gynaecology and Obstetrics, 27(1988), 365-370.

CHUKWUDI, U. M. – OKPANMA, A. C. – NWAKWUO, G. C. – DOZIE, I. N., «*Determinants of delay in seeking malaria treatment for children under-five years in parts of South Eastern Nigeria*», Journal of Community Health, 39(2014), 1171-1178.

CHUKWUOCHA, U. M., «Malaria Control in Nigeria», Journal of Primary Healthcare: Open Access, 2(2012), in https://doi.org/10.4172/2167-1079.1000118 [5-7-2016].

DAODU, O. – CROCKETT, M. – FALADE, A. G., «Supportive Care in the Management of Severe Pneumonia in Nigerian Children using Oxygen Concentrators», JSM Allergy Asthma, 2(2017), 1008.

DEPOJU, A. – OGUNJUYIGBE, O. – ADEPOJU, A., Adolescent Sexual and Reproductive Health in Nigeria, Behavioural Patterns and Needs, iUniverse, United States of America 2006.

DOCTOR, H. V. – BAIRAGI, R. – FINDLEY, S. E. – HELLERINGER, S. – DAHIRU, T., «Northern Nigeria Maternal, Newborn and Child Health Programme: Selected Analyses from Population-Based Baseline Survey», The Open Demography Journal, 4(2011), 11-21.

DURU, C. B. – EMELUMADU, O. F. – IWU, A. C. – OHALE, I. – AGUNWA, C. C. – NWAIGBO, E. – NDUKWU, E. N., «Prevalence, Pattern and Determinants of Contraceptive Use among Women of Reproductive Age (15-49) In Rural Communities in Imo State, Nigeria», International Journal of Science and Healthcare Research, 3(2018), ISSN: 2455-7587.

EBOH, D., Strategic Concept for Managing Healthcare in Nigeria. Africa's Health and Social Care Management, TamaRe House Publishers Ltd, UK 2008.

EBOMOYI, E., «Prevalence of female circumcision in two Nigerian communities», Sex Role, 17(1987), 139-151.

EDEME, R. K., «Public health Expenditure and Health Outcome in Nigeria», African Journal of Biomedical and Life Sciences, 5(2017), 96-102, in https://doi.org/10.11648/j.ajbls.20170505.13 [21-8-2018].

EFE, S. I., «Health care problem and management in Nigeria», Journal of Geography and Regional Planning, 6(2013), 244-254, in https://doi.org/10.5897/jgrp2013.0366 [10-10-2016].

EFFAH, J., «Culture and Reproductive Rights», Constitutional Rights Journal, 1995, 27.

EFODUH, O., «The Economic Development of Nigeria from 1914 to 2014», Academia. edu, citing C. N. NWACHUKWU, «The History of Agriculture in Nigeria from the Colonial Era to the Present Day: Pointing all agricultural programmes», in http://www.onlinenigeria.com/articles/ad.asp?blurb=268, [20-1-2017].

EHIGIEBA, A. E. – IGHEDOSA, S. U. – EMORE, O. F. – ONAFOWOKAN, O., «The Management Challenges of the Complications of Illegally Induced Abortions in Benin-City, Nigeria», African Journals Online (AJOL), 7(2004), 95-97. http://dx.doi.org/10.4314/smj2.v7i3.12878 [12-7-2018].

EHIRI, J. E. – OYO-ITA, A. E. – E. C. ANYANWU, E. C. – M. M. MEREMIKWU, M. M. – IKPEME, M. B., «Quality of Child health services in primary health care facilities in south-east Nigeria», Child: Care, Health and Development, 31(2005),181-191, in https://doi.org/10.1111/j.1365-2214.2004.00493.x [27-11-2017].

EJEMBI, C. L. – ALTI-MAZU, M. – CHIRDAN, O. – EZEH, H. O. – SHEIDU, S. – DAHIRU, T., «Utilization of maternal health services by rural Hausa women in Zaria environs, northern Nigeria: has primary health care made a difference?», Journal of Community Medicine & Primary Health Care, 16(2004), 47-54, in https://doi.org/10.4314/jcmphc.v16i2.32414 [27-7-2016].

EKE, C. B. – IBEKWE, R. C. – MUONEKE, V. C. – CHINAWA, J. M. – IBEKWE, M. U – UKOHA, O. M. – IBE, B. C., «End users' perception of quality of care of children attending children's outpatients clinic of University of Nigeria Teaching Hospital Ituku-Ozalla Enugu», BMC Research Notes, 7(2014), 800-805.

EKO, E. J.,«Implication of Economic Recession on the Health Care Delivery System in Nigeria», Social Sciences 6(2017), 14-18, in https://doi.org/10.11648/j.ss.20170601.13 [17/1-2018].

EKWEMPU, C. C., «The influence of antenatal care on pregnancy outcome», Tropical Journal Obstetrics Gynaecology, 1(1988), 67-71.

EME, I. O. – UCHE, O. A. – UCHE, I. B., «Building a Solid Health Care System in Nigeria: Challenges and Prospects», Academic Journal of Interdisciplinary Studies, 3(2014), 501-510, in https://doi.org/10.5901/ajis.2014.v3n6p501 [1-8-2016].

EMELUMADU, O. F. – ONYEONORO, U. U. – UKAEGBU, A. U. – EZEANYA, N. N. –IFEADIKE, C. O. – OKEZIE, O. K., «Perception of quality of maternal healthcare services among women utilizing antenatal services in selected primary health facilities in Anambra State», Southeast Nigeria, Nigerian Medical Journal, 55(2014), 148-155.

EMMANUEL, A. – ACHEMA, G. – OMALE, O., «Contraceptive choices of married market women in a north central state of Nigeria», International Journal of Nursing and Health Science, 1(2014), 41-45.

EMMANUEL, N. K. – GLADYS, E. N. – COSMAS, U. U., «Consumer knowledge and availability of maternal and child health services: a challenge for achieving MDG 4 and 5 in southeast Nigeria», BMC Health Services Research, 13(2013). http://www.biomedcentral.com/1472-6963/13/53 [7-8-2018].

ENABUELE, O. – ENABUELE, J. E., «Nigeria's National Health Act: An assessment of health professionals' knowledge and perception», Nigerian Medical Journal, 57(2016), 260-265, in https://doi.org/10.4103/0300-1652.190594 [15-9-2016].

ENEJI, A., «Health care Expenditure, Health Status and National Productivity in Nigeria (1999-2012)», Journal of Economics and International Finance, 5(2013), 258-272, in https://doi.org/10.5897/JEIF2013.0523 [21-0-2018].

ENVULADU, E. A. – AGBO, H. A. – MOHAMMED, A. – CHIA, L. – KIGBU, J. H – ZOAKAH, A. I., «Utilization of modern contraceptives among female traders in Jos South LGA of Plateau state, Nigeria», International Journal of Medicine and Biomedical Research, 1(2012), 224-231, in https://doi.org/10.14194/ijmbr.1310 [17-8-2018].

ERAH, P. O., «The changing roles of pharmacy in hospital and community pharmacy practice in Nigeria», Tropical Journal of pharmaceutical Research, 2(2003), 195-196.

ERAH, P. – OJIEABU, W., «Success of the control of tuberculosis in Nigeria: a review», International Journal of Health Research, 2(2009). http://dx.doi.org/10.4314/ijhr.v2i1.55382 [17-2-2016].

EZEH, O. K. – AGHO, K. E. – DIBLEY, M. J. – HALL, J. – PAGE, A. N., «The Impact of Water and Sanitation on Childhood Mortality in Nigeria: Evidence from Demographic and Health Surveys, 2003-2013», International Journal of Environmental Research and Public Health, 11(2014), 56-72, in https://doi.org/10.3390/ijerph110909256 [8-6-2016].

EZEANI, C. O., «Evolving a human rights based code of ethics for medical practitioners caring for women in Nigeria», Tropical Journal and Obstetrics and Gynaecology, 19(2002), 26-28.

EZECHI, O. C. – FASUBAA, O. B. – DARE, F. O., «Abortion related deaths in South Western Nigeria», Nigerian Journal of Medicine, 8(1999), 112-114.

__________,«Contraceptive promotion and utilization, Solution to problem of illegally induced abortion in countries with restrictive law», Nigerian Quarterly Journal of Hospital Medicine, 9(1999), 167-168.

EZENYEAKU, C. – EZEBIALU, I. U. – UMEOBIKA, J. C. – EZENYEAKU, C. A., «Desire to practice postpartum contraception among antenatal women at Awka, Southeast Nigeria», International Journal of Reproduction, Contraception, Obstetrics & Gynecology, 7(2018), 1682, in https://doi.org/10.18203/2320-1770.ijrcog20181895 [16-8-2018].

EZUGWU, E. C. – NKWO, P. – AGU, U. – ASOGWA, A. O., «Contraceptive use among HIV-positive women in Enugu, southeast Nigeria», International Journal of Gynaecology and Obstetrics, 126(2014), in http://dx.doi.org/10.1016/j.ijgo.2013.12.014 [15-8-2108].

FAPOHUNDA, B. M. – OROBATON, N. G., «When Women Delivery with No One Present in Nigeria: Who, What, Where and So What?», PLoS ONE, 8(2013), e69569, in https://doi.org/10.1371/journal.pone.0069569 [30-8-2018].

FASUBAA, O. B. – AKINDELE, S. T. – ADELEKAN, A. – OKWUOKENYE, H., «A politico-medical perspective of induced abortion in a semi-urban community of Ile-Ife, Nigeria», Journal of Obstetrics and Gynaecology, 22(2002), 51-57.

FASUBAA, O. B. – OLUGBENGA, O. D., «Impact of post-abortion counselling in semi-urban town of Western Nigeria», Journal of Obstetrics and Gynaecology, 24(2004), 300-305.

FASUBAA, O. B. – AKINDELE, S. T. – EZECHI, O. C., «Illegal induces abortion in Nigeria, An examination of its consequences and policy implications for social welfare and health policy makers», Journal of Human Ecology, 14(2003), 433-443.

FATUNGASE, K. O. – AMORAN, O. E. – ALAUSA, K. O., «The effect of health education intervention on the home management of malaria among the caregivers of children aged under 5 years in Ogun State, Nigeria», European Journal of Medical Research, 17(2012), 11, in https://doi/10.1186/2047/783x-17-11 [27-7-2018].

FAWOLE, O. I. – AJUWON, A. J. – OSUNGBADE, K. O. – FAWEYA, O. C., «Prevalence of violence against young female hawkers in three cities in south-western Nigeria», Health Education, 102(2002), 230-238.

FAWOLE, A. A. – ABOYEJI, A. P. – AKANDE T. M., «A Review of the Complications from Unsafe Abortions in Illorin, Nigeria», Tropical Journal of Health Sciences, 13(2006), 1-4, in http://dx.doi/10.4314/tjhc.v13i1.36699 [13-7-2018].

FOLAYAN, M. O. – HAIRE, B. – HARRISON, A. – ODETOYINGBO, M. – FATUSI, O. – BROWN, B., «Ethical Issues in Adolescents Sexual and Reproductive Health Research in Nigeria», Developing world bioethics, 15(2015), 191-198.

GALADANCI, H. S. – EJEMBI, C. L. – ILIYASU, Z. – ALAGH, B. – UMAR, U. S., «Maternal health in Northern Nigeria – a far cry from ideal», British Journal of Obstetrics and Gynaecology, 114(2007), 448-452. http://dx.doi.org/10.1111/j.1471-0528.2007.01229.x [16-11-2016].

HENSHAW, S. K. – SINGH, S. – O-.ADENIRAN, B. A. – ADEWOLE, I. F. – IWERE, N., «The incidence of induced abortion in Nigeria», International Family Planning Perspectives, 24(1998), 156-164.

HIROSE, A. – YISA, I. O. – AMINU, A. – AFOLABI, N. – OLASUNMBO, M. – OLUKA, G. – MUHAMMAD, K. –HUSSEIN, J., «Technical quality of delivery care in private- and public-sector health facilities in Enugu and Lagos States, Nigeria», Health Policy and Planning, 33(2018), 666-674.

IBADIN, S. H. – ADAM, V. Y. – ADELEYE, O. – OKOJIE, O. H.,«Birth preparedness and complication readiness among pregnant women in a rural community in southern Nigeria», South African Journal of Obstetrics and Gynaecology, 22(2016), 47, in https://doi.org/10.7196/sajog.2016.v22i2.1088 [12-10-2016].

IBAMA, S. A. – DENNIS, P., «Role of Community Health Practitioners in National Development: The Nigeria Situation», International Journal of Clinical Medicine, 7(2016), 511-518, in https://doi.org/10.4236/ijcm.2016.77056 [13-5-2017].

IBRAHIM, M. I. – OKORO, R. U., «Profile of contraceptive acceptors in UDUTH, Sokoto, Nigeria», Nigerian Medical Practitioner, 13(1997), 9-13.

IBRAHIM, I. A., «Socio-demographic Determinants of Complicated Unsafe Abortions in Semi-urban Nigerian Town: A Four-year Review», West Indian Medical Journal, 61(2012), 163.

IDONIJE, B. O. – OLUBA, O. M. – OTAMERE, H. O., «A study on knowledge, attitude and practice of contraception among secondary school students in Ekpoma, Nigeria», Journal of Physics Conference Series, 2(2011), 22-27.

IDOWU, A. – AREMU, O. A. – FUNMITO, F. – POPOOLA, G., «Knowledge, attitude and practice of contraception by female junior secondary school students in an urban community of Oyo-state, South west, Nigeria», International Journal of Reproduction, Contraception, Obstetrics and Gynaecology, 6(2017), 4759, in https://doi.org/10.18203/2320-1770.ijrcog20174983 [16-8-2018].

IDOWU, A., «Birth Preparedness and Complication Readiness among Women Attending Antenatal Clinics in Ogbomoso, South West, Nigeria», International Journal of MCH and AIDS, 4(2015), 47-56, in https://doi.org/10.21106/ijma.55 [15-10-2016].

IFEANYICHUKWU, O. – OBEHI, O. – RICHARD, K., «Birth Preparedness and Complication Readiness: Attitude and Level of Preparedness among Pregnant Women in Benin City, Edo State, Nigeria», British Journal of

Medicine and Research, 15(2016), 1-14, in https://doi.org/10.9734/bjmmr/2016/25127 [16-10-2016].

IGE, O. – FASHINA, A. – ASUZU, M., «Evaluation of the tuberculosis control programme in a southwestern State, Nigeria», Journal of Community Medicine & Primary Health Care, 22(1-2), in https://doi.org/10.4314/jcmphc.v22i1-2.68333 [20-10-2016].

IKEANYI, M. E. – OKONKWO, C. A., «Complicated illegal induced abortions at a tertiary health institution in Nigeria», Pakistan Journal Medical Sciences, 30(2014), 1398-1402.

IKECHEBULU, J. I., «Assisted reproductive techniques (ART), the state of art in Nigeria», Journal of College of Medical Sciences, 8(2003), 1-6.

ILOH, G. U. P. – OFOEDU, J. N. – ODU, F. U. – IFEDIGBO, C. V. – IWUAMANAM, K. D., «Evaluation of patients' satisfactions with quality of care provided at the National Health Insurance Scheme clinic of a tertiary hospital in South-Eastern Nigeria», Nigeria Journal of clinical practice, 15(2013), 469-474.

INNOCENT, E. O. – UCHE, O. A. – UCHE, I. B., «Building a solid health care system in Nigeria: challenges and prospects», Academic Journal of Interdisciplinary Studies, 3(2014), 501.

ISAH, H., «Prescription pattern among primary care providers in Catholic-owned primary health care facilities in Northern Ecclesiastical provinces of Abuja, Jos, and Kaduna, Nigeria: Preliminary findings», in https://doi.org/10.4314/jophas.v5i2.48470 [12-07-2018].

ISTIFANUS, A. J., «A Comparative Analysis of Health Indicators of Nigeria and Rwanda: A Nigerian Volunteers' Perspective», American Journal of Public Health Research, 1(2013), 177-182, in https://doi.org/10.12691/ajphr-1-7-6 [13-12-2016].

IWEZE, E. A., The patent medicine store: hospital for the urban poor, in P. K. MAKINWA – O. A. OZO (eds.), The Urban Poor in Nigeria, Ibadan, Nigeria 1987, 317-322.

IYANIWURA, C., «Adults perspective of adolescent reproductive health behaviour in a sub-urban town in Nigeria», Nigerian Journal of Medicine, 15(2006), 255-259, in https://doi.org/10.4314/njm.v15i3.37224 [20-6-2016].

IYIOHA, I. O., «Pathologies, Transplants and Indigenous Norms: An Introduction to Nigerian Health Law and Policy», in I. O. IYIOHA I. O. IYIOHA – R. NWABUEZE (eds.), Comparative Health Law and Policy – Critical Perspectives on Nigerian Global Health law, ASHGATE, England 2015.

IZUGBARA, C. O., «Representations of sexual abstinence among rural Nigerian adolescent males», Sexuality Research and Social Policy, 4(2007), 74-87.

—————————————, «The Socio-cultural context of adolescents' notions of sex and sexuality in rural South-eastern Nigeria», *Sexualities*, 8(2005), 600-617.

JAMEELAH, Y. – TAIWO, O. – YUSSUFF, R. O., «Public Health Expenditure and health outcome in Nigeria: the impact of governance», *European Scientific Journal*, 8(2012), e – ISSN 1857 – 7431.

JEGEDE, A. S., «Problems and prospects of health care delivery in Nigeria: issues in political economy and social inequality», *Currents and Perspectives in Sociology*, Malthouse Press Limited, Ibadan 2002, 212-226.

JEGEDE, A. S. – FAYEMINO, A. S., «Cultural and Ethical Challenges of Assisted Reproductive Technologies in the Management of Infertility among the Yoruba of South-western Nigeria», *African Journal of Reproductive Health*, 14(2010), 114-127.

JEREMIAH, I. – KALIO, D. G. B. – AKANI, C., «The Pattern of Female Genitale Mutilation in Port Harcourt, Southern Nigeria», *International Journal of Tropical Disease & Health*, 4(2014), 469-476.

JOHNSON, O. E. – ADIAKPAN, N. W. – ASUZU, M. C., «Drug availability and health facility usage in Bamako Initiative and a non-Bamako Initiative Local Government Areas of Akwa Ibom State, South-South Nigeria», *Journal of Community Medicine and Primary Health Care*, 27(2015), 73-82.

LENZER, J., «Appeals court rules that Nigerian families can sue Pfizer in US», *BMJ*, 338(2009), 458, in https://doi.org/10.1136/bmj.b458 [14-8-2018].

KAYONDA, S. O., «Assisted reproductive in Nigeria: Placing the law above medical technology», *Comparative International Law Journal of South Africa*, 34(2001), 258-279.

K.-NIMAKOH, M. – C.-OLAH, M. – MCCANN, T. V., «Access barriers to obstetric care at health facilities in sub-Sahara Africa—a systematic review», *Systematic Reviews*, 6(2017), 110. https://doi.org/10.1186/s13643-017-0503-x [31-7-2018].

KRAUSE, E. – BRANDNER, S. – MUELLER, M. D. – KUHN, A., «Out of Eastern African: Defibulation and sexual function in woman with female genital mutilation», *The Journal of Sexual Medicine*, 8(2011), 1420-1425.

L.-ABASS, B. A., «Poverty and maternal mortality in Nigeria: towards a more viable ethics of modern medical practice», *International Journal for Equity in Health*, 7(2008), in https://doi.org/10.1186/1475-9276-7-11 [14-8-2018].

LARSEN, U. – OKONOFUA, F. E., «Female Circumcision and Obstetric Complication», *International Journal of Gynaecology & Obstetrics*, 77(2002), 255-265. http://dx.doi/10.1016/s0020-7292(02)00028-0 [12-7-2018].

LAWANSON, A. O. – OPELOYERU, O. S., «Equity in healthcare financing», Journal of Hospital Administration, 5(2016), 53-59, in http://dx.doi.org/10.5430/jha.v5n5p53 [7-11-2017].

LAWRENCE, A. L. – JIMMY, J. A. – OKOYE, V. – ABDULRAHEEM, A. – IGBANS, R. O. – UZERE, M., «Birth Preparedness and Complication Readiness among Pregnant Women in Okpatu Community, Enugu State, Nigeria», International Journal of Innovation and Applied Studies, 11(2015), 644-649.

MACKLIN, R., «Bioethics, Vulnerability and Protection», Bioethics, 17(2003), 5-6.

M.-ADEBUSOYE, P., «Sexual behaviour, reproductive knowledge and contraceptive use among young urban Nigerians», International Family Planning Perspective, 18(1992), 66-70.

MALAKOFF, D., «Nigerian Families Sue Pfizer, Testing the Reach of U.S. Law», Science, 293(2001), 1742, in https://doi.org/10.1126/science.293.5536.1742 [14-82018].

MANDARA, M. U., «Female genital mutilation in Nigeria», International Journal of Gynecology & Obstetrics, 84(2004), 291-298, in https://doi.org/10.1016/j.ijgo.2003.06.001 [10-12-2016].

MANGHAM, L. J. – CUNDILL, B. – EZEOKE, O. – NWALA, E. – UZOCHUKWU, B. S. C., «Treatment of uncomplicated malaria at public health facilities and medicine retailers in south-eastern Nigeria», Malaria Journal, 10(2011), 155.

MCDIKKOH, D. M. N., The Nigerian health system's debacle and failure! Xlibris Corporation, United States of America 2010.

MITSUNAGA, T. M. – LARSEN, U. M. – OKONOFUA, F. E. «Risk factors for complications of induced abortions in Nigeria», Journal of Women's Health, 14(2005), 515–528. http://doi/10.1089/jwh.2005.14.515 [12-7-2018].

MONYE, F., «An Appraisal of the National Health Insurance Scheme of Nigeria», Commonwealth Law Bulletin, 32:3, 415-427.

MOORE, B. M. – A.-HART, B. A. – GEORGE, I. O., «Utilization of health care services by pregnant mothers during delivery: a community based study in Nigeria», East African Journal of Public Health, 8(2011), 49-51.

N.-UDAKU, B. C., From What We Should Do To Who We Should Be – Negotiating Theological Reflections and Praxis in the Context of HIV/AIDS Among the Igbos of Nigeria, AuthorHouse United States of America 2001, 244.

NDUGBU, K. U., «The Prevading Public Health Implications of Female Genital Mutilation Among Women (20-40 Years) in a Rural Community in South-eastern Nigeria», Journal of Women's Health Care, 7(2018), 414. http://dx.doi.org/10.4172/2167-0420.1000414. [13-7-2018].

NGHARGBU, R. – OLANIYAN, O., «Inequity in Maternal and Child Health Care Utilization in Nigeria», *African Development Review*, 29(2017), 630-647, in https://doi.org/10.1111/1467-8268.12301 [10-2-2018].

NNAMUCHI, O., «'Circumcision' or 'Mutilation'? Voluntary or Forced Excision? Extricating the Ethical and Legal Issues in Female Genital Ritual», *Journal of Law and Health*, 25(2012), 83-119.

NNEBUE, C. C. – CHIMA, U. – DURU, C. B. – LUKA, A. L. – OLAOYIN, T. O., «Determinants of age at sexual initiation among Nigerian adolescents: a study of secondary school students in a Military Barrack in Nigeria», *The American Journal of Medical Science*, 4(2016), 1-7.

NNEBUE, C. – EBENEBE, U. – ADOGU, P. – ADINMA, E. – IFEADIKE, C. – NWABUEZE, A.,«Adequacy of resources for provision of maternal health services at the primary health care level in Nnewi, Nigeria», *Nigerian Medical Journal*, 55(2014), 235-241, in https://doi.org/10.4103/0300-1652.132056 [19-06-2017].

NNEBUE, C. – EBENEBE, U. – DURU, C. – EGENTI, N. – EMELUMADU, O. – IBEH, C.,«Availability and continuity of care for maternal health services in the primary health centres in Nnewi, Nigeria (January – March 2010)», *International Journal of Preventive Medicine*, 7(2016), 44, in https://doi.org/10.4103/2008-7802.177885 [8-10-2017].

NUHU, B. – BABAYO, T. – HADIZA, I. – KELLY, D. T., «Knowledge and Perceptions of Maternal Health in Kaduna State, Northern Nigeria», *African Journal of Reproductive Health*, 14(2010), 71-76.

NWACHUKWU, C. N. – ORJI, A. F. – UGBOGU, O. C., «Health Care Waste Management – Public Health Benefits, and the Need for Effective Environmental Regulatory Surveillance in Federal Republic of Nigeria», in https://doi.org/10.5772/53196 [25-9-2017].

NWAEZE, I. L. – ENABOR, O. O. – OLUWASOLA, T. A. O. – AIMAKU, C. O., «Perception and satisfaction with quality of antenatal care services among pregnant women at the University College Hospital, Ibadan», Nigeria, *Annals of Ibadan Postgraduate Medicine*, 11(2013), 22-28.

NWAIWU, O. – OYELADE, O. B., «Traditional herbal medicines used in neonates and infants less than six months old in Lagos Nigeria», *Nigerian Journal of Paediatrics*, 43(2016), 40, in https://doi.org/10.4314/njp.v43i1.8 [15-8-2018].

NWAKOBY, B. N., «The influence of new maternal care facilities in rural Nigeria», *Health Policy and Planning*, 7(1992), 269-278.

O.-Adeniran, B. A. – Adewole, I. F. – Iwere, N., – P. Mahmoud, «Promoting Sexual and Reproductive Health and Rights in Nigeria through Change in Medical School Curriculum», African Journal of Reproductive Health, 8(2004), 85-91.

O.-Adeniran, B. A. – Long, C. M. – Adewole, I. F., «Advocacy for Reform of the Abortion Law in Nigeria», Journal of Reproductive Health Matters, 12(2004), 209-217.

O.-Aghoja, L., «Sexual and reproductive health: Concepts and current status among Nigerians», African Journal of Medical and Health Science, 12(2013), 103-113, in https://doi.org/10.4103/2384-5589.134906 [25-8-2017].

O.-Bello, A. I. – Abodunrin, O. L. – Adeomi, A. A., «Contraceptive Practice Among Women in Rural Communities in South-West Nigeria», Global Journal of Medical Research, 11(2011), 1-8.

Obi, S., «Female genital mutilation in southeast Nigeria», International Journal of Gynaecology & Obstetrics, 84(2004), 183-184, in https://doi.org/10.1016/j.ijgo.2003.08.014 [18-3-2018].

Odetola, T. D., «Health care utilization among rural women of child-bearing age: a Nigerian experience», Pan African Medical Journal, 20(2015), 151, in https://doi.org/10.11604/pamj.2015.20.151.5845 [31-7-2018].

Odeyemi, I. A., «Community-based health insurance programmes and the National Health Insurance Scheme of Nigeria: challenges to uptake and integration», International Journal for equity health, 13(2014), 13-20.

Odia, O. J., «The Relation between Law, Religion, Culture and Medical Ethics in Nigeria», Global Bioethics, 25(2014), 164-169, in http://doi.org/10.1080/11287462.2014.937949 [12-7-2018].

Odimegwu, C. O., «Family planning attitude and use in Nigeria», International perspective on sexual and reproductive health, 25(1999), 86-91.

Odujinrin, O. M., «Sexual activity, contraceptive practice and abortion among adolescents in Lagos, Nigeria», International Journal of Gynaecology and Obstetrics, 34(1991), 361-366.

Odunbunmi, S.A., Primary Health Care in Nigeria: Structure and Performance, LAMBERT Academic Publishing, Saarbrucken, Germany 2012.

Odusanya, O. O., «Drug use indicators at a secondary health care facility in Lagos, Nigeria», Journal of Community Medicine & Primary Health Care, 16(2014), 21-24.

Ofili, A. – Okojie, O., «Assessment of the role of traditional birth attendants in maternal health care in Oredo Local Government Area, Edo State, Nigeria», Journal of Community Medicine and Primary Health Care, 17(2005), 55-60.

Ogu, R. N. – E.-Emmanuel, B. C., «Nigeria Government Expenditure, Economic Productivity and the prevention of Maternal Mortality: A Call to Action», Journal of Economics, Management and Trade, 21(2018), 1-9.

Ogbeidi, M. M., «Political Leadership and Corruption in Nigeria Since 1960: A Socio-economic Analysis», Journal of Nigeria Studies, 1(2012), 1-25.

Okafor, S. I., «Spatial Aspects of Health Care Provision in Nigeria», in R. Akhtar (ed.), Health Care Patterns and Planning in Developing Countries, Greenwood Press, New York 1991.

Okafor, C. – Onuigbo, R. A., «Rethinking Public Administration Professionalism in Nigeria», African Research Review, 9(2015), 333-347.

Okagbue, I., «Pregnancy termination and the law in Nigeria», Studies in Family Planning, 21(1990), 197-208, in https://doi.org/10.2307/1966614 [12-1-2017].

Okeke, T. – Anyaehie, U. – Ezenyeaku, C., «An overview of female genital mutilation in Nigeria», Annals of Medical and Health Sciences Research, 2(2012), 70-73, in https://doi.org/10.4103/2141-9248.96942 [20-12-2017].

Okeke, T. A. – Okeibunor, J. C., «Rural-urban Differences in Health-seeking for the Treatment of Childhood Malaria in South-east Nigeria», Health policy, 95(2009), 62-68, in https://doi.org/10.1016/j.healthpol.2009.11.005 [3-8-2018].

Okojie, S. E., «Induced Illegal Abortion in Benin City, Nigeria, International Journal of Gynaecology & Obstetrics», 14(1976), 571-521, in http://dx.doi.org/10.1002/j.1879-3479.1976.tb00098.x [13-7-2018].

Okonofua, F. E., Abortion, in F. E. Okonofua – K. Odunsi, (eds.), Contemporary Obstetrics and Gynaecology for developing countries, Women's health and Action Research Centre 2003, 179-201.

––––––––––––––––, «Unwanted pregnancy, unsafe abortion among Adolescents», Tropical Journal of Obstetrics and Gynaecology, 19(2002), 515-517.

Okonofua, F. E. – Shittu, S. O. – Oronsaye, F. – Ogunsakin, D. – Ogbomwan, S. – Zayyan, A., «Attitudes and practices of private medical providers towards family planning and abortion services in Nigeria», Acta Obstetetricia Gynecologica Scandinavica, 84(2005), 270-280.

Okonofua, F. E. – Onwudiegwu, U. – Odunsin, A., «Illegal induced abortion, A study of 74 cases in Ile-Ife, Nigeria», Tropical Doctor, 22(1992), 75-78

Okonofua, F. E. – Abejide, A. – Makanjuola, R. A., «Maternal mortality in Ile-Ife Nigeria: a study of risk factors», Studies in Family Planning, 23(1992), 319–324.

OKONKWO, A. D. – OKONKWO, U. P., «Patent medicine vendors, community pharmacists and STI management in Abuja, Nigeria», African Health Science, 10(2010), 253-265.

OKONTA, P. I., «Ethics of clinical trials in Nigeria», Nigerian Medical Journal, 55(2014), 188-194.

OLATUBI, M. I., – OYEDIRAN, O. O., – ADUBI, I. O., – OGIDAN, O. C., «Health Care Expenditure in Nigeria and National Productivity: A Review», South Asian Journal of Social Studies and Economics, 1(2018), 1-7).

OLAKUNDE, B. O., «Public health care financing in Nigeria: Which way forward?», Annals of Nigerian Medicine, 6(2012), 4-10, in https://doi.org/10.4103/0331-3131.100199 [15-4-2017].

OLANIRAN, A. – SMITH, H. – UNKELS, R. – B.-ZEEV, S. – VAN DEN BROEK, N., «Who is a community health worker? – a systematic review of definitions»,Global Health Action, 10(2017), in https://doi.org/10.1080/16549716.2017.1272223 [16-5-2017].

OLATUBI, M. I. – OYEDIRAN, O. O. – ADUBI, I. O. – OGIDAN, O. C., «Health Care Expenditure in Nigeria and National Productivity: A Review», South Asian Journal of Social Studies and Economics, 1(2018), 1-7.

OLERIBE, O. O. – OLADIPO, O. A. – EZIEME, I. P. – ELIZABETH, M. M. – T.-ROBINSON, S. D., «From decentralization to commonization of HIV healthcare resources: Keys to reduction in health disparity and equitable distribution of health services in Nigeria», Pan African Medical Journal, 24(2016), in https://doi.org/10.11604/pamj.2016.24.266.6286 [21-8-2018].

OLORUNNIYI, O. F. – MORENIKEJI, O. A., «The extent of use of herbal medicine in malaria management in Ido/Osi local government area of Ekiti state, Nigeria», Journal of Medicinal Plant Research, 7(2013), 3171-3178.

OLORUNSAIYE, C. Z. – DEGGE, H., «Variations in the uptake of Routine Immunization in Nigeria: Examining Determinants of Inequitable Access», Journal Global Health Communication, 2(1), (2016), 19-29, in http://dx.doi.org/10.1080/23762004.2016.1206780 [3-5-2017].

OLUSEGUN, L. O. – IBE, T. R. – IKOROK, M. M., «Curbing maternal and child mortality: The Nigerian experience», International Journal of Nursing and Midwifery, 4(2012), 33-39, in https://doi.org/10.5897/ijnm11.030 [10-9-2016].

OLUKOGA, A. – BACHMANN, M. – HARRIS, G. – OLUKOGA, T. – OLUWADIYA, K., «Analysis of the perception of institutional function for health sector reform in Nigeria», International Health, 2(2010), 150-155.

OLUWABAMIDE, A. J. – UMOH, J. O., «An assessment of the relevance of religion to health care delivery in Nigeria: case of Akwa Ibom State», Journal of Sociology and Anthropology, 2(2011), 47-52.

OLUWOLE, E. O. – KUYINU, Y. A. – GOODMAN, O. O. – ODUGBEMI, B. A. – AKINYINKA, M. R., «Factors Influencing the Uptake of Modern Family Planning Methods among Women of Reproductive Age in Rural Community in Lagos State», International Journal of Tropical Disease & Health, 11(2016), 1-11.

OMONZEJELE, P. F., «African concepts of health, disease, and treatment: an ethical inquiry, Explore», Journal of Science and Healing, 4(2008), 120-126.

OMONZEJELE, P. F., «The Right to Healthcare in African Countries: Nigeria in View-A Moral Appraisal», Etno Med, 4(2010), 37-42.

ONAH, H. E. – IKEAKO, L. C. – ILOABACHIE, G. C., «Factors associated with the use of maternity services in Enugu, south-eastern Nigeria», Social Science & Medicine, 63 (7), (2006), 1870-1878.

ONWUJEKWE, O. – HANSON, K. – UZOCHUKWU, B. – EZEOKE, O. – EZE, S. – DIKE, N., «Geographic inequities in provision and utilization of malaria treatment services in southeast Nigeria: diagnosis, providers and drugs», Health Policy, 94(2010), 144-149, in https://doi/10.1016/j.healthpol.2009.09.010 [29-7-2018].

ONWUJEKWE, O. E. – ONOKA, C. A. – UZOCHUKWU, B. S. C. – OBIKEZE, E. N. – EZUMAH, N., «Issues in equitable health financing in South Eastern Nigeria: Socio-economic and geographic differences in households' illness expenditure and policymakers' views on the financial protection of the poor», Journal of International Development, 21(2009), 185-199.

ONWUJEKWE, O. – OJUKWU, J. – SHU, E. – UZOCHUKWU, B., «Inequities in valuation of benefits, choice and drugs, and mode of payment for malaria treatment services provided by community health workers in Nigeria», The American Journal of Tropical Medicine and Hygiene, 77(2007), 16-27.

ONWUJEKWE, O. E. – UZOCHUKWU, B., «Socio-economic and geographic differentials in costs and payment strategies for primary healthcare services in Southeast Nigeria», Health Policy, 71(2005), 383-397.

ONWUJEKWE, O. E. – UZOCHUKWU, B. S. C. – OBIKEZE, E. N. –OKORONKWO, I. – OCHONMA, O. G. – ONOKA, C. A. – MADUBUKO, G. – OKOLI, C., «Investigating determinants of out-of-pocket spending and strategies for coping with payments for healthcare in southeast Nigeria», BMC Health Services Research, 10(2010), 67.

ONWUJEKWE, O. – OBIKEZE, E. – UZOCHUKWU, B. – OKORONKWO, I. – ONWUJEKWE, O. C., «Improving quality of malaria treatment services: assessing inequities in consumers' perceptions and providers' behaviour in Nigeria», International Journal for Equity in Health, 9(2010), 22, in https://doi.org/10.1186/1475-9276-9-22 [10-8-2016].

OPHORI, E. A. – TULA, M. Y. – AZIH, A. V. – OKOJIE, R. – IKPO, P. E., «Current trends of immunization in Nigeria: Prospects and challenges», Tropical Medicine and Health, 42 (2), 67-75. https://doi.org/10.2149/tmh.2013-13 [10-07-2016].

ORIMADEGUN, A. E. – ILESANMI, K. S., «Mothers' understanding of childhood malaria and practices in rural communities of Ise-Orun, Nigeria: implications for malaria control», Journal of Family Medicine and Primary Care, 4(2015), 226-231.

ORJI, E. O. – ESIMAI, O. A., «Sexual behaviour and contraceptive use among secondary school students in Ilesa South West Nigeria», Journal of Obstetrics & Gynaecology, 25(2005), 269-272.

OSAIN, M., «Nigerian health care system: Need for integrating adequate medical intelligence and surveillance systems», Journal of Pharmacy and Bioallied Sciences, 3(2011), 470-478.

OSHINAME, F. O. – BRIEGER, W. R., «Primary care training for patent medicine vendors in rural Nigeria», Social Science & Medicine, 35(1992), 1477-1484.

OSUNGBADE, K. O. – AYINDE, O. O., «Maternal Complication prevention: evidence from a case-control study in southwest Nigeria», African Journal of Primary Health Care & Family Medicine, 6(2014), 656, in http://doi.org/10.4102/phcfm.v6i1.656 [20-5-2017].

OTOVWE, A. –SARKI, E., «Utilization of Primary Health Care Services in Jaba Local Government Area of Kaduna State Nigeria», Journal of Health Science, 27(2017), 339. https://dx.doi.org/10.4314/ejhs.v27i45 [31-7-2018].

OTOIDE, V., «Targeting adolescents for family planning and post abortion care», Tropical Journal of Obstetrics and Gynaecology, 21(2004), 65-68.

OVADJE, L. – NRIAGU, J., «Multi-dimensional knowledge of malaria among Nigerian caregivers: implications for insecticide-treated net use by children», Malaria Journal, 15(2016), in https://doi.org/10.1186/s12936-016-1557-2 [10-12-2016].

OYENIYI, S. O. – OLOYEDE, J. O., «A Comparative Analysis of Safe Water and Sanitation in Selected Urban and Rural Areas of Osun State, Nigeria», Donnish Journal of Research in Environmental Studies, 3(2016) 8-16.

OYEWALE, T. O. – MAVUNDLA, T. R., «Socioeconomic factors contributing to exclusion of women from maternal health benefit in Abuja, Nigeria», Curationis, 38(2015), 1-11, in https://doi.org/10.4102/curationis.v38i1.1272 [16-8-2018].

OYEKALE, A. S. – OYEKALE, T. O., «Healthcare waste management practices and safety indicators in Nigeria», BMC Public Health, 17(2017), 740. https://doi.org/10.1186/s12889-017-4794-6 [30-7-2018].

OYIBO, P. G., «Out-of-pocket payment for health services: constraints and implications for government employees in Abakaliki, Ebonyi State, south east Nigeria», African Health Sciences, 11(2011), 481-485.

OZUMBA, B. C., «Acquired Gynaetresia in Eastern Nigeria», International Journal of Gynaecology & Obstetrics, 37(1992), 105-109.

RAJI, M., «Awareness and utilization of family planning commodities in a rural community of North West Nigeria», Caliphate Medical Journal, 1(2013), 103-108.

SALLY, H., «Time to right the wrongs: Improving Basic Health Care in Nigeria», The Lancet, 359(2002), 2030-2035.

SAMBO, M. – EJEMBI, C. – ADAMU, Y. – ALIYU, A., «Out-of-pocket health expenditure for under-five illnesses in a semi-urban community in Northern Nigeria», Journal of Community Medicine and Primary Health Care, 16(2004), in https://doi.org/10.4314/jcmphc.v16i1.32404 [12-11-2016].

SANGOWAWA, A. O. – AMODU, O. K. – OLANIYAN, S. A. – AMODU, F. A. – OLUMESE, P. E. – OMOTADE, O. O., «Factors associated with a poor treatment outcome among children treated for malaria in Ibadan, southwest Nigeria», Epidemiology Research International, 2014, in http://dx.org/10.1155/2014/974693 [6-8-2017].

SEDE, P. I. – OHEMENG, W., «Socio-economic determinants of life expectancy in Nigeria (1980-2011)», Health Economics Review, 5(2015). https://doi.org/10.1186/s13561-014-0037-z [7-2-2015].

SEDGH, G. – BANKOLE, A. – O-.ADENIRAN, B. – ADEWOLE, I. F. – SINGH, S. – HUSSAIN, R., «Unwanted pregnancy and associated factors among Nigerian women», International Family Planning Perspectives, 32(2006), 175-184.

SHARMA, V. – LEIGHT, J. – ABDULAZIZ, F. – GIROUX, N. – BJORKMAN, N. M., «Illness recognition, decision-making, and care-seeking for maternal and newborn complications: a qualitative study in Jigawa State, Northern Nigeria», Journal of Health, Population and Nutrition, 36(2017), 59-63, in https://doi.org/10.1186/s41043-017-0124-y [15-8-2018].

SHEHU, A. U. – JOSHUA, I. A. – UMAR, Z., «Knowledge of contraception and contraceptive choices among human immunodeficiency virus-positive women attending antiretroviral clinics in Zaria, Nigeria», 3(2016), 84, in https://doi.org/10.4103/2384-5147.184355 [15-08-2018].

SMITH, D. J., «Imagining HIV/AIDS: Morality and perception of personal risk in Nigeria», Medical Anthropology, 22(2003), 343-372.

———————————, «Youth, sin and sex in Nigeria: Christianity and HIV/AIDS-related beliefs and behaviour among rural-urban migrants», Culture, Health, & Sex, 6(2004), 425-437.

STOCK, R., «Distance and the utilization of health facilities in rural Nigeria», Social Science & Medicine, 17(1983), 563-570.

SUNDAY, B. – UZOCHUKWU, C. – OSSAI, E.N. – OKEKE, C. C. – NDU, A. C. – ONWUJEKWE, O. E., «Malaria Knowledge and Practices in Enugu State, Qualitative Study», International Journal of Health Policy and Management, 7(2018), 895-866.

TEMITOPE, A., «Effect of Health Investment on Economic Growth in Nigeria», IOSR Journal of Economics and Finance, 1(2013), 39-47

T.-WEST, C. I. – BIGGS, N., «Effectiveness of trained community volunteers in improving knowledge and management of childhood malaria in a rural area of River State, Nigeria», Nigerian Journal of Clinical Practice, 18(2015), 651-658. https://doi/10.4103/1119-3077.158971 [29-7-2018].

TEMITOPE, A., «Effect of Health Investment on Economic Growth in Nigeria», IOSR Journal of Economics and Finance, 1(2013), 39-47.

TIMOTHY, G. – IRINOYE, O. – YUNUSA, U. – DALHATU, A. – AHMED, S. – SUBERU, A., «Balancing Demand and Efficiency in Nigerian Health Care Delivery System», European Journal of Business and Management, 6 (23), 2014, 50-56.

TITUS, O. B. – ADEBISOLA, O. A. – ADENIJI, A. O., «Healthcare access and utilization among rural households in Nigeria», Journal of Development and Agricultural Economics, 7(2015), 195-203.

TOBIN, E. A. – OFILI, A. N. – ENEBELI, N. – ENUEZE, O., «Assessment of birth preparedness and complication readiness among pregnant women attending Primary Health Care Centres in Edo State, Nigeria», Annals of Nigerian Medicine, 8(2014), 76-81, in https://doi.org/10.4103/0331-3131.153358 [27-5-2017].

UCHENDU, O. C. – ILESANMI, O. S. – OLUMIDE, A. E., «Factors influencing the choice of health care providing facility among workers in a local government secretariat in south western Nigeria», Annals of Ibadan Postgraduate Medicine 11(2013), 87-95.

UGBOMA, H. A. – AKANNI, C. I. – BABATUNDE, S., «Prevalence and mediatisation of female genital mutilation», Nigerian Journal of Medicine, 13(2004), 254-258.

Ukwuma, M. C., Multiparity and Childbirth Complications in Rural Women of Northeast Nigerian Origin, «IOSR Journal of Pharmacy and Biological Sciences», 2(2012), 1-4.

UNUIGBE, J. A. – ORHUE, A. A. – ORONSAYE, A. U., «Maternal mortality at the University of Benin Teaching Hospital Benin City, Nigeria», Tropical Journal of Obstetrics and Gynaecology, 1(1988), 13-18.

USHIE, B. A. – UGAL, D. B. – INGWU, J. A., «Overdependence on For-Profit Pharmacies: A Descriptive Survey of User Evaluation of Medicines Availability in Public Hospitals in Selected Nigerian States», PLoS ONE 11(2016), e0165707, in https://doi.org/10.1371/journal.pone.0165707 [30-7-2018].

UZOCHUKWU, B. – ONWUJEKWE, O., «Healthcare reform involving the introduction of user fees and drug revolving funds: influence on health workers' behaviour in southeast Nigeria», Health Policy, 75(2005), 1-8, in https://doi.org/10.1016/j.healthpol.2005.01.019 [1-8-2018].

UZOCHUKWU, B. S. C. – UGHASORO, M. D. – ETIABA, E. – OKWUOSA, C. – ENVULADU, E. – ONWUJEKWE, O. E., «Health care financing in Nigeria: Implications for achieving universal health coverage», Nigerian Journal of Clinical Practice, 18(2015), 437-444, in https://doi.org/10.4103/1119-3077.154196 [27-11-2017].

WELCOME, M. O., «The Nigerian health care system: Need for integrating adequate medical intelligence and surveillance systems», Journal of Pharmacy and Bioallied Sciences, 3(2011), 470-478, in https://doi.org/10.4103/0975-7406.90100 [6 8 2016].

WOLLUM, A. – BURSTEIN, R. – FULLMAN, N. – D.-LINDGREN, L. – GAKIDOU, E., «Benchmarking health system performance across states in Nigeria: a systematic analysis of levels and trends in key maternal and child health interventions and outcomes», 2000-2013, BMC Medicine, 13(2015), 208, in https://doi/10.1186/s12916-015-0438-9 [6-8-2018].

YAHA, S. – BISHWAJIT, G. – UTHMAN, O. A. – AMOUZOU, A., «Why some women fail to give birth at health facilities: A comparative study between Ethiopia and Nigeria», PLoS ONE, 13(2018), e0196896, in https://doi.org/10.1371/journal.pone.0196896 [29-8-2018].

YAQUB, J. O. – OJAPINWA, T. V. – YUSSUFF, R. O., «Public Health Expenditure and health outcome in Nigeria: the impact of governance», European Scientific Journal, 8(2012), e – ISSN: 1857 – 7431.

YAYA, S. – EKHOLUENETALE, M. – TUDEME, G. – VAIBHAV, S. – BISHWAJIT, G. – KADIO, B., «Prevalence and determinants of childhood mortality in Nigeria», BMC Public Health, 17(2017), 1, in https://doi.org/10.1186/s12889-017-4420-7 [14-8-2018].

YUNUSA, E. – AWOSAN, K. – TUNAU, K. – MAINASARA, R. – DANGUSAU, A. – GARBA, M., «Knowledge, Perception and Practice of Birth Preparedness and Complication Readiness among Pregnant Women Attending a Tertiary Healthcare Facility in Sokoto, Nigeria», Asian Journal of Medicine and Health, 7(2017), 1-12, in https://doi.org/10.9734/ajmah/2017/36705 [10-1-2018].

6. Ethics, Healthcare and Medicine (Other authors)

A.-FALLOUJI, M. A. – McBRIEN, M. P., Circumcision, Postgraduate surgery, Butterworth-Heinemann, Oxford 2000[4].

AKHTAR, R., «Socioeconomic and Political Aspects of Health Care» in R. Akhtar (ed.), Health Care Patterns and Planning in Developing Countries, Greenwood Press, New York 1991.

BEAUCHAMP, T. L. – CHILDRESS, J. F., Principles of Biomedical Ethics, Oxford University Press, Inc., New York 2001[5].

BEAUREGARD, D., «Virtue in Bioethics», in E. J. Furton – P. J. Cataldo – A. S. Moraczewski (eds.) Catholic Health Care Ethics. A Manual for Practitioners, The National Catholic Bioethics Center, Philadelphia 2009[2], 27-29.

BHUTTA, Z. A., «Childhood pneumonia in developing countries», BMJ, 333(2006), 612-613, in https://doi.org/10.1136/bmj.38975.602836.be [6-9-2016].

BOGNAR, G. – HIROSE, I., The Ethics of Health Care Rationing – An Introduction, Routledge, London and New York 2014, 25-26.

BRAVEMAN, P. A. – KUMAYIKA, S. – FIELDING, J. – LaVEIST, T. – BORRELL, L. N. – MANDERSCHEID, R. – TROUTMAN, A., «Health Disparities and Health Equity: The Issue Is Justice», American Journal of Public Health, 101 (2011), 149-155.

BRAVEMAN, P.,*Defining equity in health, Journal of Epidemiology & Community Health*, 57(2003), 254-258, in https://doi.org/10.1136/jech.57.4.254 [3-12-2017].

BUTTRAM, R. T – FOLGER, R – SHEPPARD, B. H., «*Equity, Equality and Need: Three Faces of Social Justice*», in *Conflict, Cooperation, and Justice: Essays Inspired by the Work of Morton Deutsch*, B. B. BUNKER – M. DEUTSCH (eds.), *Jossey-Bass Inc. Publishers*, San Francisco 1995.

CALLAHAN, D., «*Religion and the Secularization of Bioethics*», *The Hasting Center Report*, 4(1990), 2-4.

CAIRNCROSS, S. – HUNT, C. – BOISSON, S. – BOSTOEN, K. – CURTIS, V. – CH FUNG, I. – SCHMIDT, W. P., «*Water, Sanitation and hygiene for the prevention of diarrhoea*», *International Journal of Epidemiology*», 39(1), (2010), 193-205.

CAIRNCROSS, S. – PETACH, H., «*The risk of unimproved water and sanitation and the global burden of disease*», *Journal of Water Sanitation and Hygiene for Development*, 3(2013), 479-480, in https://doi.org/10.2166/washdev.2013.054 [15-10-2016].

CAIRNCROSS, S. – HUNT, C. – BOISSON, S. – BOSTOEN, K. – CURTIS, V. – FUNG, I. C. – SCHMIDT, W. P., «*Water, sanitation and hygiene for the prevention of diarrhoea*»,*International Journal of Epidemiology*, 39(2010), i193-i205, in https://doi.org/10.1093/ije/dyq035 [17-10-2016].

CAPP, S. – SAVAGE, S. – CLARKE, V., «*Exploring distributive justice in health care*», *Australian Health Review*, 24 (2001), 40-44.

CAPONE, R. A., «*AMA Reconsiders opposition to physician-assisted suicide*», in *Ethics & Medics*, 41(2016), 1-3.

CHRISTOPHER, A. S – CARUSO, D., «*American Medical Association (AMA)*», *Journal of Ethics*, 17(2015), 958-965. https://doi.org/10.1001/journalofethics.2015.17.10.msoc1-1510 [02-01-2018].

COHEN, D., «*Medical Ethics and Economics in Health Care*», *Journal of Medical Ethics*, 15(1989), 54-55, in https://doi.org/10.1136/jme.15.1.54-a [15-12-2016].

COOK, J. R., «*Ethical Concerns in Female Genital Cutting*», *African Journal of Reproductive Health*, 12(2008), 7-11 [13-7-2018].

COOKSON, R. – DOLAN, P., «*Principles of justice in health care rationing*», *Journal of Medical Ethics*, 26(2000), 323-329, in https://doi.org/10.1136/jme.26.5.323 [20-11-2016].

CROPLEY, L., *The effect of health education intervention on child malaria treatment seeking practices among mothers in rural refugee village in Belize, Central America*, Health Promotion International, 19(2004), 445-452.

CULYER, A. J., «*Economics and Ethics in Health Care*», Journal of Medical Ethics, 27(2001), 217-222, in *https://doi.org/10.1136/jme.27.4.217* [15-10-2016].

CURTIS, S., *Health and Inequality: Geographical Perspectives*, Sage, London 2004.

DEUTSCH, M., «*Justice and Conflict*», in *The Handbook of Conflict Resolution: Theory and Practice*,M. DEUTSCH – P. T. COLEMAN (eds.), Jossey-Bass Inc. Publishers, San Francisco 2000.

DONCHIN, A. – PURDY, L. M., *Embodying Bioethics, Recent Feminist Advances*, Roman & Littlefield publishers, Maryland 1999.

EVANS, J. G., «*The rationing debate: Rationing health care by age: The case against*», BMJ, 314(1997), 822-822, in *https://doi.org/10.1136/bmj.314.7083.822* [21-11-2017].

FAGGIONI, M. P., *La Vita Nelle Nostre Mani, Manuale di Bioetica teologica*, Edizione Camilliane, Torino 2006².

_______________, «*Le Mutilazioni Genitali Feminili*», in M. C. BASILE (ed.), *Vita, Ragione, Dialogo, Scritti in Onore Elio Sgreccia*, Edizioni Cantagalli, Siena 2012.

FISHER, A., «*The ethics of health care (Lecture delivered to the annual sympotium of the Guild of Catholic Doctors on April 24, 1993)*», Catholic Medical Quarterly, 44(1993), 13-20.

FLAMIGNI, C. –MASSARENTI, A. – MORI, M. – PETRONI, A., «*Manifesto di Bioetica Laica*», "Il Sole24Ore" – 9 giugno 1996.

FORNERO, G., *Bioetica laica*, Bruno Mondadori, Milano 2005.

FRATTALLONE, R., *Persona*, in S. LEONE – S. PRIVITERA (eds.), *Nuovo Dizionario di Bioetica*, Città Nuova, Firenze 2004,856-863.

GALLAGHER, D. M., «*The Common Good*», in E. J. Furton – P. J. Cataldo – A. S. Moraczewski (eds.), *Catholic Health Care Ethics. A Manual for Practitioners*, The National Catholic Bioethics Center, Philadelphia 2009².

GATELY, P. – BECK, A. – JONES, D. A., *Healthcare Allocation & Justice, Applying Catholic Social Teaching*, Incorporated Catholic Truth Society, London 2011.

GILLAM, S. – YATES, J. – BADRINATH, P., «*Health needs assessment*», in S. Gillam – J. Yates – P. Badrinath (eds.), *Essential Public Health: Theory and Practice*, Cambridge University Press, Cambridge 2012, 104-114.

GILLON, R., «Medical ethics: four principles plus attention to scope», *BMJ*, 309(1994), 184-184, in *https://doi.org/10.1136/bmj.309.6948.184* [10-6- 2017].

————————, «Defending the four principles approach to biomedical ethics», *Journal of Medical Ethics*, 21(1995), 323-324, in *https://doi.org/10.1136/jme.21.6.323* [12-6-2017].

GRONEBAUM, M., *John Rawls' Theory of Justice: Justice as fairness*, Grin, Norderstedt Germany 2013, I-II.

HADDAD, L. B., – NOUR, N. M., *Unsafe abortion: Unnecessary Maternal Mortality*, Reviews in Obstetrics and Gynaecology, 2(2009), 122-126.

HARRIS, J., «The rationing debate: Maximising the health of the whole community. The case against: what the principle objective of NHS should be», British Medical Journal, 314(1997), 669-672, in *https://doi.org/10.1136/bmj.314.7081.669* [23-7-2017].

HEHIR, J. B., «Policy Arguments in a Public Church: Catholic Social Ethics and Bioethics», *The Journal of Medicine and Philosophy*, 17(1992), 347-364.

HOPE, T., *Medical Ethics. A very short introduction*, Oxford University Press 2004.

HURLEY, J., «Ethics, economics, and public financing of health care», *Journal of Medical Ethics*, 27(2001), 234-239, in *http://dx.doi.org/10.1136/jme.27.4.234* [22-12-2017].

HSIAO, T., «Why Recreational Drug Use Is Immoral» in *The National Catholic Bioethics Quarterly*, E. J. FURTON (ed.), Philadelphia, 17(2017), 605-614.

INGRID, R., *The Capability Approach: a theoretical survey*, Journal of Human Development, 6(2005), 93-117.

JEFFERY, R., *The Impact of Socio-economic and Political Factors on the Provision of Health Care in India*, in R. AKHTAR (ed.) Health Care Patterns and Planning in Developing Countries, Greenwood Press, New York 1991, 99-114.

JENNINGS, B., «Frameworks for Ethics in Public Health», Acta Bioethica 9(2003), in *https://doi.org/10.4067/s1726-569x2003000200003* [30 08 2016].

JOSEPH, J. – GEORGE, J., «Female Genital Mutilation», International Journal of Science and Research, 4(2015), 2113-2118, in *https://doi.org/10.21275/v4i11.nov151641* [10-2-2018].

KEEHAN, C., *Catholic Social Teaching and Just Health Care Policy*, Journal of Catholic Social Thoughts, 7(2010), 7-15, in *https://doi.org/10.5840/jcathsoc20107113* [10-1-2017].

KIDANE, G., – R. H. MORROW, «Teaching mothers to provide home treatment of malaria in Tigray, Ethiopia: A randomized trial», The Lancet, 365(2000), 550-555.

KILAMA, W. L., «Ethical perspective on malaria research for Africa», *Acta Tropica*, 95(2005), 276-284.

KUTZIN, J., «Health financing for universal coverage and health system performance: concepts and implications for policy», *Bulletin of the World Health Organization*, 91(2013), 602-611, in *https://doi.org/10.2471/blt.12.113985* [27-11-2016].

LAMM, R. D., «Saint Martin of Tours in a New World of Medical Ethics», *Cambridge Quarterly of Healthcare Ethics*, 3.2 (1994), 159-167.

LANGO, J. W., «Global Health, Human Rights, and Distributive Justice», in *Medicine and Social Justice*, Oxford University Press, Oxford, 2012,231-244, in *https://doi.org/10.1093/acprof:osobl/9780199744206.003.0019* [6-8-2017].

LEGET, C. – HOEDEMAEKERS, R., «Teaching medical students about fair distribution of healthcare resources», *Journal of Medical Ethics*, 33(2017), 737-741, in *http://dx.doi.org/10.1136/jme.2006.017095* [22-12-2017].

LELKENS, J. P. M., *AIDS: il preservativo non preserva. Documentazioni di una truffa*, in *Studi Cattolici*, 405(1994), Milano, 718 – 723.

LENZER, J., *Appeals court rules that Nigerian families can sue Pfizer in US*, BMJ, 338(2009), 458, in *https://doi.org/10.1136/bmj.b458* [14-8-2018].

—————————, *Secret report surfaces showing that Pfizer was at fault in Nigerian drug tests*, BMJ, 332(2006), 1233. *https://doi.org/10.1136/bmj.332.7552.1233-a* [14-8-2018].

—————————, *Nigerian judge orders arrests of Pfizer officials*, BMJ, 336(2008), 11. *https://doi.org/10.1136/bmj.39444.446725.DB* [14-8-2018].

LORENZO, C. – GARRAFA, V. – SOLBAKK, J. H. – VIDAL, S., «Hidden risks associated with clinical trial in developing countries», *Journal of Medical Ethics*, 36(2010), 111-115.

MALAKOFF, D., *Nigerian Families Sue Pfizer, Testing the Reach of U.S. Law*, Science, 293(2001), 1742, in *https://doi.org/10.1126/science.293.5536.1742* [14-82018].

MAHONEY, M. E., «Medical Rights and Public Welfare», *Proceeding of the American Philosophical Society*, 135(1991), 22-29.

MAY, W. E., *Catholic Bioethics and the human life*, Our Sunday Visitor Inc., Huntington, Indiana 2000.

MAYNARD, A., «Ethics and health care 'underfunding'», *Journal of Medical Ethics*,27(2001), 223-227, in *https://doi.org/10.1136/jme.27.4.223* [16-1-2016].

MCELWEE, J. J., "*African Archbishop Frankly Criticizes Western Attitude at Synod*", *National Catholic Reporter*, October 8, 2014.

MCKLIN, R., Liberty, «*Utility and Justice, An Ethical Approach to Unwanted Pregnancy*», *International Journal of Gynaecology & Obstetrics*, 3(1989), 37.

——————, «*Bioethics, Vulnerability and Protection*», *Bioethics*, 17(2003), 5-6.

MORACZEWSKI, A. S., «*The Fetus and Human Embryo - Abortion*», in E. J. FURTON – P. J. CATALDO – A. S. MORACZEWSKI (eds.), *Catholic Health Care Ethics. A Manual for Practitioners*, The National Catholic Bioethics Center, Philadelphia 2009².

——————, «*The Human Person and the Church's Teaching Authority*», in E. J. Furton – P. J. Cataldo – A. S. Moraczewski (eds.) *Catholic Health Care Ethics. A Manual for Practitioners*, The National Catholic Bioethics Center, Philadelphia 2009².

NAJERA, J. A., «*Malaria control: Achievements, problems and strategies*», *Parassitologia*, 43(2001), 1-89.

NAUMANN, J. F. – FINN, R. W., «*Principles of Catholic Social Teaching and Health Care Reform*», in *https://www.catholiceducation.org/en/religion-and-philosophy/social-justice/principles-of-catholic-social-teaching-and-health-care-reform.html* [20-07-2017].

NELSON, W., «*The Very Idea of Pure Procedural Justice*», *Ethics*, 90(1980), 502-511.

OMOREGBE, J., *Ethics A Systematic and Historical Study*, Joja Educational Publishers, Lagos 1989.

OUTKA, G., «*Social Justice and Equal Access to Health Care*», in *On Moral medicine*, S. E. Lammers, A. Verhey, (eds.) William B. Eerdmans Publishing Company, Grand Rapids, Michigan 1988.

PELLEGRINO, E. D., «*Foreward*», in E. J. Furton – P. J. Cataldo – A. S. Moraczewski (eds.) *Catholic Health Care Ethics. A Manual for Practitioners*, The National Catholic Bioethics Centre, Philadelphia 2009².

PETRINI, C., «*Theoretical Models and Operational Frameworks in Public Health Ethics*», *International Journal of Environmental Research and Public Health*, 7(2010), 189-202, in *https://doi.org/10.3390/ijerph7010189* [17-8-2018].

PINTO, B., «*Nigeria During and After the Oil Boom: A Comparison with Indonesia*», *The World Bank Economic Review*, 1(1987), 419-445, in *https://doi.org/10.1093/wber/1.3.419.* [6-8-2016].

PRAH, R. J., «Health Capability: Conceptualization and Operationalization», *American Journal of Public Health*, 100(2010), 41-49, in *https://doi. org/10.2105/ajph.2008.143651* [3-3-2018].

PRINCIPI, N. – ESPOSITO, S., «Management of severe community-acquired pneumonia of children in developing and developed countries», *Thorax*, 66(2011), 815-822, in *https://doi.org/10.1136/thx.2010.142604* [9-11-2016].

RAWLS, J., *A Theory of Justice (Revised edition)*, The Belknap Press of Harvard University Press Cambridge, Massachusetts 1999.

ROBEYNS, I., «The Capability Approach: a theoretical survey», *Journal of Human Development*, 6(2005), 93-117, in *https://doi. org/10.1080/146498805200034266* [15-6-2017].

ROBBINS, A., «The World Health Report 2000: Health Systems: Improving Performance», in *Public Health Reports*, 116 (2001), 268-269.

ROEMER, M. I., *National Health System of the World*, Oxford University Press, 1991.

RUGER, J. P., «Health Capability: Conceptualization and Operationalization», *American Journal of Public of Health*, 100(2010), 41-49.

RUSHTON, G., «Use of Location-Allocation Models for Improving the Geographical Accessibility of Rural Services in Developing Countries», in R. AKHTAR (ed.) *Health Care Patterns and Planning in Developing Countries*, Greenwood Press, New York 1991, 147-170.

SCHLAG, M., *The Dignity of the Human Person as the Core and Foundation of Catholic Social Teaching*, in M. Schlag (ed.), *Handbook of Catholic Social Thought*, Catholic University of America Press, Washington, DC 2017, 21-23.

SCRANDIS, D. A., «Jacques Maritain on the Rights of Man and the Common Good» in *The National Catholic Bioethics Quarterly*, E. J. Furton (ed.), Philadelphia, 17(2017), 615-621.

S.-ESTELLE, A. – FERGUSON, L. – GRUSKIN, S., *Applying Human Rights-Based Approaches to Public Health: Lessons Learned from Maternal, Newborn and Child Health Programs*, African Population Studies, 29(2015), 1713-1728, in *https://doi.org/10.11564/29-1-720* [5-5-2017].

SELGELID, M. J., «Capabilities and Incapabilities of the Capabilities Approach to Health Justice», *Bioethics*, 30(2016), 25-33, in *https://doi.org/10.1111/ bioe.12222* [19-5-2017].

SGRECCIA, E., *Personalist Bioethics: Foundations and Application*, translated by Di Camillo J. A. – Miller M. J., The National Catholic Bioethics, Philadelphia 2012.

SHANN, F., «*Etiology of severe pneumonia in children in developing countries*», *The Pediatric Infectious Disease Journal*, 5(1986), 247-252, in *https://doi.org/10.1097/00006454-198603000-00017* [10-7-2016].

SHELTON, R. L., «*Human rights and distributive justice in health care delivery*», *Journal of medical ethics*, 4(1978), 165-171, in *https://doi.org/10.1136/jme.4.4.165* [15-9-2017].

SMART, J. J. C. – WILLIAMS, B., *Utilitarianism for & Against*, Cambridge University Press, New York 1973.

SMITH, G. P., «*Distributive Justice and Health Care*», *Journal of Contemporary Health Law & Policy*, 18(2001-2002), 421-430.

SUAUDEAU, J., *Sesso sicuro* in *Lexicon*, 795-817.

SUMMER, J., «*Principle of Healthcare Ethics*», in E. E. MORRISON (ed.) *Health Care Ethics: Critical Issues for the 21st Century*, Jones and Bartlett Publishers, Sudbury MA 2009^2.

SOARES, M. O., «*Is the QALY blind, deaf and dumb to equity? NICE's considerations over equity*», *British Medical Bulletin*, 101(2012), 17-31.

STEVENS, A. – GILLAM, S., «*Needs assessment from theory to practice*», *Biomedical Journal*, 316(1998), 1448-1452, in *https://doi.org/10.1136/bmj.316.7142.1448* [7-2-2017].

THAM, J., «*Human Dignity in Dignitas Personae: Philosophical and Theological Reflections*», in G. Miranda (ed.), *Studia Bioethica*, 2(2009), 12-18.

THOMAS, W., (ed.), *A Dictionary of Medical Ethics and Practice*, John Wright & Sons Ltd, Bristol 1977.

THOMPSON, I. E., «*Fundamental ethical principles in health care*», *British Medical Journal (Clinical Research Ed.)*, 29(1987), 1461-1465.

TRUJILLO, A. L. – CLOWES, B., *The Case Against Condom – The Scientific and Moral Basis for the Teaching of the Catholic Church on Preventing the Spread of Disease*, Human Life International, USA 2006.

VOGEL, R. J., *Financing Health Care in Sub-Saharan Africa*, Greenwood Press, Michigan 1993.

WAAGE, J. – YAP, C. – BELL, S. – LEVY, C. – MACE, G. – PEGRAM, T. – UNTERHALTER, E. – DASANDI, N. – HUDSON, D. – KOCK, R. – MAYHEW, S. – MARX, C. – POOLE, N., «*Governing the UN Sustainable Development Goals: interactions, infrastructures, and institutions* ». *THE LANCET Global Health*, 3(2015) PE251-E252, in *http://doi.org/10.106/S2214-109X(15)70112-9* [9-07-2019].

WHITEHEAD, M., «*The Concepts and principles of equity in health*», International *Journal of Health Services*, 22(1992), 429-445, in https://doi.org/10.2190/986l-lhq6-2vte-yrrn [28-5-2018].

WILLIAMS, A., «*Economics, QALYs and medical ethics — A health economist's perspective*», Social Science & Medicine, 3(1996), 221-226, in https://doi.org/10.1007/bf02197671 [19-10-2017].

——————, «*The rationing debate: Rationing health care by age: The case for*», BMJ, 314(1997), 820-820, in https://doi.org/10.1136/bmj.314.7083.820 [20-10-2017].

WOUTERS, O. J. – NACI, H. – SAMANI, N. J., «*QALYs in cost-effectiveness analysis: an overview for cardiologists*», Heart, 101(2015), in https://doi.org/10.1136/heartjnl-2015-308255 [3-1-2018].

YAHYA, M. B. – PUMPAIBOOL, T., «*Factors Affecting Women Willingness to Pay for Maternal, Neonatal and Child Health Services (MNCH) in Gombe State, Nigeria*», Journal of Women's Health Care, 6(2017), 404, in http://dx.doi.org/10.4172/2167-0420.1000404 [13-7-2018].

7. **Public Documents**

COMMONWEALTH SECRETARY-GENERAL (2017), «*Female Genital Mutilation*», in *Judicial Bench Book on Violence Against Women in Commonwealth East Africa*, OECD Publishing, Paris 2017, 221-232, in https://doi.org/10.14217/9695a522-en [18-2-2018].

CONSTITUTION OF THE FEDERAL REPUBLIC OF NIGERIA [Nigeria], Act n. 24, 5 May 1999, in http://www.refworld.org/docid/44e344fa4.html [16-05-2018].

Declaration of Alma-Ata International Conference on Primary Health Care, Alma-Ata, USSR, 6–12 September 1978, Development, 47(2004), 159-161, in https://doi.org/10.1057/palgrave.development.1100047 [10-12-2016].

FEDERAL MINISTRY OF HEALTH, ABUJA, NIGERIA, National Reproductive Health Strategic Framework and Plan, 2002-2006, Federal Ministry of Health Abuja 2002, 19, in http://www.policyproject.com/pubs/countryreports/nig_rhstrat.pdf [10-04-2018].

——————, *The National Antimalaria Treatment Policy; National Malaria and Vector Control Division*, Abuja, Nigeria: FMOH; 2005, 17-26.

——————, *National Strategic Health Development Plan (NSHDP)*, 2010 -2015, 11, in http://www.health.gov.ng/doc/NSHDP.pdf [25-11-2017].

__________, *National Strategic Plan for Roll Back Malaria in Nigeria 2001 – Abuja; Federal Ministry of Health, Nigeria (2001).*

__________, *Nigeria May 2001, National Reproductive Health Policy and Strategy to achieve quality Reproductive and Sexual Health for all Nigerians.*

__________, *Inventory of Health Facilities in Nigeria, Abuja, Federal Ministry of Health, 2005.*

__________, *Draft National Health Policy 2006,*

__________, *Secondary Draft National Child Health Policy, Abuja, Nigeria 2006.*

__________, *2010-2015, National Strategic Health Development Plan (NSHDP), in* www.health.gov.ng/doc/NSHDP.pdf *[7-8-2018].*

__________, *Revised National Health Policy, Abuja Nigeria, Federal Ministry of Health (FMOH), 2004.*

__________, *National HIV/AIDS Reproductive Health Survey, 2007.*

__________, *National HIV/AIDS Reproductive Health Survey 2003, 2005, 2007.*

__________, *Guidelines for Young Persons' Participation in Research and Access to Sexual and Reproductive Health Services in Nigeria 2014.*

FEDERAL REPUBLIC OF NIGERIA, NATIONAL AGENCY FOR THE CONTROL OF AIDS *(NACA 2015), Global Aid Response Country Progress Report, Nigeria (GARPR 2015), Abuja, Nigeria.*

__________, *Millennium Development Goals Report 2010, Abuja, Nigeria, Government of the Federal Republic of Nigeria, 2010.*

__________, *National Human Resources for Health Strategic Plan 2008 to 2012, 15.*

GHANA STATISTISTICAL SERVICE & ICF MACRO *(2015), Ghana demographic and health survey 2014, Accra, Ghana.*

INTERNATIONAL RELIGIOUS FREEDOM REPORT FOR 2018, *United States Department of State, Bureau of Democracy, Human Rights, and Labor in* https:// www.state.gov/wp-content/uploads/2019/05/NIGERIA-2018-INTERNATIONAL-RELIGIOUS-FREEDOM-REPORT.pdf. *[06-12-2019].*

NATIONAL ACTION COMMITEE ON HIV/AIDS, *National strategic framework for action (2005-2009), 2005.*

NATIONAL ASSEMBLY, *National Health Act, 2014: Explanatory Memorandum, in* http://www.nassnig.org/document/download/7990. *[25-11-2017].*

NATIONAL CODE OF HEALTH RESEARCH ETHICS 2006, NATIONAL HEALTH RESEARCH ETHICS COMMITTEE OF NIGERIA (NHREC), Federal Ministry of Health, Abuja Nigeria.

NATIONAL POPULATION COMMISSION (NPC) NIGERIA, and ICF MACRO, Nigeria demographic and health survey 2008, Abuja Nigeria, National Population Commission Nigeria and ICF Macro, 2009.

NATIONAL POPULATION COMMISSION, NATIONAL MALARIA CONTROL PROGRAMME, Nigeria Malaria Indicator Survey 2010 Final Report, Abuja, Nigeria 2012.

NATIONAL MALARIA ELIMINATION PROGRAMME (NMEP), NATIONAL POPULATION COMMISSION (NPopC), NATIONAL BUREAU OF STATISTICS (NBS), AND ICF INTERNATIONAL 2016, NIGERIA MALARIA INDICATOR SURVEY 2015, Key Indicators, Abuja, Nigeria, and Rockville, Maryland, USA: NMEP, NPopC, and ICF International.

NATIONAL POPULATION COMMISSION, 2013, Nigeria Demographic and Health Survey, in http://www.population.gov.ng/index.php/2013-nigeria-demographic-and-health-survey [11-12-2017].

NATIONAL PRIMARY HEALTH CARE DEVELOPMENT AGENCY (2009), National immunization policy (rev.), Abuja, Nigeria: Federal Ministry of Health.

NIGERIAN HIGH COMMISSION, Nigerian Fact Sheet 2001, published by Nigerian High Commission, New Delhi.

Nigerian Demographic Health Survey, Abuja, Nigeria 2013.

NIGERIAN HEALTH SECTOR, Market Study Report, March 2015.

OIL AND GAS 2005, AFRICAN DEVELOPMENT BANK, Murrow Prints.

PRESIDENT'S MALARIA INITIATIVE, Nigeria: Malaria Operational Plan FY 2017.

THE NIGERIAN PETROLEUM INDUSTRY in http://www.economywatch.com/worldeconomy/nigeria/ [18- 12- 2016].

The statement of National Association of Pro-Life Nurses on health care Legislation, in www.nursesforlife.org/napnstatement.pdf [27-07-2017].

UNICEF, Final Report, Impact Evaluation of Water, Sanitation, and Hygiene (WASH) within the UNICEF Country Programme of Cooperation, Government of Nigeria and UNICEF, 2009-2013, 29 August 2014, Abuja, Nigeria.

__________, Childhood under threat. The State of the world's children. United Nation Children Fund (2006).

__________, Ending Preventable Child Deaths from Pneumonia and Diarrhoea by 2025 – The integrated Global Action Plan for Pneumonia and Diarrhoea (GAPPD), UNICEF, (2013).

UNICEF/WHO, *Diarrhoea: Why Children are still Dying and What Can Be Done*, UNICEF/WHO; Geneva, Switzerland 2009.

__________, *Report of the Joint Monitoring Programme: Progress on Sanitation and Drinking Water*, New York, USA 2013.

UNIVERSAL DECLARATION OF HUMAN RIGHTS, United Nations General Assembly Resolution 217 A (III), United Nations, New York, NY 1948.

UNITED NATIONS, HUMAN RIGHTS OFFICE OF THE HIGH COMMISSIONER, *Special Rapporteur on the right to health*, in *http://www.who.int/mediacentre/factssheets/fs323/en/* [02-01-2018].

UNITED NATIONS, DEPARTMENT OF ECONOMIC AND SOCIAL AFFAIRS (2015), *Transforming our world: The 2030 agenda for sustainable development*, in *https://sustainabledevelopment.un.org/post2015/transformingourworld* [6-6-2016].

__________, «Pneumonia and diarrhoea, Tackling the deadliest diseases for the world's poorest children», in *http://www.childinfo.org/publication* [10-6-2017].

__________, «The children, Maternal and child health», in *https://www.unicef.org/nigeria/children_1926.html* [20-5-2016].

UNITED NATIONS GENERAL ASSEMBLY SPECIAL SESSION (UNGASS), *Nigeria Report, 2007* in *http://data.unaids.org/pub/Report/2008/nigeria_2008_country_progress_report_en.pdf.* [10-8-2018].

UNITED NATIONS DEPARTMENT OF ECONOMIC AND SOCIAL AFFAIRS, (2015). *Transforming our world: The 2030 agenda for sustainable development*, in *https://sustainabledevelopment.un.org/post2015/transformingourworld* [10-03-2017].

WORLD BANK, *Reproductive Health at a Glance*, in *http://web.worldbank.org/WBSITE/EXTERNAL/TOPICS/EXTHEALTHNUTRTIONAND POPULATION/EXTPHAAG/0,contentMDK:20722992~menuPK:64229817~piPK:64229743--theSitePK:672263,00html* [9-8-2018].

__________, *Nigeria Economic Report, 1 May 2013*.

__________, *Child Survival in Nigeria: Situation, Response, and Prospects–Key Issues*, POLICY Project/Nigeria, October 2002, in *www.policyproject.com/pubs/countryreports/nig_csrevised.pdf* [1-8-2018].

WORLD HEALTH ORGANIZATION, (1992), *The Report of WHO Review, 10. ID., Practical chemotherapy of malaria. Report of scientific group. Technical Report Series*, 1998; n. 981.

__________, *Female Genital Mutilation: An overview. Geneva: World Health Organization*; 1998.

__________________, *The World health report, Health Systems: improving performance*, Geneva: WHO 2000.

__________________, *Gender and Women's Health Department, Female genital mutilation, Fact sheets No. 241, 2000*.

__________________, *"Effectiveness of Male Latex Condoms in Protecting against Pregnancy and Sexually Transmitted Infections", in Information Fact Sheet*, n. 243, June 2000.

__________________, *The World Health Report, Health Systems: Improving Performance*, Geneva, Switzerland, 2000.

__________________, *Antenatal care randomised trial: Manual for the implementation of the new model. Geneva: WHO, 2001*.

__________________, *2006. Health Workers: A Global Profile*.

__________________, *The World Health Report 2006—working together for health*, Geneva, World Health Organization, 2006.

__________________, *«Global tuberculosis control — epidemiology of Tuberculosis: Prospects for control», Seminars in Respiratory and Critical Care medicine*, 29, (2008), 481.

__________________, *World Health Report 2010—health systems financing: the path to universal coverage*, Geneva, World Health Organization, 2010.

__________________, *Progress and impact series: focus on Nigeria*, Geneva, World Health Organization, 2012.

__________________, *(2013b), «Progress towards poliomyelitis eradication in Nigeria, January 2012 — September 2013», Weekly Epidemiological Record*, 51-52(88), 545-556.)

__________________, *World Health Organization Statistics 2015*.

__________________, *Global tuberculosis report 2016*, Geneva: World health Organization, 2016.

__________________, *Nigeria, in Global Health Workforce Alliance*, Geneva, World Health Organization, 2016.

__________________, *Maternal Mortality. Factsheet 348, 2014, in http://www.who.int/mediacecentre/factsheets/fs348/en [10-5-2016]*.

__________________, *Health Expenditure Indicators, WHO: Geneva, 2015, in http://apps.who.int/nha/database/select/indicators/en [7-5-2016]*.

__________________, *(2015a). 1 in5 children in Africa do not have access to life saving vaccines, in http://www.afro.who.int/en/media-centre/afro-feature/item/7620-1-in-5-children-in-africa-do-not-have-access-to-life-saving-vaccines.html [20-12-2016]*.

__________, *Primary Care Systems Profiles & Performance (PRIMASYS)*, in *http://www.who.int/alliance-hpsr/projects/AHPSR-Nigeria-300916. pdf* [11-12-2017].

__________, *Global Health Observatory data repository: Health expenditure per capita, by country, 1995-2014 – Nigeria*, in *htt://apps.who.int/gho/data/ view.main.HEALTHEXPCAPNGA* [11-12-2017].

__________, *Global Health Observatory Data Repository Nigeria: statistics summary (2002–present). http://apps.who.int/gho/data/node.country. country-NGA* [23-11-2017].

__________, *Abuja Declaration: Ten Years On*, in *http://www.who.int/ healthsystems/publications/Abuja10.pdf* [2-12-2017].

__________, *Female Genital Mutilation: An overview. Geneva: World Health Organization, 1998*, in *http://apps.who.int/iris/bitstream/handle/10665 /42042/9241561912_eng.pdf;jsessionid=EC3FD2FFF95F272DAE 7FC30D2DE4B07E?sequence=1* [11-04-2018].

__________, *Traditional Medicine Strategy, 2002-2005, 7*, in *http://www. wpro.who.int/health_technology/book_who_traditional_medicine_ strategy_2002_2005.pdf* [07-05-2018].

__________, *«Primary Care Systems Profiles & Performance (PRIMASYS), July 2015»*, in *http://www.who.int/alliance-hpsr/projects/AHPSR-Nigeria-300916.pdf* [11-12-2017].

__________, *Unsafe abortion: Global and Regional Estimates of the Incidence of Unsafe Abortion and Associated Mortality in 2003, Geneva, World Health Organization 2007[5]*, in *http://www.who.int/reproductivehealth/ publications/unsafeabortion_2003/ua_estimates03.pdf.* [9-8-2018].

__________, *The prevention and management of unsafe abortion, Report of a Technical Working Group*, in *http://whqlibdoc.who.int/hq1992/WHO_ MSM_92.5.pdf* [9-8-2018].

WHO, UNICEF, UNFPA, *World Bank Group and the United Nations Population Division, Trends in maternal mortality: 1990-2015, Geneva: World Health Organization; 2015*, in *http://www.who.int/gho/maternal_health/ countries/nga.pdf* [7-4-2017].

8. **Other Sources**

A.-ALLEN, K., *Nigerian Democracy and Democratic Experience, A Historical, Political, Economic, Social and Religious Analysis*, Kayode Asoga-Allen, Great Britain 2016.

ANGER, B., «Poverty Eradication, Millennium Development Goals and Sustainable Development in Nigeria», *Journal of Sustainable Development*, 3(2010), 138-144.

ANSARI, A. H., «Distributive Justice in Islam: An Expository Study of Zakah for Achieving a Sustainable Society», *Australian Journal of Basic and Applied Sciences*, 5(2011), 383-393.

ATANDA, J. A. – ALIYU, A. Y., (eds.) *Proceedings of the National Conference on Nigeria Since Independence: Political Development*, Zaria, Gaskiya Corporation, 1985.

AWOFESO, O., «Political Islam and Democracy in Nigeria: Compatibility or Incompatibility?» In *International Journal of Interdisciplinary Research Method*, 3(2016), 24-33.

BARKAN, J. D. – GBOYEGA, A. – STEVENS, M., *State and Local Governance in Nigeria, Public Sector and Capacity Building Program: Africa Region*, August 2, 2001.

BEGUM, S. – RAHIM, A., «A Conceptual Framework of Distributive Justice in Islamic Economics», *AL ALBAB – Borneo Journal of Religious Studies (BJRS)*, 1(2015), 19-38.

FRIED, J., *Cultural Anthropology*, Harper's College Press, New York 1976.

GESLER, W. M. – KEARNS, A., *Culture/Place/Health*, Routledge, London 2002.

GREGORY, D. – JOHNSTON, R. – PRATT, G. – WATTS, M. J. – WHATMORE, S. (eds.), «Health and Health care», in *The Dictionary of Human Geography*, Wiley-Blackwell, Oxford 2009[5], 325-326.

HARING, B., *The Law of Christ*, The Newman Press, Westminster 1996.

HONDERICH, T. (ed.), *The Oxford Companion to Philosophy*, Oxford University Press Inc., New York 1995.

KHAN, M. M. –BHATTI, M. I., «Islamic Economics: Divine Vision of Distributive Justice», in *Developments in Islamic Banking*, Palgrave Macmillan, London 2008, 7-37.

LEWIS, N. D. – DYCK, I. – McLAFFERTY, S., (eds.), *Geographies of women's health: place diversity and differences*, Routledge, London 2001.

MAUTNER, T. (ed.), *The Penguin Dictionary of Philosophy*, Penguin Books, London 1999.

MAYER, A. E., «Legge Islamica» in D. M. COSI – L. SAIBENE – R. SCAGNO (eds.), *Enciclopedia delle Religioni*, Città Nuova, Milano 2004, 398-414.

PHILLIPS, D., *Nigeria*, Chelsea House Publishers, Philadelphia 2004.

OKOYEUZU, R. C. – EGBO, O. P. – ONWUMERE, J. U. J., «Shaping the Nigerian Economy: The Role of Women» *Acta Universitatis Danubius Œconomia*, 4(2012), 15-24.

OLERIBE, O. O. – T.-ROBINSON, S. D., «Before Sustainable Development Goals (SDG): why Nigeria failed to achieve the Millennium Development Goals (MDGs) », *The Pan African Medical Journal*, 24(2016), 156.

UCHWNDU, V., *The Igbos of South East Nigeria*, London, Rinehart & Winston 1965.

WALKER, M. – UNTERHALTER, E., «The Capability Approach: Its Potential work in Education», in M. Walker – E. Unterhalter (eds.), *Amartya Sen's Capability Approach and Social Justice in Education*, Palgrave Macmillan, New York 2007.

WIREDU, K., *Morality and Religion in Akan Thought*, in H. Odera, D. Wasola (eds.), *Philosophy and Cultures*, Book Wise Publishers, Nairobi 1983.